D0142723

STEM CELL RESEARCH DEVELOPMENTS

Stem Cell Research Developments

Calvin A. Fong
Editor

Nova Biomedical Books
New York

Copyright © 2007 by Nova Science Publishers, Inc.

All rights reserved. No part of this book may be reproduced, stored in a retrieval system or transmitted in any form or by any means: electronic, electrostatic, magnetic, tape, mechanical photocopying, recording or otherwise without the written permission of the Publisher.

For permission to use material from this book please contact us:
Telephone 631-231-7269; Fax 631-231-8175
Web Site: http://www.novapublishers.com

NOTICE TO THE READER

The Publisher has taken reasonable care in the preparation of this book, but makes no expressed or implied warranty of any kind and assumes no responsibility for any errors or omissions. No liability is assumed for incidental or consequential damages in connection with or arising out of information contained in this book. The Publisher shall not be liable for any special, consequential, or exemplary damages resulting, in whole or in part, from the readers' use of, or reliance upon, this material.

Independent verification should be sought for any data, advice or recommendations contained in this book. In addition, no responsibility is assumed by the publisher for any injury and/or damage to persons or property arising from any methods, products, instructions, ideas or otherwise contained in this publication.

This publication is designed to provide accurate and authoritative information with regard to the subject matter covered herein. It is sold with the clear understanding that the Publisher is not engaged in rendering legal or any other professional services. If legal or any other expert assistance is required, the services of a competent person should be sought. FROM A DECLARATION OF PARTICIPANTS JOINTLY ADOPTED BY A COMMITTEE OF THE AMERICAN BAR ASSOCIATION AND A COMMITTEE OF PUBLISHERS.

LIBRARY OF CONGRESS CATALOGING-IN-PUBLICATION DATA
Stem cell research developments / editor, Calvin A. Fong.
     p. ; cm.
Includes bibliographical references and index.
ISBN-13: 978-1-60021-601-5 (hardcover)
ISBN-10: 1-60021-601-3 (hardcover)
1. Stem cells. 2. Stem cells--Research. I. Fong, Calvin A.
 [DNLM: 1. Stem Cells. 2. Biomedical Research. QU 325 S818 2007]
QH588.S83S7397   2007
616'.02774--dc22   2007004868

Published by Nova Science Publishers, Inc. ✦ New York

Contents

Preface

Stem cells are primal cells common to all multi-cellular organisms that retain the ability to renew themselves through cell division and can differentiate into a wide range of specialised cell types.

The two broad categories of mammalian stem cells exist: embryonic stem cells, derived from blastocysts, and adult stem cells, which are found in adult tissues. In a developing embryo, stem cells are able to differentiate into all of the specialised embryonic tissues. In adult organisms, stem cells and progenitor cells act as a repair system for the body, replenishing specialised cells.

As stem cells can be readily grown and transformed into specialised tissues such as muscles or nerves through cell culture, their use in medical therapies has been proposed. In particular, embryonic cell lines, autologous embryonic stem cells generated therapeutic cloning, and highly plastic adult stem cells from the umbilical cord blood or bone marrow are touted as promising candidates.

Among the many applications of stem cell research are nervous system diseases, diabetes, heart disease, autoimmune diseases as well as Parkinson's disease, end-stage kidney disease, liver failure, cancer, spinal cord injury, multiple sclerosis, Parkinson's disease, and Alzheimer's disease. Stem cells are self-renewing, unspecialized cells that can give rise to multiple types all of specialized cells of the body. Stem cell research also involves complex ethical and legal considerations since they involve adult, fetal tissue and embryonic sources. This book presents new and important research in this field.

Chapter 1 - Currently, stem cell therapy and regenerative medicine programmes represent one of the main research areas in biology and medicine and, in the future, could be an opportunity for the treatment of several diseases that until this moment have been incurable like diabetes mellitus, neurodegenerative disorders, osteo-articular diseases, etc.

At the moment, a wide variety of research centres have begun many investigation programmes about stem cell cultures with both human adult stem cells (hASCs) and human embryonic stem cells (hESCs). Because of the pluripotency of both kinds of progenitor cells (above all hESCs) [1], these biological products are the best source to obtain stem cell lines for cell-based therapies.

In summary, I think that we are still near the starting point in stem cell research. Since Thomson et al [1] derived the first stem cell lines, the knowledge of the mechanisms of cell differentiation have advanced little. Although important advances are being produced, several problems remain and these should be resolved before the generalization of human transplantation of stem cell lines.

Chapter 2 - Vascular disease-induced heart attack and stroke remain one of the major causes of mortality in the Western world. A common characteristic of all types of vascular diseases, including native atherosclerosis, angioplasty-induced restenosis, vein graft atherosclerosis and transplant arteriosclerosis, is endothelial dysfunction/damage followed by an inflammatory response and smooth muscle accumulation in the intima. Although the mechanisms of disease development are not fully elucidated, recent findings indicate an impact of stem and progenitor cells to the pathogenesis of atherosclerosis as well as the endogenous endothelial repair process.

It has been demonstrated that endothelial progenitor cells present in the blood have an ability to repair damaged arterial wall endothelium, and that smooth muscle cells in the lesions are derived, at least in part, from stem cells existing in circulation and the vessel wall. Accumulating evidence indicates that the number and function of endothelial progenitor cells have a diagnostic and prognostic value for vascular diseases. In addition, embryonic stem cells, adult mesenchymal stem cells and bone marrow stem/progenitor cells, have been identified as contributors to angiogenesis and hence have therapeutic potential to revascularise ischaemic tissues.

In the present review we will briefly summarize the recent findings in stem cell research relating to vascular disease, focusing on the role of stem/progenitor cells in the pathogenesis of vascular disease and the mechanism of stem/progenitor cell differentiation and maturation. We will also discuss the therapeutic potential of stem and progenitor cells for various vascular diseases by examining data from animal models and human clinical studies.

Chapter 3 - Various members of the Gata family transcription factors play a crucial role in the regulation of T lymphocyte development from hematopoietic stem cells (HSCs). In this review, we will summarize recent interesting findings on how multiple stages of the T cell developmental program are controlled by Gata family transcription factors. In the adult bone marrow Gata1, 2 and 3 transcripts are present in a subpopulation of HSCs that is commonly defined as LSK (Lin⁻Sca-1^{hi}c-kit^{hi}) cells. Both Gata2 and Gata3 are also expressed in the sub-aorta region in mid-gestation stage embryos. It has been shown that Gata2 gene dosage affects the expansion of HSCs in this intra-embryonic hematopoietic site. By contrast, the Gata3 expression pattern suggests that it might regulate embryonic HSC production through effects on the microenvironment. While Gata2 expression also regulates adult HSC function in the bone marrow, Gata3 positive cells mark a previously undescribed Lin⁻ subpopulation in the bone marrow and in early uncommitted thymocytes, suggesting a role for Gata3 in T lineage specification from hematopoietic multipotent progenitors. Although the findings that the generation of T-lineage cells is absolutely dependent on Gata3 and that Gata3 is expressed throughout thymic T cell development suggest a role of Gata3 in T-lineage commitment, direct evidence demonstrating Gata3 as a T-lineage commitment factor is still lacking. The analysis of overexpression and conditionally deficient mouse mutants showed that in the thymus Gata3 (i) is essential for β-selection upon successful T cell receptor (TCR) β chain gene rearrangement, (ii) can negatively regulate TCR signals via E2A and CD5, and (iii) is absolutely required for CD4 single positive T cell development. In the spleen, Gata3 is active in CD4$^+$ T helper-2 (Th2) T cells and is crucial for the induction of Th2 cytokine expression. The essential role of Gata factors in the regulation of cell division and differentiation is also underscored by various findings implicating Gata family members, including Gata2 and Gata3, in the etiology of specific leukemias. Knowledge on the control of T cell development by Gata factors facilitates improvement of clinical strategies for the generation of various T cell subtypes from HSCs, e.g. in the context of bone marrow or stem cell transplantation, or for the specific expansion of particular mature T cell subpopulations for immuno-based therapies.

Chapter 4 - Shp-2 is a cytoplasmic protein tyrosine phosphatase that contains two SH2 domains and a tyrosine phosphatase domain. This phosphatase exhibits either a positive or negative regulatory role in a number of cytokine receptor signaling pathways, including several that are critical in stem cell regulation. For instance, it is involved in LIF receptor signaling and has a positive regulatory role in embryonic stem (ES) cell differentiation and proliferation. Maintenance of balance between activation of the JAK-STAT and Shp-2-Ras-MAPK pathways is critical to sustain the pluripotency of ES cells. Shp-2 is necessary for hematopoiesis in a mouse model expressing a mutant residual protein ($Shp-2^{\Delta/\Delta}$). We recently used siRNA to reduce Shp-2 expression and examined the consequences on ES cell-derived hematopoietic development and observed Shp-2 expression is essential for ES cell derived-hemangioblast, primitive, and definitive hematopoietic progenitor development. We further demonstrated that reduction of Shp-2 expression using siRNA blocked the bFGF-induced increase in hemangioblast development. Recently, it has been demonstrated that trophoblast stem cells require FGF4 for self-renewal and to prevent differentiation. Shp-2 prevents apoptosis in trophoblast stem cells, by activation of Erk and subsequent phosphorylation and destabilization of the pro-apoptotic protein Bim. In neural stem/progenitor cell, a recent study reveal that Shp-2-binding sites on FRS2α play an important role in NSPC proliferation but are dispensable for NSPC self-renewing capacity after FGF2 stimulation. In this review, the role of Shp-2 signaling in cytokine receptor and various stem cells, including both embryonic stem cells and adult stem cells is extensively reviewed and appropriately discussed.

Chapter 5 - Neurodegenerative diseases and the nervous system's inability to repair following injury, create a growing need for the replacement of neural tissue. The non-immunogenic environment of the nervous system lends itself to accepting cell grafts more readily than the majority of the organs in the body. Stem cells may integrate into the host tissue and act beneficially in ways additional to adding to neuron numbers. Replacing a damaged cell with a phenotypically exact cell may not be necessary or most practical. An immature cell or neural stem cell (NSC) may be beneficial by exerting a trophic support for the mobilization of endogenous progenitors in the niche. In fact, a specified heterogeneous mix of cells may provide one or more roles for regeneration. Therefore, NSCs from a variety of sources may hold great potential for integration into a damaged human nervous system environment, promoting cognitive and behavioral recovery. NSCs have been derived from a variety of sources; fetal, embryonic, and adult stem cells and are cultured in different ways. Beyond deciphering the mechanisms, the availability and safety of implementing stem cell therapies, amongst such diverse stem cell types are among the many considerations that need to be accounted for. There is a need to solve these issues to be able to start implementing life saving therapies.

Chapter 6 - The main purposes of this chapter are to serve as a compilation of all contradictory data on circulating stem cells, and to describe new methods for their isolation and differentiation in animal models.

A population of round cells and spindle cells, morphologically similar to fibroblasts, isolated from the peripheral blood mononuclear cell Buffy coat in a liquid culture medium without any stimulating factors was described in the eighties. In 1997 Bucala called them fibrocytes, and they were immunophenotyped as CD34+, Collagen I+, and Vimentin+. These are powerful antigen-presenting cells -more even than monocytes and dendritic cells- and play an important role in wound repair.

In the last few years, due to the fact that research using human embryonic stem cells raises serious ethical issues, mesenchymal stem cells (MSC) have become the center of attention, even more so when regenerative medicine became a reality. Their presence among bone marrow stromal cells was know, but they were recently found as circulating MSC. These round to elongated cells were first typified as CD14-, CD45-, and CD34-, although there is little consensus because other research teams were unable to repeat these results. However, it is widely accepted that MSCs, also known as mesenchymal progenitor cells, can differentiate into osteocytes, chondrocytes, or adipocytes, and are CD34-, CD45-, CD14-, CD44+, CD13+, CD29+ and CD90+.

In 2003 a monocyte-derived subset of CD45+, CD14+, and CD34+ was isolated from human peripheral blood; hence, monocytes became relevant in stem cell research. These cells were differentiated into mature macrophages, epithelial cells, endothelial cells, hepatocytes, and neurons by Zhao and cols.

Our studies in several animal species using liquid media without stimulating factors, and semisolid media enriched with recombinant human cytokines show growth patterns very similar to those obtained in human beings, with a preponderant CD34+ fibroblast- like cell population. Another relevant finding in these assays that has to be highlighted is the stimulation achieved using only recombinant human cytokines (CSF,IL-3,IL-6, G-CSF, GM-CSF, EPO).

Even though there is a wealth of emerging new data, it is clear that starting with the same fibroblastic population different immunophenotypes (pertaining to CD45/CD14/CD34) could be obtained, and completely different tissues could be generated. Despite cursory knowledge in identification and differentiation of these circulating stem cells, several results of ongoing clinical trials will yield advances in regenerative medicine.

Chapter 7 - Neural stem cells (NSC) are present in the embryonic and adult vertebrate brain. The study of the role of extra cellular factors in the generation, maintenance and differentiation of NSC is complex because: 1) Although embryonic NSC belong to a glial lineage their morphology, proliferation potential, multi potentiality and membrane markers expression evolve during embryogenesis and differ from the adult NSC. 2) The extra cellular environment that surrounds NSC is not static and changes throughout development. 3) A number of proteins expressed at multiple stages of central nervous system (CNS) development appear to function in a "context-dependent" manner. In the light of this complexity it is not surprising that the definition of the NSC niche poses a difficult problem. Here a qualitative theoretical model is proposed to explain how expression of specific proteins that alter the signalling responses of activated receptors, which themselves may not be spatially restricted to the putative NSC niche area (the ventricular zone, VZ) may help define a functional rather than an architectural niche. Such a model may be applied or extended to proteins that are involved in the internalization, processing and degradation of receptors not restricted to the VZ, thereby affecting their signalling in a spatially controlled manner, which compartmentalizes the signalling output rather than the receptor expression pattern. Experimental data on Caveolin1 will be discussed as an example of a possible functionally defining niche protein.

Chapter 8 - Neuronal transplantation has provided a direction for treating neurodegenerative diseases. Recent studies have started to induce various stem cells to transform into neurons in vitro. Here we have demonstrated human umbilical mesenchymal cells in Wharton's jelly behave as stem cells. Human umbilical mesenchymal cells are easily available and capable of rapid expansion in vitro. We are the first to differentiate a large quantity of neuronal-like cells derived from human umbilical mesenchymal cells in neuronal conditioned medium, which may be of great value in treating neurological diseases. Human umbilical mesenchymal cells started to express neuron-specific proteins, such as NeuN and neurofilament treatment with neuronal conditioned medium for 3 days. At the sixth day of culture in neuronal conditioned medium, the human umbilical mesenchymal cells have exhibited retraction of cell body, elaboration of process, clustering of cells and induction of functional mRNA and proteins, such as the subunits of kainate receptor and glutamate decarboxylase. At the ninth-twelfth days, the percentage of human umbilical mesenchymal cells expressed neurofilament could be as high as 87% and glutamate evoked an inward current. At this stage, cells were differentiated into mature neurons with post-mitosis phase. These results have proven its application in clinical transplantation in future without a risk of being transformed to neuronal tumor.

Human umbilical mesenchymal stem cells in Wharton's jelly were induced to transform into dopaminergic neurons *in vitro* through stepwise culturing in neuron condition medium (NCM), SHH, and FGF8. The success rate was 12.7% as characterized by positive staining for tyrosine hydroxylase (TH), the rate limiting catecholaminergic synthesizing enzyme and dopamine being released into the culture medium. Transplantation of such cells into the striatum of rats previously made Parkinsonian by unilateral striatal lesioning with the dopaminergic neurotoxin 6-hydroxydopamine (6-OHDA) partially corrected the lesion-induced amphetamine-evoked rotation. Viability of the transplanted cells, at least 4 months after transplantation, was identified by positive TH staining and migration of 1.4 mm both rostrally and caudaully. The results suggest that human umbilical mesenchymal stem cells have the potential for treatment of Parkinson's disease.

Chapter 9 - At present, it is widely believed that all primary follicles in adult human ovaries originate from the fetal period of life, since their numbers decline in aging females and fetal genetic abnormalities increase with advancement of maternal age. However, during 20 years of prime reproductive period (PRP; women between 18-38 years of age) the numbers of primary follicles do not show significant decline and fetal genetic abnormalities are rare, but their incidence begins to increase gradually thereafter. Our observations clearly demonstrate that during the PRP, but not thereafter, newly emerging germ and granulosa cells form new primary follicles, which replace aging follicles undergoing atresia (follicular renewal). The bipotent source of new germ and granulosa cells are ovarian surface epithelium

(OSE) stem cells differentiating during adulthood by mesenchymal-epithelial transition from tunica albuginea mesenchymal cells. During follicular renewal, the OSE-derived germ cells enter peripheral blood circulation and assemble with granulosa cell nests associated with ovarian vessels. The follicular renewal during the PRP ensures that there are always fresh eggs available for the development of healthy progeny. *In vitro*, the OSE stem cells differentiate into distinct cell types (fibroblasts, epithelial, granulosa, and neural type cells) and oocytes. This suggests that OSE cells represent a new type of totipotent adult stem cells, which could be considered for autologous IVF treatment of premature or natural ovarian failure, and possibly for the local or systemic applications in distinct approaches of autologous regenerative medicine.

Chapter 10 - Cells of the gastric mucosa undergo constant renewal. This process is thought to be regulated by multipotent stem cells, which give rise to all gastric epithelial cell lineages and can regenerate whole gastric glands by production of committed precursor cells. Molecular studies are beginning to reveal the pathways that regulate the proliferation and differentiation of gastrointestinal stem cells. The Wnt/β-catenin signaling pathway and downstream molecules such as APC, Tcf-4, fkh-6, Cdx-1, and Cdx-2 play an important role in the differentiation and proliferation of gastrointestinal epithelial cells. Recent evidence indicates that gastric stem cells occupy a niche in the isthmus gastric glands, which might regulate the function of gastric stem cells through mesenchymal-epithelial interactions. Due to the lack of reliable stem cell markers at the single-cell level, the precise nature of gastric stem cells is difficult to define and characterize precisely, and data about numbers and positions of gastric stem cells remain unclear. Identification of the stem cell marker, Musashi-1, in both the intestine and stomach will provide a clear insight into the properties of gastric stem cells in humans.

In: Stem Cell Research Developments
Editor: Calvin A. Fong, pp. 1-3

ISBN: 978-1-60021-601-5
© 2007 Nova Science Publishers, Inc.

Commentary

Current Problems in Stem Cell Therapy: Are We Ready for Human Transplantation?

Fernando Cobo

Stem Cell Bank of Andalucia (Spanish Central Node), Hospital Universitario Virgen de las Nieves, Granada, Spain

Currently, stem cell therapy and regenerative medicine programmes represent one of the main research areas in biology and medicine and, in the future, could be an opportunity for the treatment of several diseases that until this moment have been incurable like diabetes mellitus, neurodegenerative disorders, osteo-articular diseases, etc.

At the moment, a wide variety of research centres have begun many investigation programmes about stem cell cultures with both human adult stem cells (hASCs) and human embryonic stem cells (hESCs). Because of the pluripotency of both kinds of progenitor cells (above all hESCs) [1], these biological products are the best source to obtain stem cell lines for cell-based therapies.

The isolation, the proliferation and the plasticity of hESCs are higher than hASCs. hESCs have an extremely wide developmental capacity as well as a high growth rate. These cells can be propagated in very large numbers, up to a few billion cells in a standard laboratory. Another advantage of hESCs is the relative ease with which they genetically modify by a broad range of techniques such as viral infection, electroporation and transfection. However, the problems related with ethical aspects are limited to hESCs; due to this, several researchers prefer the work with hASCs. Moreover, due to the limited number of available hES cell lines, there is an urgent need for the generation and characterization of more cell lines. Furthermore, there is also a need to establish the appropriate and robust methods for maintenance and expansion of hESCs.

hASCs have already been used for the treatment of several diseases. For example, cardiomyocytes have been used for the treatment of myocardial acute infarction in several clinical trials [2-4]. However, the results of these clinical trials have been very different and this has been due, in my opinion, to the lack of standardization with respect to the methods of cell selection, cell obtention, cell culture, human application and other factors. Thus, the lack of standardization leads to different results [5]. In this sense, the grafted population must be homogeneously purified to contain only the beneficial cells because other cell types may cause deleterious effects.

Until now, all these transplants are being done in the patients themselves (autologous transplant); in these kinds of situations there is no problem with respect to both infection transmission and cell transplant rejection. However, in the future, the trend of cell therapy programmes is to do massive transplants to the human being. In this situation, there will be two problems: firstly, the possibility of pathogen transmission through the cell products, so the screening of some microorganisms capable of transmitting and producing infections will be necessary, and secondly the possibility of transplant rejection due to HLA incompatibility. There are two possible strategies to avoid this rejection: the choice of the best HLA matching from HLA defined hESC line banks and the establishment of immunotolerance by pre-injection or co-injection of hematopoietic cells derived from the same donor [6].

Another important problem in stem cell research is the presence of animal products in stem cell cultures; the use of murine "feeder" layers that are necessary to help in the growth of embryonic stem cells can produce the transmission of murine viruses to the recipient [7]. All the hESCs lines currently approved in the United States were derived on mouse "feeder" layers and were exposed to a variety of other poorly defined animal products. Thus, while the technology does not avoid the presence of these animal products, a screening of these viruses will be necessary before the transplant is carried out. Moreover, the use of bovine foetal serum could produce prion particle transmission, so tests for these microorganims should be carried out in all the serum batches. In this sense, recently Ludwig et al [8] have developed a new culture medium without the presence of animal products. By means of this conditioned medium, the authors have obtained two new stem cell lines, but these lines have developed chromosomal alterations; thus, these lines are unsuitable for transplantation. The high capacity of proliferation of embryonic stem cells could also produce chromosomal alterations, and the possibility of tumoral degeneration [9], so control in the derivation and the differentiation of these cells is necessary.

Finally, it is also remarkable to know the future problems about disease recurrence, absence of activity or organ/tissue integration of cells, and both patient and disease selection that will appear. The answers to these questions will come with the long term monitoring of patients.

In summary, I think that we are still near the starting point in stem cell research. Since Thomson et al [1] derived the first stem cell lines, the knowledge of the mechanisms of cell differentiation have advanced little. Although important advances are being produced, several problems remain and these should be resolved before the generalization of human transplantation of stem cell lines.

REFERENCES

[1]   Thomson JA, Itskovitz-Eldor J, Shapiro SS, Waknitz MA, Swiergiel JJ, MarshallVS, Jones JM. Embryonic stem cell lines derived from human blastocysts. *Science.* 1998; 282: 1145-1147.

[2]   Lunde K, Solheim S, Aakhus S, Arnesen H, Abdelnoor M, Egeland T, et al. Intracoronary injection of mononuclear bone marrow cells in acute myocardial infarction. *N. Engl. J. Med.* 2006; 355: 1199-1209.

[3]   Schächinger V, Erbs S, Elsässer A, Haberbosch W, Hambrecht R, Hölschermann H, et al. Intracoronary bone marrow-derived progenitor cells in acute myocardial infarction. *N. Engl. J. Med.* 2006; 355: 1210-1221.

[4]   Assmus B, Honold J, Schächinger V, Britten MB, Fischer-Rasokat V, Lehmann R, et al. Transcoronary transplantation of progenitor cells after myocardial infarction. *N. Engl. J. Med.* 2006; 355: 1222-1232.

[5]   Rosenzweig A. Cardiac cell therapy- Mixed results from mixed cells. *N. Engl. J. Med.* 2006; 355: 1274-1277.

[6]   Cabrera CM, Cobo F, Nieto A, Concha A. Strategies for preventing immunologic rejection of transplanted human embryonic stem cells. *Cytotherapy.* 2006; 8: 517-518.

[7]   Cobo F, Talavera P, Concha A. Diagnostic approaches for viruses and prions in stem cell banks. *Virology.* 2006; 347: 1-10.

[8]   Ludwig TE, Levenstein ME, Jones JM, Berggren WT, Mitchen ER, Frane JL, et al. Derivation of human embryonic stem cells in defined conditions. *Nat. Biotechnol.* 2006; 24: 185-187.

[9]   Martinez-Climent JA, Andreu EJ, Prosper F. Somatic stem cells and the origin of cancer. *Clin. Transl. Oncol.* 2006; 8: 647-663.

In: Stem Cell Research Developments   ISBN: 978-1-60021-601-5
Editor: Calvin A. Fong, pp. 5-63   © 2007 Nova Science Publishers, Inc.

Chapter I

Stem Cells, Progenitor Cells and Vascular Diseases

Qingzhong Xiao[1], Neil Roberts[2],
Marjan Jahangiri[2] and Qingbo Xu[1]*

[1] Cardiovascular Division, King's College London,
University of London, London, SE5 9NU, UK
[2] Department of Cardiac Surgery, St George's University of London,
SW17, 0RE, UK

ABSTRACT

Vascular disease-induced heart attack and stroke remain one of the major causes of mortality in the Western world. A common characteristic of all types of vascular diseases, including native atherosclerosis, angioplasty-induced restenosis, vein graft atherosclerosis and transpant arteriosclerosis, is endothelial dysfunction/damage followed by an inflammatory response and smooth muscle accumulation in the intima. Although the mechanisms of disease development are not fully elucidated, recent findings indicate an impact of stem and progenitor cells to the pathogenesis of atherosclerosis as well as the endogenous endothelial repair process.

It has been demonstrated that endothelial progenitor cells present in the blood have an ability to repair damaged arterial wall endothelium, and that smooth muscle cells in the lesions are derived, at least in part, from stem cells existing in circulation and the vessel wall. Accumulating evidence indicates that the number and function of endothelial progenitor cells have a diagnostic and prognostic value for vascular diseases. In addition, embryonic stem cells, adult mesenchymal stem cells and bone marrow stem/progenitor cells, have been identified as contributors to angiogenesis and hence have therapeutic potential to revascularise ischaemic tissues.

In the present review we will briefly summarize the recent findings in stem cell research relating to vascular disease, focusing on the role of stem/progenitor cells in the

---
* Correspondence to Professor Qingbo Xu: Cardiovascular Division; King's College London; 125 Coldharbour Lane; London, SE5 9NU, UK; Tel. +44 20 7848 5322; Fax. +44 20 7848 5296; Email: qingbo.xu@kcl.ac.uk

pathogenesis of vascular disease and the mechanism of stem/progenitor cell differentiation and maturation. We will also discuss the therapeutic potential of stem and progenitor cells for various vascular diseases by examining data from animal models and human clinical studies.

Keywords: stem cells, progenitor cells, smooth muscle cells, endothelial cells, vascular disease, atherosclerosis.

INTRODUCTION

One of the most promising areas in basic research today involves the use of stem/progenitor cells because they have the ability to differentiate into somatic cells of all tissue types, which can be used for tissue engineering and repair of damaged organs. Much of the initial work on stem/progenitor cells focused on their regenerative ability following organ injury, whereas now there is increasing interest in their role in the pathogenesis of disease processes. This is true in vascular diseases, where investigation of stem/progenitor cells was initially directed at their ability to contribute to angiogenesis, the revascularisation of ischaemic tissues, and the repair of injured aorta[1-4], rather than their role in the development of vascular disease. Recent growing evidence has provided much insight into the role of stem/progenitor cells in various vascular diseases, the mechanism of stem/progenitor cell differentiation, as well as the potential mechanism of transplanted cell-mediated repair, which will be briefly summarized in this review.

THE FUNCTIONAL ROLE OF STEM/PROGENITOR CELLS IN THE PATHOGENESIS OF VASCULAR DISEASES

Atherosclerosis is a severe pathological condition that underlies several important adverse vascular diseases including coronary artery disease (CAD), stroke, and peripheral arterial disease (PAD), responsible for over 55% of all deaths in Western civilization. Atherosclerosis is an inflammatory disease, in which risk factors such as hyperlipidemia, hypertension, diabetes, smoking and infections can directly or indirectly stimulate the arterial endothelium, resulting in its dysfunction, damage or both. Once the integrity of the endothelium is interrupted, lipid penetration and mononuclear-cell adhesion might be initiated.

Traditionally, it was believed that the damaged endothelial cells would be replaced by neighboring endothelial replication, and smooth muscle cells from the media would migrate into the intima to constitute atherosclerotic lesions. There is no doubt that the atherosclerotic lesion is characterised by the neointimal accumulation of smooth muscle cells along with macrophages and lipids, but the source of these smooth muscle cells is now thought to be, at least in part, from stem/progenitor cells rather than purely migrating from the vessel wall media.

Accumulating evidence demonstrates that stem/progenitor cells in the circulation and adventitia contribute to endothelial repair and smooth muscle cell accumulation. Stem /progenitor cells from blood and the adventitia migrate into the intima, where they proliferate and differentiate into neo-smooth muscle cells to form neointima[5]. The evidence to support this theory comes from a variety of animal models of arteriosclerosis each investigating the process of a particular type of the disease. The different forms of arteriosclerosis should be understood to allow accurate interpretation of the results of the experiments in the literature.

Native Atherosclerosis

Native atherosclerosis, which varies in severity according to vascular site, anatomy, vessel diameter, blood pressure and function, is a spontaneous, specific, complex, and chronic degenerative disease of blood vessels, ubiquitous in humans and widespread in lower animals. Atherosclerosis is a chronic disease that begins in fetal life, slowly progresses during childhood and adolescence, and then accelerates in fits and spurts in adult life to result in plaque erosion or rupture, effecting morbid or fatal clinical events. Animal models are designed to be preliminary tools for better understanding of complicated pathogenesis, improvement in diagnosis, prevention, and therapy of arteriosclerosis in humans.

Attracted by the advancement of molecular biology in the past two decades, a number of investigators have begun to use specific target gene-knockout mice as experimental systems for arteriosclerosis research. Sixteen years ago, no strains of mice were available that spontaneously developed complex atherosclerotic lesions, although small lesions of the fatty streak type could be induced in strain C57BL/6 mice by feeding them high-fat/high-cholesterol diets.

The advent of gene targeting to modify genes in a predetermined manner changed the situation dramatically by allowing the generation of mice having targeted inactivation of the apolipoprotein E (*ApoE*) gene in 1992 and of the LDL receptor (*LdlR*) gene in 1993. Both these animals, under appropriate conditions, develop complex atherosclerotic lesions and provide practical atherosclerotic mouse models[6].

Such mouse models have considerable advantages over other animal systems in that they overcome the need to administer a cholesterol diet, and have been widely used in atherosclerosis research to answer many critical questions about the pathogenesis of atherosclerosis.

On the other hand, researchers have identified and shown that some cells, with multilineage differentiation potential, existed in the artery wall[7, 8]. They found that calcifying vascular cells, a subpopulation of cells from the arterial wall and cardiac valves, have the ability to undergo osteoblastic differentiation and mineralization, as well as other mesenchymal lineage differentiation. Tintut and colleagues[8] have tested calcifying vascular cells for lineage plasticity. Their results showed that these cells have the capacity for chondrogenic, leiomyogenic (smooth muscle), and stromogenic (marrow stromal) lineages in addition to the osteogenic potential shown previously. Adipogenic potential was limited even with use of specialized induction media. These cells expressed the same surface CD antigens shown on marrow-derived mesenchymal stem cells, and they have substantial self-renewal capacity.

Their findings suggest that the arterial wall contains mesenchymal stem cells with lineage plasticity and a unique differentiation repertoire. Based on these important findings, an interesting hypothesis has arisen in the scientific community investigating atherosclerosis pathogenesis, that stem/progenitor cells harbored in arterial wall or localized in the bone marrow and peripheral blood might participate in the pathogenesis of vascular disease.

Atherosclerosis-related gene knock-out mouse models have been applied to explore the potential role of stem/progenitor cells in the pathogenesis of atherosclerosis. Sata and colleagues demonstrated that hematopoietic stem cells derived from bone marrow can differentiate into vascular cells that participate in the pathogenesis of atherosclerosis[9]. In their study, 8-wk-old male ApoE-/- mice (C57BL/6J background) were lethally irradiated with a total dose of 900 rads. On the following day, 3×10^6 unfractionated bone-marrow cells from a GFP mouse (C57BL/6J background) or a ROSA26 mouse (C57BL/6J background) were injected into ApoE-/- mice. The recipient mice were fed a western-type diet (0.15% cholesterol, 15% butter) starting at 4 weeks after bone marrow transplantation (BMT). After 8 weeks on the western-type diet, the aorta was carefully isolated, examined under a xenon fiber optic light source and snap-frozen in OCT compound. They found that GFP+ cells accumulated in atherosclerotic plaques developing in the aorta of BMTGFP$\xrightarrow{}$ApoE-/- mice and a significant amount (42.5 $\pm$8.3%) of the α-SMA+ cells in the lesions were GFP+. Immunofluorescence double staining documented that the bone marrow-derived smooth-muscle cells expressed smooth-muscle myosin heavy chain, calponin, h-caldesmon and α-SMA. Furthermore, using electron microscopy, they identified smooth muscle cells with muscle fibers in the atherosclerotic plaques of BMTLacZ$\xrightarrow{}$ApoE-/- mice. Immunogold-labeling revealed that the smooth muscle cells expressed LacZ. The smooth muscle cells had a larger cell body and possessed synthetic and secretory organelles, associated with a decrease in the myofilament content, in contrast to medial smooth muscle cells in the aorta of a wild-type mouse. These results indicate that bone-marrow cells give rise to the smooth muscle cells observed in atherosclerotic plaques. However, a recent paper from Falk's group[10] found no evidence of bone marrow origin of smooth muscle cells in atherosclerotic lesions in apoE-/- mice. Similarly, they analyzed plaques in lethally irradiated apoE–/– mice reconstituted with sex-mismatched bone marrow cells from eGFP+apoE–/– mice, which ubiquitously express enhanced green fluorescent protein (eGFP), but did not find a single smooth muscle cell of donor bone marrow origin among (approx) 10 000 smooth muscle cell profiles analyzed. They then transplanted arterial segments between eGFP+apoE–/– and apoE–/– mice (isotransplantation except for the eGFP transgene) and induced atherosclerosis focally within the graft by a recently invented collar technique. No eGFP+ smooth muscle cells were found in plaques that developed in apoE–/– artery segments grafted into eGFP+apoE–/– mice. Concordantly, 96% of smooth muscle cells were eGFP+ in plaques induced in eGFP+apoE–/– artery segments grafted into apoE–/– mice. These experiments indicate that smooth muscle cells in atherosclerotic plaques are exclusively derived from the local vessel wall in apoE–/– mice. How can we explain these controversial results? Our opinion is that their criteria for smooth muscle cells are different, and that data interpretation for "double positive" cells varies. Smooth muscle cells within the lesions have at least two different phenotypes, e.g. pre-mature smooth muscle cells expressing alpha-actin, but not other markers, which might be derived from bone marrow, and mature smooth muscle cells from the vessel wall stem/progenitor cells. To prove this hypothesis, futher studies are needed.

Concerning endothelial repair, Rauscher and colleagues[11] explored the effect of ageing on endothelial progenitor cells in ApoE deficient mice. They found that old ApoE deficient mouse bone marrow transfusion did not prevent atherosclerosis in the high fat diet fed ApoE$^{-/-}$ mice, whilst young bone marrow infusion did. They further examined the old and young marrow and found reduced vascular progenitor cell markers in the old marrow with no change in the number of hematopoetic stem cell markers or generalised murine stem cell markers. They concluded that old ApoE deficient mice had suffered from exhaustive consumption of their endothelial progenitor cells and that this had contributed to their development of atherosclerosis by deficient vascular repair mechanism.

Zulli and colleagues[12] found that CD34 Class III positive stem cells are present both overlying and within atherosclerotic plaques in a rabbit model. Such cells also react with antibodies to α-SMA, RAM-11, prolyl-4 hydroxylase and the pan-leukocytic marker, CD45, which indicates that macrophages and smooth muscle cells within atherosclerotic plaques might well be from CD34-positive bone marrow cells.

In human clinical trials, our group has provided the first evidence that vascular progenitor cells exist within atherosclerotic lesions, and identified an increased number of progenitor cells in the adventitia of human atherosclerotic vessels[13]. These cells might be a source for the smooth muscle cells, macrophages and endothelial cells that form atherosclerotic lesions. In this study, a range of normal and atherosclerotic human arteries were collected from patients undergoing coronary artery bypass surgery. Segments of internal mammary artery (normal controls), and segments of proximal ascending aorta with visible fatty streak were analysed. Immunofluorescence was used to detect a panel of progenitor cell markers. A small number of progenitor cells were identified within neointimal lesions and the adventitia with variable expression of CD34, stem cell antigen (Sca-1), c-kit and VEGF receptor 2 (VEGFR2) markers, but no CD133 expression. On average there was a two- to three-fold increase in progenitor cell number in the adventitia of atherosclerotic vessels compared with normal controls, with a significant difference ($p < 0.05$) in the frequency of cells expressing VEGFR2. This suggests further that vascular stem/progenitor cells act a functional role in the development of human native atherosclerosis.

Angioplasty-Induced Restenosis

Postangioplasty restenosis is a major problem confronting interventional cardiology. Over 400,000 angioplasties are performed every year in the United States, and 30-50% of these will experience postangioplasty restenosis. In recent years the use of stents (bare metal and drug eluting) has increased because of restenosis after simple balloon angioplasty. In-stent restenosis, however, affects 25-35% of patients undergoing this procedure. These rates remain unacceptably high, and although many approaches have been tried, no pharmacological therapy has yet proved to be safe and effective in preventing postangioplasty or poststent restenosis. This is partly due to the fact that there remains uncertainty about the underlying basis of post-angioplasty restenosis[14].

Traditionally, restenosis was thought to be caused by proliferation of smooth muscle cells originating from the medial wall of the atherosclerotic lesion, which formed an intimal mass that compromised the lumen. Continued proliferation and production of extracellular matrix by intimal cells derived from the medial wall formed the "restenosis" lesion which was responsible for lumen loss[15-17]. However, this concept needs to be reconsidered since two reports demonstrated that restenosis may be caused not by the development of an intimal lesion, but by abnormal vascular remodeling of the artery in response to balloon overstretch injury[18, 19]. Experimental angioplasty studies in rabbits and pigs failed to show a significant relationship between the size of the intima and the loss in lumenal diameter measured morphometrically or angiographically. Instead, it was suggested that "restenotic" vessels failed to remodel or enlarge in response to lesion formation[18], or they showed an overall constriction of the artery at the injury site, measured as a change in the diameter of the external elastic lamina[19]. In both cases the impact of the neointimal mass on lumen loss was minor compared to the effect that alteration in the overall size of the artery had on the luminal area. Clinical studies have further confirmed and extended these observations[20]. In this clinical trial, serial (postintervention and follow-up) intravascular ultrasound imaging was used to study 212 native coronary lesions in 209 patients after percutaneous transluminal coronary angioplasty, directional coronary atherectomy, rotational atherectomy, or excimer laser angioplasty. Data from this trial indicated that restenosis appears to be determined primarily by the direction and magnitude of vessel wall remodeling , and that an increase in external elastic membrane is adaptive, whereas a decrease in external elastic membrane contributes to restenosis[20].

Given the above findings, the concept that stem/progenitor cells might participate in or respond to the process of restenosis was put forward. Studies show that bone-marrow-derived progenitors have the potential contribution to arterial remodeling[21]. Shoji and colleagues extensively characterized cellular constituents during neointimal hyperplasia after mechanical vascular injury. They observed that the injured artery remained dilated with a thin media containing very few cells after 2 hours of injury, with fibrin and platelet deposition at the luminal side. One week after the injury, CD45-positive hematopoietic cells accumulated at the luminal side. These CD45-positive cells gradually disappeared, whereas neointimal hyperplasia was formed with α-SMA positive cells. In bone marrow chimeric mice, bone-marrow-derived cells substantially contributed to neointimal hyperplasia after wire injury. This finding provided some insight into the functional role of bone-marrow-derived progenitor cells contributing to vascular repair and remodeling. Human coronary atherectomy tissue from in-stent restenosis, postangioplasty restenosis, and primary atherosclerotic lesions, as well as postmortem coronary artery cross sections from young individuals without atherosclerosis, were examined by Hibbert and colleagues[22]. They found that all in-stent restenosis (ISR) and some postangioplasty restenosis (PR) tissue specimens contained cells that immunolabeled for the primitive cell marker c-kit and α-SMA, whereas the intima and media of PR lesions and normal arteries were devoid of c-kit-immunopositive cells.

Meanwhile, the abundance of peripheral blood mononuclear cell-derived cultured angiogenic cells (CAC) was assessed in 10 patients with in-stent restenosis, 6 patients with angiographically verified patent stents, and 6 individuals with no clinical evidence of coronary artery disease. CAC levels were lower in the in-stent restenosis patients than in the non-in-stent restenosis controls, and both of these groups had fewer CAC than non-coronary artery disease patients. These findings suggest a unique pathogenesis for in-stent restenosis and postangioplasty restenosis lesions that involves c-kit-immunopositive smooth muscle cells. The paucity of CAC in patients with ISR may contribute to the pathogenesis of ISR, perhaps because of attenuated reendothelialization. In another study[23], atherectomy specimens from 17 patients with coronary in-stent restenosis (n=10; time post-stenting 5+/-3 months) and with peripheral in-stent restenosis (n=7; 7+/-3 months) versus those from 10 patients with primary lesions were immunohistochemically examined for the presence of CD34, AC133 and α-SMA, followed by computer-assisted morphometry. They found that α-SMA cells occupied 67% of intimal cells in in-stent restenosis, and expression of endothelial progenitor cells was significantly increased in in-stent restenosis samples compared to primary lesions. This data indicates the recruitment, and potential role, of primarily extravascular stem/progenitor cells within neointimal formation in human in-stent restenosis.

Intact endothelialization machinery is essential to facilitate vessel healing after stent placement and to prevent restenosis. Circulating endothelial progenitor cells have been demonstrated in the peripheral blood and shown to display endothelial functional properties, along with the ability to traffic to damaged vasculature. It is reasoned that robust in-stent intimal growth could be partially related to impaired endothelialization resulting from reduced circulating endothelial progenitor cell number or function. In a small clinical trial, George and colleagues[24] examined endothelial progenitor cell numbers in sixteen patients with angiographically-demonstrated in-stent restenosis, and compared them with patients with a similar clinical presentation but with exhibited patent stents (n=11). They found that circulating endothelial progenitor cell number in patients with diffuse in-stent restenosis was reduced, and functional ability to adhere to fibronectin impaired, in patients with restenosis, which provides a potential mechanism mediating the development of in-sent restenosis. Most recently evidence provided by Matsuo and colleagues further suggested that endothelial progenitor cells might be involved in the development of in-stent restenosis[25]. In this clinical trial, endothelial progenitor cell numbers and endothelial progenitor cell-colony formation units were analyzed in 46 patients who underwent coronary stenting. Angiogenic growth factors secreted by endothelial progenitor cells, such as vascular endothelial growth factor (VEGF), basic fibroblast growth factor (b-FGF), hepatocyte growth factor (HGF), and macrophage chemoattractant protein (MCP-1) from the culture medium were also measured by enzyme-linked immunosorbent assay. They found that patients with in-stent restenosis (defined as >40% stenosis, n=16) had a decreased number of CFU (p<0.05), and increased senescent cells (p<0.05), compared to patients without restenosis (n=30). However, no significant difference of secretion of angiogenic growth factors (VEGF, HGF, b-FGF, and MCP-1) between the two groups was observed. On multivariate analysis, an increased number of senescent endothelial progenitor cell was an independent factor associated with in-stent restenosis (OR 1.10, 95% CI 1.01 to 1.20).

On the contrary, data from a follow-up clinical trial indicates that an increase in circulating CD34+ cells after coronary stenting constitutes an independent risk factor predicting in-stent restenosis[26]. The rate of restenosis (75% vs 11%, p = 0.015) and the extent of diameter stenosis at 8.1 +/- 2.6 months of follow-up (56.9 +/- 26.9% vs 26.5 +/- 16.5%, p = 0.012) were higher in patients with a postprocedural increase in CD34+ cells than in those with a decrease in CD34+ cells. Postprocedural CD34+ cell counts were increased in patients with restenosis but decreased in those without restenosis (p = 0.002). A robust correlation was seen between the change in CD34+ cells and late lumen loss (r = 0.65, p <0.005). In a multivariate regression model, the change in CD34+ cells, lesion length, and preprocedural minimal lumen diameter independently predicted for late lumen loss.

This controversial data from different groups suggests that the role of endothelial progenitor cells in the pathogenesis of angioplasty-induced restenosis is more complex than assumed previously. Knowledge of the mechanism of in-stent restenosis is still far from complete, so additional experimental and clinical data is very much required.

Vein Graft Atherosclerosis

Vascular grafts are widely used in aortocoronary bypass graft surgery and peripheral vascular reconstruction. The small caliber long saphenous vein is the most commonly used conduit, but occlusion of the vein grafts are as high as 50% at 10 years post bypass operations. Three pathological processes are primarily responsible for graft occlusion: thrombosis (early closure), intimal hyperplasia (a few months to a few years), and atherosclerosis (usually after 1 year). Understanding the pathogenesis of vein graft atherosclerosis is often extrapolated from studies on native atherosclerosis in arteries, but the features of the lesions and the pathogenic processes of graft-induced atherosclerosis differ from spontaneous atherosclerosis. Therefore, appropriate mouse models of vein grafts are needed to study this disease process[27]. Our group developed a mouse vein graft model of atherosclerosis several years ago[28]. This mouse model allows us to take advantage of transgenic, knockout, or mutant animals. In our mouse model, autologous or isogeneic vessels of the external jugular or vena cava veins were end-to-end grafted into carotid arteries of C57BL/6J mice. Vessel wall thickening was observed as early as 1 week after surgery and progressed to 4-, 10-, 15-, and 18-fold original thickness in grafted veins at age 2, 4, 8, and 16 weeks, respectively. The lumen of grafted veins was significantly narrowed because of neointima hyperplasia. Histological and immunohistochemical analyses revealed three lesion processes: marked loss of smooth muscle cells in vein segments between 1 and 2 weeks after grafting, massive infiltration of mononuclear cells (CD11b/181) in the vessel wall between 2 and 4 weeks, and a significant proliferation of vascular smooth muscle cells (α-actin) to constitute neointimal lesions between 4 and 16 weeks. In a previous study, we have also shown that there is an early event of endothelial apoptosis and cell death in vein grafts[29], probably due to the sudden changes in mechanical stress when veins are exposed to systemic blood pressure.

Acumulating evidence shows that nonmedial smooth muscle cells may contribute to vascular diseases[9, 30-35] and that smooth muscle cells in atherosclerotic lesions differ from those of the media[36, 37]. We observed that smooth muscle cells in mouse vein grafts appear in the neointima earlier than in the media after massive cell death, which is an early cellular event in the grafted vessels[29]. A recent study demonstrated that smooth muscle progenitors were present in circulating blood[38], although their origins are unknown. A cell population isolated from human blood mononuclear cells was identified, that, when cultured in vitro with platelet-derived growth factor-BB (PDGF-BB) gave rise to cells expressing smooth muscle cell markers[38]. In addition, endothelial cell (EC) and smooth muscle cell progenitors were isolated from human cord blood, which had the capacity to express mature EC and smooth muscle cell markers[39]. These cells were expanded and differentiated ex vivo before transplantation to SCID mice where they could home to sites of tumor angiogenesis. Progenitor cells in the circulation appear capable of homing, differentiating, and integrating into the existing vasculature.

We have also shown that about 60% of smooth muscle cells in atherosclerotic lesions of vein grafts are derived from the donor vessel wall and 40% from recipients, possibly from circulating blood[40]. These findings strongly suggest the possibility of progenitor cells being the source of smooth muscle cell accumulation in vein-graft arteriosclerotic lesions.

Based on double staining for α-actin and smooth muscle cell markers, reports from other groups[9, 35] suggest that a proportion of smooth muscle cells within lesions might be derived from bone marrow cells. A study of human coronary atherosclerosis found that smooth muscle cells in atherosclerotic lesions can originate from cells administered at bone marrow transplantation[41]. Sex-mismatched bone marrow transfer was used to identify donor bone marrow cells that had been incorporated at the site of atherosclerosis. However, it was noted that aspirated bone marrow contains some peripheral blood cells and this could also be the source of the donor-derived smooth muscle cell progenitor cells.

Using the transgenic mouse vein-graft model, our previous findings in SM22-LacZ mice expressing LacZ gene only in smooth muscle cells did not support the contribution of bone marrow cells to smooth muscle cell formation[32]. With the use of this approach, bone marrow was transplanted from SM-LacZ mice into aortic allograft recipients so that any bone marrow cells from the SM-LacZ mice, which differentiated to smooth muscle cells, would stain positive for β-gal activity. However, the allograft did not show X-gal staining of neointimal cells so we concluded that there was no evidence of bone marrow cell contribution to neointimal smooth muscle cell formation. Thus, additional sources of progenitor cells for smooth muscle cells in lesions could exist, and we continue to search for these progenitor cells.

We have also demonstrated that a population of vascular progenitor cells are present in the adventitia, which can differentiate into smooth muscle cells that contribute to atherosclerosis[42]. In this study, we have shown that cells expressing a range of progenitor cell markers are found in the adventitia of mouse aorta. After isolating the Sca-1+ progenitor cell population from the adventitia we have confirmed that these cells can be cultured and differentiated to smooth muscle cells and ECs in vitro. When these Sca-1+ cells were added to the adventitia they displayed in vivo migration to the neointima and acquired a smooth muscle cell phenotype. We have directly identified that progenitor cells from the adventitia can migrate and differentiate to smooth muscle cells in vivo and contribute to neointima formation. This suggests that stem/progenitor cells from the circulation and adventitia can both contribute to arteriosclerosis (figure 1; adapted from Margariti et al [43]).

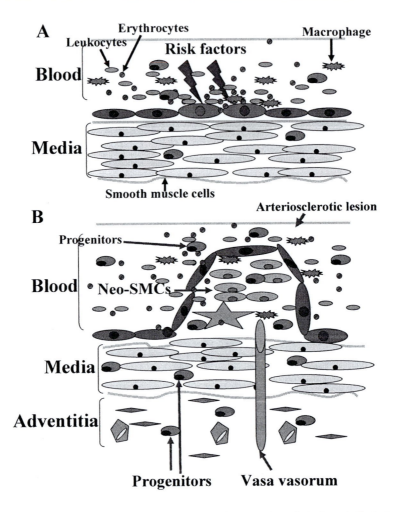

Figure 1. Stem/progenitor cells contribute to the formation of arteroscloerotic lesion. A. Endothelial cells were slowly degenerated by disturbed blood flow or damaged by some risk factors such as free radicals, hyperlipidemia and toxins. B. Stem/progenitor cells existing in circulation and adventitia were mobilized and recruited to damaged site, further differentiate into neo-smooth muscle cells (Neo-SMC) which participated in neointima formation. Damaged endothelial cells were replaced by new endothelial cells differentiated from stem/progenitor cells. Meanwhile, angiogenesis within atherosclerotic lesions occur because lesions become enlarged, creating a hypoxic environment. These microvessels or vasa vasorum play a part in transport vascular stem or progenitor cells from the media and adventitia into the lesion. This process repeats many times, leading to the formation of atheroma.

The model we propose is that progenitor cells from the circulation, or other sources such as the adventitia, can home to the specific site of vessel injury and differentiate either to ECs and re-endothelialize the vessel lumen, or migrate to the subendothelial compartment and differentiate to smooth muscle cells. Neointimal smooth muscle cells may therfore be derived from different sources in response to different stimuli[44].

Using our vein-graft mouse model in transgenic mice carrying LacZ genes driven by an endothelial TIE2 promoter, and hence expressing β-galactosidase only in endothelial cells, we demonstrated that endothelial cells of vein grafts are regenerated from circulating progenitor cells and not migration of neighboring mature endothelial cells[45]. By further creating chimeric mice via bone marrow transplantation, we also determined that of the circulating progenitor cells that regenerated the vein graft endothelium, only one third were derived from bone marrow cells. In ApoE deficient mice we documented a reduced number of circulating progenitor cells and also a reduced regeneration of the endothelium of vein grafts[45], which correlated with enhanced atherosclerosis. Using this vein-graft model with Inducible NO synthase (iNOS)-deficiency (iNOS$^{-/-}$) mice, we have demonstrated that iNOS deficiency accelerates neointima lesion formation by abrogating endothelial progenitor cell repair and facilitating mononuclear cell infiltration and smooth muscle cell accumulation. This indicates that iNOS is a crucial enzyme that attenuates lesion development in vein grafts by stimulating endothelial progenitor cell homing and differentiation[46]. We have shown that neointimal lesions can be reduced in this model by local application of aspirin[47] and VEGF[46], but have yet to demonstrate a reduction in atherosclerosis by infusion or mobilisation of endothelial progenitor cells.

Transplant Arteriosclerosis

Transplantation atherosclerosis is commonly used in reference to changes in coronary arteries in cardiac transplants and in vessels associated with chronic rejection of transplanted kidneys and other organs. Transplant-accelerated arteriosclerosis in coronary arteries is the major limitation to long-term survival of patients with heart transplantation. The pathogenesis of this disease is not fully understood. Accompanying the vein-graft mouse model, our group developed another mouse model to explore the pathogenesis of transplant atherosclerosis[48]. In this model, common carotid arteries or aortic vessels were end-to-end allografted into carotid arteries between C57BL/6J and BALB/c mice. Neointimal lesions were observed as early as 2 weeks after surgery and had progressed at 4 and 6 weeks postoperatively. The lumen of grafted arteries was significantly narrowed due to neointima hyperplasia 4 weeks after transplantation. Using this model, we have examined the role of intercellular adhesion molecule-1 (ICAM-1) in the development of transplant arteriosclerosis in ICAM-1–deficient (ICAM-1$^{-/-}$) mice, and demonstrated that ICAM-1 is critical in the development of allograft arteriosclerosis via mediation of leukocyte adhesion to, and infiltration into, the vessel wall. Neointimal lesions of artery grafts from ICAM-1$^{-/-}$C57BL/6J to BALB/c mice were reduced up to 60% compared with wild-type controls, and the major cellular component of neointimal lesions 4 weeks after surgery was found to be α-actin–positive smooth muscle cells, which were significantly reduced in lesions of ICAM-1$^{-/-}$ artery grafts. This model has been proven to be useful for understanding the mechanism of transplant arteriosclerosis and clarification of cell origins in arteriosclerotic lesions of allografts. It was believed that donor vessel cells contributed to the formation of arteriosclerotic lesions in allografts. However, this concept has been challenged by the results of mouse models from several laboratories that suggest smooth muscle cells within the intimal lesions are completely derived from recipients[9, 32, 33, 35].

Using an allograft model with transgenic mice, previous studies[9, 35] have shown that approximately 10 to 20% of α-actin+ cells in the neointimal lesions of allografts were co-localized with β-galactosidase+ (β-gal) cells in a chimeric mouse expressing β-gal in bone marrow cells. It was reasonable to conclude that host bone-marrow cells are, at least in part, a source of smooth muscle-like cells in transplant neointimal lesions. To clearly classify the cell origins of smooth muscle cell in transplant atherosclerotic lesions, our group use a simplified model of artery allografts in different transgenic mice to identify the source of smooth muscle cells in transplant atherosclerosis[33]. Aortic segments donated by BALB/c mice allografted to ROSA26 (C57B/6) mice expressing β-gal in all tissues showed that neointimal cells derived exclusively from host cells. Also, when aortic segments taken from ROSA26 and SM22-LacZ transgenic mice were allografted into the carotid arteries of BALB/c mice, no β-gal-positive cells were detected in the aortic segment, indicating that neointimal cells were not derived from donor vessels. Interestingly, when aortic segments from BALB/c mice were grafted into irradiated mice (B6/ROSA26 BM) that had only β-gal activity in bone marrow cells or marrow-derived cells, then β-gal–positive cells in lesions were observed. However, no β-gal activity was found in lesions of vessels allografted into B6/SM22-lacZ chimeric mice. To confirm the contribution of bone marrow cells as a possible source of smooth muscle cells in allograft atherosclerosis, aortic segments of BALB/c mice were grafted into SM22-LacZ/apoE$^{-/-}$ or apoE$^{-/-}$ chimeric mice with SM22-LacZ bone marrow. β-gal–positive smooth muscle cells were abundant in atherosclerotic lesions of vessels allografted to SM22-LacZ/apoE$^{-/-}$ mice, but were lacking in lesions of apoE$^{-/-}$ chimeric mice with SM22-LacZ bone marrow. Furthermore, LacZ mRNA in allografts from apoE$^{-/-}$ chimeric mice with SM22-LacZ bone marrow was not detectable, indicating that bone marrow cells are not a source of smooth muscle cells in allografts.

Recipient origin of smooth muscle cell in neointimal or transplant atherosclerotic lesion has been confirmed by Johnson and colleagues[49]. They used aortic interposition grafts between fully histoincompatible rat strains (Brown Norway and Lewis) to investigate the origin of neointimal cells. In their study, three transplant paradigms were used: BN to Lew, Lew to BN and BN to Lew with immunosuppression. Neointimal cells were isolated from aortic transplant tissue through an EDTA wash/mechanical stripping technique and examined by polymerase chain reaction analysis with strain-specific primers. Their data has shown that the neointimal cells are of recipient, and not donor origin. Thus, our studies, together with other findings, provide strong evidence that smooth muscle cells of neointimal and atherosclerotic lesions in allografts are derived from the recipients and that non-bone marrow-derived progenitor cells are a possible source of smooth muscle cells in atherosclerotic lesions.

This mouse model has also been used to define the origin of endothelial cells in transplant vessels. Our group demonstrated that regenerated endothelial cells of arterial allografts are originated from recipient circulating blood, rather than from remaining endothelial cells of donor vessels using a different transgenic mouse (Tie2-LacZ)[50]. Aortic segments were allografted between Balb/c and Tie2-LacZ (C57BL/6) mice expressing β-gal only in endothelial cells. β-gal+ cells in Tie2-LacZ vessels grafted to Balb/c mice completely disappeared, whereas the positive cells found in Balb/c aorta allografted into Tie2-LacZ mice 4 weeks after surgery indicated a host origin of the regenerated endothelial cells. We also demonstrated that endothelial cells are regenerated by circulating progenitor cells, not by cells from the anastamosed artery.

To clarify whether the bone marrow cells contributed to endothelial regeneration, we created chimeric mice, having bone marrow cells donated by Tie2-LacZ animals, which resulted in a β-gal+ cells on the aortic surface. When Balb/c aorta was allografted into carotid artery of Balb/c chimeric mice with bone marrow derived from Tie2-LacZ mice, β-gal activity was seen on the surface of allografts 4 weeks after surgery. Meanwhile, much more β-gal+ cells were observed on the surface of allografts when Balb/c aorta was allografted into carotid artery of Tie2-LacZ chimeric mice with bone marrow derived from wild type mice. Quantitative analysis of the percentage of β-gal-positive cells on the surface of allografts showed that about one third (35±19%) of regenerated endothelial cells were derived from bone marrow cells, and approximately 60% of regenerated endothelial cells come from non-bone marrow tissues. Furthermore, our group demonstrated that endothelial cells of microvessels within allografts were derived from recipient, and that β-gal+ cells of microvessels in transplant arteriosclerosis were derived from bone marrow progenitors.

Thus, our group provides strong evidence that endothelial cells of neointimal lesions in allografts are derived from circulating progenitor cells and that bone marrow-derived progenitors are responsible for angiogenesis of the allograft, that is, the formation of microvessels in transplant arteriosclerosis. Data from another group have also shown that the neointimal α-actin-positive vascular smooth muscle cells in rat aortic or cardiac allografts are of recipient and not of donor origin, and in aortic but not in cardiac allografts, recipient-derived endothelial cells (ECs) replaced donor endothelium[31].

These data suggests that circulating progenitor cells are sources of cells that contribute to neointimal lesions of allografts. This means that all cells of lesions are derived from the recipients, rather than donor vessel wall per se. Interestingly, this result was confirmed to be true for transplant arteriosclerosis in humans, ie, recipient origins of smooth muscle cells[51, 52] and endothelial cells[53], indicating a possibility of direct data translation from the mouse model to the human.

THERAPEUTIC POTENTIAL OF STEM/PROGENITOR CELLS FOR VARIOUS VASCULAR DISEASES

Therapeutic strategies for cardiovascular disease include the early prevention of endothelial cell death and endothelial dysfunction, the prevention of atherosclerotic plaque progression, and effective therapy of myocardial infarction and congestive heart failure. Various therapeutic attempts using pharmacological agents have been developed to positively influence and modulate vascular function and regenerate endothelial cells. In the last several years, an exciting achievement has been obtained in the field of cardiovascular research, in which stem/progenitor cells were reported to differentiate into vascular endothelial cells, smooth muscle cells and cardiomyocytes, representing a potentialy promising cell source for cardiovascular tissue repair.

Angiogenesis and Vasculogenesis

The adult vasculature is formed by two distinct mechanisms: vasculogenesis and angiogenesis. The illumination of stem/progenitor cells contribute to angiogenesis and vasculogenesis as shown in figure 2. Vasculogenesis, a process whereby vessels are formed *de novo* from endothelial cell (EC) precursors, known as angioblasts. During vasculogenesis, angioblasts proliferate and come together to form an initial network of vessels, also known as the primary capillary plexus. Sprouting and branching of new vessels from pre-existing vessels in the process of angiogenesis remodel the capillary plexus. Normal angiogenesis, a well balanced process, is important in the embryo to promote the primary vascular tree as well as an adequate vasculature from developing organs. Vasculogenesis, the *in situ* assembly of capillaries from undifferentiated endothelial precursor cells, and angiogenesis, the sprouting of capillaries from pre-existing blood vessels, have been extensively studied in embryonic stem cells of mouse[54, 55] and human origin[56]. It was believed that both processes require the activity of vascular stem/progenitor cells to differentiate and form the components of the vessel wall[57]. The potential of stem cells and related cell-based therapies to treat disease and injury in humans has generated great excitement in the scientific community as well as among patients and their advocates. Especially, embryonic stem (ES) cells with pluripotency and self-renewal are now highlighted as promising cell sources for regeneration medicine, although ethical and political debates about the use of human embryos in medical research have captured the public eye and to some extent have delayed potential breakthroughs.

When leukemia inhibitory factor (LIF) is removed, ES cells spontaneously differentiate into cystlike structures, termed embryoid bodies (EBs), which contain derivatives of the 3 primitive germ layers. The appearance of blood island-like structures that consist of immature hematopoietic cells surrounded by endothelial cells suggest that ES-derived cells in EBs produce all the factors necessary for the induction of vasculogenesis[58-61].

Wartenberg and colleague induced ES cells to differentiate into EBs with a spinner flask technique and demonstrated that ES cells effectively differentiated into ECs within the three-dimensional tissue of EBs and formed capillary-like structures, which were positive for CD31 (platelet endothelial cell adhesion molecule, PECAM-1). Endothelial differentiation occurred between day 4 and day 8 of EB development. Within 7 days, 100% of EBs contained capillary-like structures. They also demonstrated that ES cell-derived EBs are a suitable in-vitro model system to study the effects of antiangiogenic agents in a three-dimensional tissue context, and provide a unique model to investigate the diffusion of anticancer agents in tissue in both the avascular and vascularized states[62].

Recently it has been shown that murine ES cells plated on matrigel, but not collagen or gelatin, could form embryoid bodies and differentiate into sprouting blood vessels without the addition of growth factors[63]. The expression of the endothelial cell marker CD31 and the smooth muscle marker α-SMA was partially colocalized and started to increase 7 days after culture on matrigel, accompanied by the induction of a number of growth factors, such as vascular endothelial growth factor (VEGF), fibroblast growth factor-2 (FGF-2), hepatocyte growth factor (HGF), transforming growth factor-β (TGF-β), and angiopoietin-1 (Ang-1), which is very important for angiogenesis and vasculogenesis.

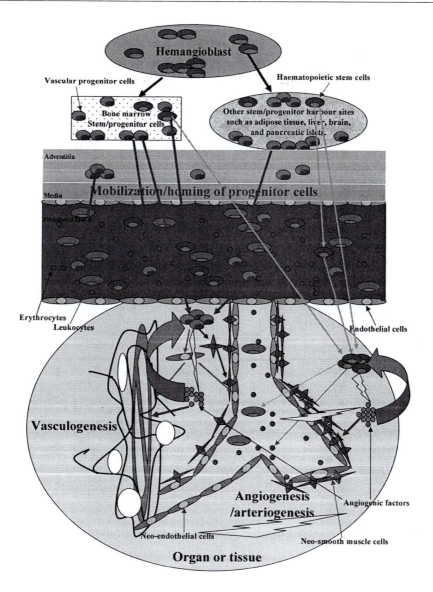

Figure 2. The illumination of stem/progenitor cells contributing to angiogenesis and vasculogenesis. Common progenitor cells for vascular progenitor cells and hematopetic stem cells, known as hemangioblasts, can give rise to vascular cells and hematopetic cells, which contribute to vasculature development. During vasculogenesis and angiogenesis, vascular progenitor cells and hematopetic stem cells come from hemangioangioblasts or moblised from bone marrow and other stem/progenitor cells harbouring site were released to circulation and target organ/tissue, then proliferate and differentiate into endothelial cells or smooth muscle cells, which come together to form an initial network of vessels, also known as the primary capillary plexus (vasculogenesis). Vessels then sprout and become stabilized by stem/progenitor cells-derived smooth muscle cells (angiogenesis/arteriogenesis). Hematopetic stem cells were differentiate into hematopetic cells including erythocytes, leukocytes, macrophage, dendritic cells, mast cells and platelet, which directly or indirectly contribute to angiogenesis through angiogenic growth factors secrection, such as VEGF, PDGF, HGF, IGF, G(M)-CSF, SDF-1, Angiopoietin-1/2, MCP-1 and IL-1. Angiogenic growth factors secreted from hematopetic cells, vascular cells, bone marrow strmal cells or injured organ/tissue, in turn, promote angiogenesis and stem/progenitor cells differentiate into vascular cells and hematopetic cells.

Other groups in China and France have demonstrated that mouse ES cells can differentiate into endothelial cells, as well as smooth muscle cells, during EB formation and further develop endothelial outgrowths after EBs are embedded into collagen in the presence of angiogenic growth factors (VEGF, basic FGF, interleukin-6 and erythropoietin), which respectively recapitulate vasculogenesis, angiogenesis, and arteriogenesis in vivo[64, 65].

The identification of endothelial progenitor cells has revolutionized the field of vascular biology. Evidence accumulated since Asahara and colleagues[1] first publication on the isolation of endothelial progenitor cells has elucidated the importance of a postnatal vasculogenesic mechanism for neovascularization and vascular remodeling.

This unique cell fraction among peripheral blood mononuclear cells (MNCs) derived from bone marrow has a similar profile to that of an embryonic angioblast, which proliferates and/or migrates in response to angiogenic growth factors and differentiates into mature endothelial cells in situ for blood vessel formation. Considering the importance of blood vessel development on organogenesis, vasculogenesis by endothelial progenitor cells may be an essential cascade for tissue and organ regeneration following pathological damage in various critical diseases[66].

Asahara's group has been major contributors in investigating the functional role of endothelial progenitor cells in postnatal vasculogenesis. To determine the origin and role of endothelial progenitor cells contributing to postnatal vasculogenesis, transgenic mice (Flk-1-LacZ or Tie-2-LacZ) were used as transplant donors. First of all, after bone marrow transplantation, chimeric mice (Balb/c/Flk-1-LacZ or Balb/c/Tie-2-LacZ) received subcutaneous implantation of mouse syngeneic colon cancer cells (MCA38), with tumor samples then harvested at 1 week. Sections stained with X-gal demonstrated that the neovasculature of the developing tumor frequently comprised Flk-1– or Tie-2–expressing endothelial progenitor cells. Secondly, in a cutaneous wound model, wounds examined at 4 days and 7 days after skin removal by punch biopsy in chimeric mice disclosed endothelial progenitor cells incorporated into foci of neovascularization at high frequency. Thirdly, lacZ-positive endothelial progenitor cells were shown to incorporate into capillaries among skeletal myocytes one week after the onset of hindlimb ischemia. Finally, data obtained from histological samples of myocardial infarction sites demonstrated incorporation of endothelial progenitor cells into foci of neovascularization at the border of the infarct after permanent ligation of the left anterior descending coronary artery. All their findings suggest that endothelial progenitor cells released from bone marrow incorporate into and thus contribute to postnatal physiological and pathological vasculogenesis[67].

Revascularization in Ischaemic Tissues

Rapid revascularization of injured, ischemic and regenerating organs is essential to restore organ function. Revascularization of adult tissues is a complex process and is modulated by the collaboration of stem/progenitor cells as well as yet unrecognized angiogenic factors. Adult bone marrow is a rich reservoir of tissue-specific pluripotent stem and progenitor cells. Accumulating evidence suggests that bone marrow-derived endothelial, hematopoietic stem and progenitor cells contribute to tissue vascularization during both embryonic and postnatal physiological processes. Previous studies have shown that bone marrow-derived cells functionally contribute to neoangiogenesis during wound healing and limb ischemia[1, 2, 67-74], postmyocardial infarction[75-79], endothelialization of vascular grafts[80-83], atherosclerosis[9], retinal and lymphoid organ neovascularization[84-86], vascularization during neonatal growth[87] and tumor growth[67, 88-92].

Wound Healing and Limb Ischemia

Vascular wound healing and limb ischemia may be mediated in part by recruitment of stem/progenitor cells. In several studies, genetically marked, bone marrow-derived endothelial progenitor cells were recruited to the ischemic limbs of mice[1, 73, 93]. Asahara and colleagues[1] isolated and demonstrated for the first time that endothelial progenitor cells from human peripheral blood had functional roles in vascular diseases. Endothelial progenitor cell isolated with anti-CD34 or anti-Flk-1 microbeads from human peripheral blood mononuclear cells can differentiate into EC in vitro. To determine if endothelial progenitor cell contribute to angiogenesis in vivo, they used mouse and rabbit models of hindlimb ischemia. For administration of human endothelial progenitor cells, C57BL/6J /129/SV background athymic nude mice were used to avoid potential graft-versus-host complications. Two days after creating unilateral hindlimb ischemia by excising one femoral artery, they injected mice with 5 - 10^5 DiI-labeled human endothelial progenitor cells into the tail vein. Histological examination 1 to 6 weeks later revealed numerous proliferative DiI-labeled cells in the neovascularized ischemic hindlimb. Nearly all labeled cells appeared integrated into capillary vessel walls. In endothelial progenitor cell-injected mice, $13.4 \pm 5.7\%$ of all CD31-positive capillaries contained DiI-labeled cells. By 6 weeks, DiI-labeled cells were clearly arranged into capillaries among preserved muscle structures and consistently colocalized with cells immunostained for CD31, Tie-2, and UEA-1 lectin. No DiI-labeled cells were observed in the uninjured limbs of endothelial progenitor cell-injected mice. Their group further demonstrated that endothelial progenitor cell derived from bone marrow can incorporate into and thus contribute to postnatal physiological and pathological neovascularization including tumor neovascularogenesis, cutaneous wound healing, hindlimb ischemia, and myocardial infarction using different transgenic mice (Tie2-LacZ or Flk-1-LacZ) and appropriate models[67]. Their findings opened a new door in vascular biology research, and after their findings were published, studies around the world began to focus on the role of endothelial progenitor cells in vascular biology and various vascular diseases.

Montesinos and colleagues[94] provided interesting evidence to show endothelial progenitor cells have a functional role in wound healing in adult mice. Four weeks after bone marrow reconstitution from donor FVB/N-Tie2-GFP transgenic mice, two full-thickness excisional wounds were performed on the dorsum of FVB/N wild-type mice and treated with either an A (2A) receptor agonist (CGS-21680) or vehicle alone. Vessel density, as measured by CD31 staining, and density of endothelial progenitor cell-derived vessels, as measured by GFP expression, was quantified in a blinded fashion using two-color fluorescence microscopy. They observed nearly a threefold increase in CD31-positive vessels and a more than 10-fold increase in GFP-positive cells in A (2A) agonist-treated 3-day old wounds, but by 6 days after wounding the differences between A (2A) agonist-treated and vehicle-treated wounds were no longer statistically significant. They concluded that an exogenous agent such as an adenosine A (2A) receptor agonist increases neovascularization in the early stages of wound repair by increasing both endothelial progenitor cell recruitment (vasculogenesis) and local vessel sprouting (angiogenesis).

This finding is consistent with another evidence reported by Galiano and colleagues[95]. They examined the effects of VEGF on skin wound healing in a diabetic mouse model and explored the potential mechanism involved in this process. They demonstrated that topical VEGF is able to improve wound healing by locally up-regulating growth factors important for tissue repair and by systemically mobilizing bone marrow-derived cells, including a population that contributes to blood vessel formation, and recruiting these cells to the local wound environment where they are able to accelerate repair.

Ex vivo endothelial progenitor cell infusion experiments further confirmed the functions of endothelial progenitor cells in wound healing. Suh and colleagues[96] use a murine dermal excision wound model to demonstrate that ex vivo endothelial progenitor cell transplantation accelerated wound re-epithelialization compared with the transplantation of mature endothelial cells in control mice. When the wounds were analyzed immunohistochemically, the endothelial progenitor cell-transplanted group exhibited significantly more monocytes/macrophages in the wound at day 5 after injury than did the EC-transplanted group. At day 14 after injury, the endothelial progenitor cell-transplanted group showed a statistically significant increase in vascular density in granulation tissue relative to that of the EC-transplanted group. Fluorescence microscopy revealed that endothelial progenitor cells preferentially moved into the wound and were directly incorporated into newly formed capillaries in granulation tissue. These results suggest that endothelial progenitor cell transplantation will be useful in dermal wound repair and skin regeneration, because endothelial progenitor cells both promote the recruitment of monocytes/macrophages into the wound and increase neovascularization.

Animal studies and preliminary results in humans suggest that endogenous endothelial progenitor cells in the circulation released from the bone marrow have therapeutic potential in the treatment of ischemia[67]. However, the resident population of endothelial progenitor cell is small in patients with vascular disease, which may potentially limit their clinical use.

Accordingly, Asahara's group demonstrated that transplantation of ex vivo expanded human endothelial progenitor cells markedly enhanced tissue neovascularization[2]. Endothelial progenitor cell were isolated from human blood, expanded in vitro for 7-10 days, and harvested for use. One day after operative excision of one femoral artery, athymic nude mice, in which angiogenesis is characteristically impaired, received an intracardiac injection of $5 - 10^5$ DiI pre-labeled culture-expanded endothelial progenitor cells. Laser Doppler perfusion imaging (Moor Instrument, Wilmington, DE) was used to record serial blood flow measurements over the course of 4 week postoperatively, and Tissue sections from the lower calf muscles of ischemic and healthy limbs were harvested on days 3 to 28 to look for incorporation of human endothelial progenitor cells. Serial examination of hindlimb perfusion by laser Doppler perfusion imaging performed at different times displayed profound differences in the limb perfusion within 28 days after induction of limb ischemia. At 3 days postoperatively, limb perfusion was severely reduced in all groups. Over the subsequent 28 days, however, substantial blood flow recovery in mice receiving human endothelial progenitor cells returned perfusion of the ischemic hindlimb to levels that were similar to those recorded in the contralateral non-ischemic hindlimb. In contrast, limb perfusion remained markedly depressed in mice receiving either HMVECs or culture media. Such improvement in hindlimb perfusion in mice receiving human endothelial progenitor cell has been previously shown to reflect neovascularization based on morphometric analyses of capillary density, endothelial progenitor cells mobilization, homing, and incorporation to injured sites.

Evidence from other groups has further enriched the concept that endogenous or exogenous stem/progenitor cells provide significant benefits to wound healing and limb ischemia. Stem/progenitor cell transplantation can contribute to revascularization of ischemic tissues. However, the optimal cell population to be transplanted has yet to be determined due to the heterogeneity of progenitor cells in bone marrow and other adult tissues. Madeddu and colleagues[97] have compared the therapeutic potential of two subsets of human cord blood CD34+ progenitors, either expressing the VEGF-A receptor 2 (KDR) or not. They found that a low number (10^3) of CD34+KDR+ cells improved limb salvage and haemodynamic recovery better than a larger dose (10^4) of CD34+KDR- cells, when the two cell types were injected into the hind muscles of immunodeficient SCID mice subjected to unilateral limb ischemia. The neovascularization induced by KDR+ cells was significantly superior to that promoted by KDR- cells. Similarly, endothelial cell apoptosis and interstitial fibrosis were significantly attenuated by KDR+ cells, which differentiated into mature human endothelial cells and skeletal muscle cells.

Meanwhile, Botta and colleagues[98] also demonstrated that the CD34+KDR+ fraction, not KDR- fraction within the CD34+ cell population is responsible for the improvement in cardiac haemodynamics and hence represents the active CD34+ cell subset.

Most recently, Friedrich et al observed the presence of CD34+ and CD34- subpopulations in CD133+ progenitor cells[99]. CD34-/133+ progenitors differentiate into CD34+/133+ endothelial progenitor cells, adhere more potently than these in response to SDF-1, and rapidly home to sites of limb ischemia in human volunteers. In CD34-/133+ endothelial progenitor cell-injected nude mice, more transplanted cells coexpressing endothelial markers homed to carotid artery damaged endothelium than in CD34+/133+-injected mice. In the former, lesions were smaller and reendothelialization higher than in the latter. These studies indicate that transplantation of a low dose of CD34+KDR+ cells promote vascular and muscle regeneration in ischemic limbs, and suggest that selective use of different cell populations may improve therapeutic intervention in regenerative medicine.

The potential function of other adult stem cells for instance, mesenchymal stem cells in wound healing and limb ischemia, has also been investigated.

Iwase and colleagues found that bone marrow-derived mesenchymal stem cell transplantation caused significantly greater improvement in hindlimb ischemia than mononuclear cell transplantation. Compared with Mononuclear cells, mesenchymal stem cells survived well in an ischaemic environment, and differentiated not only into endothelial cells but also vascular smooth muscle cells. Thus, mesenchymal stem cells transplantation may be a new therapeutic strategy for the treatment of severe peripheral vascular disease[100].

Besides bone marrow-derived mesenchymal stem cells[101-103], other origins of cells have similar ability to improve the recovery of limb ischaemia and wound healing, including umbilical cord blood[104] and adipose tissue[105].

Post-Myocardial Infarction

Myocardial infarction leads to loss of tissue and impairment of cardiac performance. It was believed that remaining myocytes around the infarcted zone are unable to reconstitute necrotic tissue, and retard post-infarcted heart deterioration after myocardial infarction.

Various stem/progenitor cells are mobilized and migrate to sites of damage, and undergo stem cell differentiation in response to target organ or tissue damage, to promote structural and functional repair. As stem cells have a high degree of cell plasticity, researchers were prompted to test whether dead myocardium could be restored by mobilizing endogenous stem/progenitor cells or transplanting bone marrow cells in infarcted mice.

Orlic and colleagues[75] sorted out c-kit positive progenitor cells from lineage-negative (Lin⁻) bone marrow cells from transgenic mice expressing enhanced green fluorescent protein (EGFP) by fluorescence-activated cell sorting. Shortly after coronary ligation, Lin⁻ c-*kit*^{POS} cells were injected in the contracting wall bordering the infarct. They observed that newly formed myocardium occupied 68% of the infarcted portion of the ventricle 9 days after transplanting the bone marrow cells, and more than half of new myocytes were EGFP positive. The developing tissue comprised proliferating myocytes and vascular structures. Their observations suggested that locally delivered bone marrow cells can generate *de novo* myocardium, ameliorating the outcome of coronary artery disease. They further suggested that bone marrow progenitors, mobilized by stem cell factor and granulocyte-colony stimulating factor, would home to the infarcted region, replicate, differentiate, and ultimately promote myocardial repair[76].

A growing number of investigators have implicated adult bone marrow progenitor cells in myocardial replication and regeneration, suggesting that bone marrow serves as a reservoir for cardiac precursor cells. However, it remained unclear which BM progenitor cells could contribute to myocardium, and whether they did so by transdifferentiation or cell fusion.

To sort out the controversy in this field, Balsam and colleagues[106] examined the ability of c-kit-enriched BM cells, Lin- c-kit+ BM cells and c-kit+ Thy1.1(lo) Lin- Sca-1+ long-term reconstituting haematopoietic stem cells to regenerate myocardium in an infarct model. Cells were isolated from transgenic mice expressing EGFP and injected directly into ischaemic myocardium of wild-type mice. Abundant EGFP+ cells were detected in the myocardium after 10 days, but by 30 days, few cells were detectable. These EGFP+ cells did not express cardiac tissue-specific markers, but rather, most of them expressed the haematopoietic marker CD45 and myeloid marker Gr-1. This data suggests that even in the microenvironment of the injured heart, c-kit-enriched BM cells, Lin- c-kit+ BM cells and c-kit+ Thy1.1(lo) Lin- Sca-1+ long-term reconstituting haematopoietic stem cells adopt only traditional haematopoietic fates, not cardiac fates.

This concept was further supported by the important finding that bone marrow haematopoietic stem cells do not transdifferentiate into cardiac myocytes in myocardial infarcts[107, 108]. Murry and colleagues[107] used both cardiomyocyte-restricted and ubiquitously expressed reporter transgenes to track the fate of haematopoietic stem cells after 145 transplants into normal and injured adult mouse hearts. In this study, the cardiac-specific α-myosin heavy chain promoter driven expression of a nuclear-localized β-galactosidase reporter was used to monitor cardiomyogenic transdifferentiation events. No transdifferentiation into cardiomyocytes was detectable when using these genetic techniques to follow cell fate, and stem-cell-engrafted hearts showed no overt increase in cardiomyocytes compared to sham-engrafted hearts. These results indicate that cell fusion occurred in the cardiac regeneration process, a common phenomena in vivo cell-cell interaction, such as cardiac and skeletal muscle cells[109], or myoblast and bone marrow stromal cells[110]. On the other side, some evidence supports the former concept that bone marrow progenitor cells differentiate into cardiac cell lineages after infarction independently of cell fusion[111, 112].

To add to this conflict, a new concept has emerged that bone marrow nonhaematopoietic stem/progenitor cells, not haematopoietic stem cells, can be mobilized and differentiate into cardiomyocytes after myocardial infarction, which contribute to cardiac regeneration, including mesenchymal stem cells[112-115], and endothelial progenitor cells[116-121].

In addition, transplantation of mature ECs derived from in vitro generated, human bone marrow−derived, multipotential adult progenitor cells has facilitated revascularization of various tissues[89, 122]. The physiological significance of stem/progenitor cells was further underscored when thoracic aortae from adult dogs, previously transplanted with genetically haploidentical bone marrow, were replaced with Dacron grafts impervious to the ingrowth of established ECs[80, 81]. In the 3-month-old grafts the newly established endothelial layer were determined to arise from the transplanted bone marrow. In humans, the evidence of contribution of endothelial progenitor cells and circulating endothelial progenitor cells to wound healing originates from patients with end-stage heart disease implanted with a left-ventricular assist device. Insertion of a left-ventricular assist device results in early recruitment of CD34+VEGFR2+ bone marrow−derived cells to the artificial coated surfaces, facilitating formation of a non-thrombogenic vascular surface[123, 124]. All the findings in the past decade highlighted the functional role of stem/progenitor cells in the physiological or pathological revascularization of adult tissues.

Reendothelization in Injured/Damaged Endothelium on the Arterial Wall

Tissue regeneration for organ recovery in adults has two physiological mechanisms. One is the replacement of differentiated cells by newly generated populations derived from residual cycling stem cells. Hematopoietic cell regeneration is a typical example of this kind of mechanism. Whole hematopoietic lineage cells are derived from a few self-renewal stem cells by regulated differentiation under the influence of appropriate cytokines and/or growth factors. The second mechanism is the self-repair of differentiated functioning cells, preserving their proliferative activity. Hepatocytes, ECs, smooth muscle cells, keratinocytes, and fibroblasts are considered to possess this ability. After physiological stimulation or injury, factors secreted from surrounding tissues stimulate cell replication and replacement.

However, regenerative activity of these fully differentiated cells is still limited because of finite proliferation by senescence and because of their inability to incorporate into remote target sites[66].

In recent years, increasing evidence indicates a repairing capacity of stem/progenitor cells[4, 5, 125, 126], especial endothelial progenitor cell[127, 128], providing a novel cell therapeutic option for various vascular diseases. Hill and colleagues demonstrated that the number of CFU-EC in vitro is a predictor for endothelial function in healthy subjects without clinical signs of atherosclerosis[129]. In patients with manifest atherosclerotic disease the number of circulating endothelial progenitor cell is significantly reduced[1, 130]. These observations raised the question whether vascular disease may be significantly influenced by circulating endothelial progenitor cell. Two scenarios are possible[131]:

Firstly, circulating endothelial progenitor cells contribute to endothelial repair mechanisms at the vascular wall thereby preventing the initiation and/or progression of atherosclerotic disease. In this case, the lack of a sufficient number of circulating endothelial progenitor cells in patients with atherosclerotic disease would be a contributing cause for the presence of atherosclerotic lesions. Secondly, the decrease of endothelial progenitor cells is an epiphenomenon and not causative for the development of atherosclerotic disease.

In order to elucidate the underlying mechanisms of endothelial progenitor cells in endothelial cell regeneration and atherogenesis, various animal models have been evaluated. The systemic transfusion of ex-vivo expanded endothelial progenitor cells can enhance reendothelialization after focal endothelial cell damage in a mouse model of endothelial denudation[128, 132]. Interestingly, not only the systemic transfusion of stem and progenitor cells but also endogenous mobilization of the organism's own stem cell pool is associated with an enhancement of reendothelialization in different models of endothelial denudation[133, 134]. The effect of recombinant human G-CSF on neointimal formation was evaluated in a balloon injury model in the rat carotid artery. Neointimal formation was markedly attenuated by G-CSF treatment (39% versus the control; $P<0.05$) due to an enhancement of re-endothelialization (1.8-fold increase vs. control; $P<0.05$) [133]. Regenerated endothelium was functionally intact as demonstrated by NO-dependent vasodilatation. Similar results have been shown by some groups in mice using statin-based mobilization of stem and progenitor cells[135-142]. Using GFP chimeras it has been demonstrated that the endogenous progenitor cell pool contributes to the restoration of the endothelium after focal wire-induced endothelial denudation[135].

Besides endothelial progenitor cells, our group demonstrated for the first time that embryonic stem (ES) cell-derived progenitor cells or mature endothelial cells (EC) have a good therapeutic potential in arterial damage or injury[4, 126]. Mouse ES cells had been differentiated into vascular progenitor cells and ultimately into mature EC in vitro. To evaluate the therapeutic potential of ES-derived sca-1$^+$ progenitor cells or EC on neointima formation after arterial injury, mice were given sham-treatment (medium) or local ES-derived sca-1$^+$ progenitor cells/EC transfer after femoral artery injury. Wire-induced injury resulted in prominent neointima formation, whereas local injection of ES-derived sca-1$^+$ progenitor cells or mature ECs markedly inhibited the neointima formation (30%-40% v.s. 70%-80%). X-gal staining was applied to trace exogenous ES cell-derived mature ECs, our data showed that β-gal positive cells were detected on the majority of the luminal surfaces, and in some areas covered all of the luminal surface, indicating that transferred ES cell-derived mature ECs were incorporated into the injured arterial site. Immunofluorescence staining confirmed double positive cells for β-gal and EC-specific markers, including CD31, CD106, CD144, and vWF. Quantitative morphometric analysis of EC-specific markers, including CD31, CD106, CD144 and vWF immunofluorescence intensity along the luminal surface showed that local ES cell-derived mature EC transfer significantly increased the reendothelialization of injured arteries up to 86%±13.6%. These results indicate that locally applied stem cell-derived endothelial cells contributed to reendothelialization and resulted in significantly reduced neointima formation at the site of arterial injury. The functionally intact endothelial monolayer was promptly formed and suppressed the recruitment of inflammatory cells, thus modulating the process of vascular remodeling and down-regulating intimal hyperplasia. Our results provide further support to the concept that differentiation of stem cells toward vascular progenitor cells or mature EC is beneficial to the therapy of vascular diseases.

Stroke

A growing number of studies highlight the potential of stem/progenitor cell transplantation as a novel therapeutic approach for stroke. A variety of cell types derived from humans and animals have been tested in experimental stroke models and in many cases some index of behavioral function has been improved[143-151]. BM-MSCs[143, 145, 146, 148, 149], human umbilical cord blood cells (HUCBC)[144, 147], peripheral blood progenitor cells[150] and adipose tissue MSCs[151] have been reported by several groups to graft into the parenchyma intracranially surrounding the lesion or, if delivered intravenously, survive, differentiate and enhance functional recovery. Umbilical cord and BM samples are comprised of many cell types including haematopoeitic and endothelial stem/progenitor cells (CD34+, CD133+), mesenchymal cells (CD34-, CD133-), as well as immature lymphocytes and monocytes. It is not clear which of these cells are most important for functional recovery after stroke since different cell populations can enhance functional recovery.

An advantage of a haematopoetic source of cells is that they avoid the ethical issues and tissue limitation associated with embryonic and fetal tissue. Human BM- and peripheral blood-derived stem/progenitor cells also offer the potential of autologous transplants, negating the need for immunosuppresion regimes. Another major advantage is that these cells have been used in the clinic for various malignant and non-malignant disorders for many years. However, very few transplanted cells are found in the brain, even when delivered IC, and of these only a small percentage expresses neural markers. It is believed that both bone marrow and cord blood cells target to the ischemic border when delivered either IC or IV, mediated by injury-induced chemokines[143-145]. It is unlikely that these transplanted cells act to replace the damaged tissue[152, 153], and it is more likely that they secrete trophic factors that enhance endogenous mechanisms of brain repair[146, 147]. The fact that functional recovery is found often with very few transplanted cells in the brain, suggests that the cells may exert an acute but persistent effect on the brain before they die; IV administered cells may not even need to enter the brain to elicit an effect, but rather act in the periphery to increase trophic factor expression in the brain[147].

POTENTIAL MECHANISM OF TRANSPLANTED CELL-MEDIATED REPAIR

Understanding how transplanted cells exert their functional and repair capability in injured or damaged endothelium is important before proceeding to clinical trials. Various mechanisms may be responsible for the transplanted cell-mediated effect.

Incorporation into the Host Endothelium

The attraction of using stem/progenitor cell-derived cells is their potential to incorporate into endothelium, replace injured or damaged endothelial cells and thus have prolonged beneficial effects. To maintain or promptly regenerate an intact endothelial monolayer after the integrity of a vessels endothelium has been disrupted is crucial for prevention of various vascular diseases. Our previous data demonstrated that locally applied ES cell-derived vascular progenitor cells or mature EC can incorporate into denuded endothelium, enhance re-endothelialization and result in significantly reduced neointimal formation in an injured artery[4, 126]. Similar phenomena were observed in different vascular injury models using cell therapy. Cultured endothelial progenitor cells were labeled with red fluorescence DiI and infused systemically into rabbits after balloon vessel injury. Tissues were harvested at 3 days after infusion of the endothelial progenitor cell and analyzed by fluorescence microscopy. DiI-labeled red fluorescent endothelial progenitor cells were found to home to the denuded arterial site and incorporate into the regenerated endothelium at sites of arterial injury. Labeled endothelial progenitor cell incorporation was also observed in the reticuloendothelial system (liver and spleen) but not in uninjured arteries, lung, kidney, and heart[154].

Fujiyama and colleagues[127] further demonstrated that bone marrow monocyte lineage cells adhere to injured endothelium and accelerate re-endothelization in a monocyte chemoattractant protein-1-dependent manner. CD34-/CD14+ monocyte lineage cells (BM-MLCs) were isolated from human bone marrow and differentiated into EC in the presence of vascular endothelial growth factor. BM-MLCs were intra-arterially transplanted into balloon-injured arteries of athymic nude rats, and, activated by monocyte chemoattractant protein-1 (MCP-1) in vivo, they adhered to injured endothelium, differentiated into EC-like cells by losing haematopoietic markers, and inhibited neointimal hyperplasia. The ability to prevent neointimal hyperplasia was more efficient than that of BM-derived CD34+ cells. MCP-dependent adhesion was not observed in PB-derived CD34-/CD14+ monocytes. Regenerated endothelium exhibited a cobblestone appearance, blocked extravasation of dye, and induced NO-dependent vasorelaxation. Thus, BM-MLCs can function as EC progenitors that are more potent than CD34+ cells, and acquire the ability to adhere to injured endothelium in a MCP-1-dependent manner, leading to reendothelialization associated with inhibition of intimal hyperplasia.

Production or Release of Various Angiogenic Growth Factors from Vascular Injury as Well as Transplanted Cells

Adult bone marrow is a rich reservoir of haematopoietic and vascular stem and progenitor cells. Mobilization and recruitment of these cells are essential for tissue revascularization. Physiological stress, secondary to tissue injury or tumor growth, results in the release of angiogenic factors, including VEGF, which promotes mobilization of stem cells to the circulation, contributing to the formation of functional vasculature. Neovascularization and increased expression of angiogenic factors including VEGF[155-157] were observed in ischaemic regions after permanent common carotid artery occlusion (CCAO) and chronic cerebral hypoperfusion. These observations have introduced the concept that vascular trauma results in the release of chemokines that recruit endothelial progenitor cells and CEPs to the neoangiogenic site, such as VEGF[155]. Another possibility of transplanted cell-mediated vascular repair is that these cells can produce various angiogenic growth factors at the site of injury or release such growth factors into the circulation, leading to endogenous stem/progenitor cell mobilization, homing to the site of injury, and participation in the vascular repair process.

Previous evidence has shown that stem/progenitor cells can produce various angiogenic growth factors in vivo or in vitro. Nagakami and colleagues[158] demonstrated that adipose tissue-derived cells (ADSC) isolated from C57Bl/6 mouse inguinal adipose tissue significantly increased EC viability, migration and tube formation mainly through secretion of vascular endothelial growth factor (VEGF) and hepatocyte growth factor (HGF). At 4 weeks after transplantation of ADSC into the ischemic mouse hindlimb, the angiogenic scores were improved in the ADSC-treated group, which were evaluated by laser Doppler imaging (LDI) to measure blood flow and by immunostaining with anti-CD31 antibody to assess capillary density. Rehman and colleagues[159] further observed that ADSC secreted 1203+/-254 pg of VEGF per 10^6 cells, 12 280+/-2944 pg of HGF per 10^6 cells, and 1247+/-346 pg of transforming growth factor-beta (TGF-β) per 10^6 cells, which could be increased 5-fold by culture in hypoxic conditions. Conditioned media obtained from hypoxic ADSCs significantly increased endothelial cell growth (P<0.001) and reduced endothelial cell apoptosis (P<0.05). These adipose tissue-derived cells demonstrate potential as angiogenic cells for use in therapy for ischemic disease, which appears to be mainly achieved by their ability to secrete angiogenic growth factors, not replacement of dead cells.

Evidence from endothelial progenitor cells further supports the concept that various angiogenic growth factors secreted from transplanted cells provide benefit to vascular repair[160]. Dimmeler's group[160] and other groups[161, 162] demonstrated that cultured endothelial progenitor cells in vitro or recruited endothelial progenitor cells in vivo exhibited a high expression of angiogenic growth factors, such as VEGF-A, VEGF-B, IGF-1, SDF-1, G-CSF, and GM-CSF, as well as nitric oxide[163], which enhanced migration of mature endothelial cells and tissue resident cardiac progenitor cells. Their results suggest that besides the physical contribution of endothelial progenitor cells to newly formed vessels, the enhanced expression of cytokines by endothelial progenitor cells may be a supportive mechanism to improve blood vessel formation and cardiac regeneration after cell therapy.

Increased Neovascularization

Increased vascularization of ischemic tissue is associated with recovery of cardiac physiological function and offers another potential mechanism for cell therapy. Transplanted cell-induced blood vessel formation has been reported with ES cell-derived cells[4, 126, 164], bone marrow stem/progenitor cells[149, 165], adipose tissue-derived stem/progenitor cells[105, 166], cord blood[163, 167, 168] and peripheral blood[169-171] stem/progenitor cells. Direct incorporation of the transplanted cells into new blood vessels has been observed in some cases including functional bone healing[169], vascular injury or damage[4, 126], stroke[164], limb ischemia[105, 163, 166-168, 170], and myocardial infraction[165, 171]. BM progenitor cells promoted angiogenesis in the ischemic border by increasing endogenous levels of the angiogenic factors, such as VEGF[149]. Transplanted cells have been reported to increase endogenous levels of other factors (VEGF-A/B, TGF, IGF-1, HGF, BNDF, SDF-1, TGF-β, and FGF) that could induce proliferation of existing vascular endothelial cells (angiogenesis) and mobilization with homing of endogenous endothelial progenitors (vasculogenesis)[161, 162].

Transplanted Cells Inhibit Smooth Muscle Cell Migration and Proliferation, and Attenuate Inflammation

Atherosclerosis is an inflammatory disease, in which some risk factors can directly or indirectly stimulate the vessel endothelium, resulting in its dysfunction, damage or both. There is no doubt that the atherosclerotic lesion is characterised by the neointimal accumulation of smooth muscle cells along with macrophages and lipids. Accordingly, an intriguing potential repair mechanism is the ability of transplanted cells to inhibit smooth muscle cell migration and proliferation, either by the attenuation of endothelium damage or reduction of the ischemia-induced inflammatory/immune response. Rapid recovery of injured or damaged endothelium and restoration of the integrity of a functional endothelial monolayer is crucial for vascular functional and structural recovery. Evidence has shown that confluent endothelial cells inhibited vascular smooth muscle cell proliferation and migration in vitro[172]. Administration of human umbilical cord blood cells (HUCBCs) reduced leukocyte infiltration into the brain[173], although it is not clear whether this was a direct effect on the inflammatory response or a secondary effect due to a reduction in infarct size. HUCBCs decrease inflammation in the brain after stroke and thereby enhance neuroprotection. HUCBCs transplantation resulted in a decrease in CD45/CD11b- and CD45/B220-positive (+) cells. This decrease was accompanied by a decrease in mRNA and protein expression of pro-inflammatory cytokines and a decrease in nuclear factor kappaB (NF-kappaB) DNA binding activity in the brain of stroke animals treated with HUCBCs.

Another group demonstrated that administration of bone marrow progenitor cells induced a substantial reduction in IL-6 level and such an effect on IL-6 blood concentration is the strongest registered so far as a result of interventions (drug or otherwise) in situations of advanced atherosclerosis in any model[174]. Furthermore, the ability of marrow cells to down-regulate IL-6 was dependent upon the specific history of the donor mice. Thus, marrow cells obtained from wild type mice on regular chow brought the IL-6 level to near background. In contrast, marrow cells from ApoE-deficient mice on a high-fat diet were significantly less able to reduce IL-6. The ability of marrow cells to induce repair, suppress inflammation, and prevent atherosclerosis all seem to be interconnected. Some reports in the literature suggest that stem cells can directly inhibit T cell activation, leading to immune response inhibition and reduction of inflammation[175, 176]. In one rabbit model, one iliac artery of hypercholesterolaemic rabbits was subjected to balloon injury and intravascular radiation with a Re-188 balloon. They then received granulocyte-macrophage colony-stimulating factor (recombinant human GM-CSF) (60 microg/d subcutaneously) daily for 1 week. Endogenous endothelial progenitor cells were rapid mobilized, which accelerated reendothelialization and reduced vascular inflammation after intravascular radiation with GM-CSF treatment[154].

Recruitment of Endogenous Stem/Progenitor Cells

Recruitment of endogenous stem/progenitor cells is essential for recovery from various vascular diseases. Specific signals stimulate the stem/progenitor cells to differentiate and move to systemic circulation (mobilization). It is believed that stem/progenitor cells are recruited and stay at the site of neovascularization (homing), where they differentiate into endothelial cells (differentiation) and proliferate (proliferation) to repair injured/damaged endothelium or form new vessels in ischemic organs/tissues. The related mechanism involved in such process, however, remains unknown.

Several chemokines and cytokines have been shown to promote the mobilization of endothelial progenitor cells[177]. VEGF, a potent angiogenic growth factor, promotes mobilization of endothelial progenitor cells in animals[68] and humans[178]. Placenta growth factor (PlGF) was shown to stimulate collateral vessel formation in ischemic organs by mobilizing and recruiting the BM-derived stem/progenitor cells via VEGFR-1[179, 180]. Other angiogenic growth factors, including angiopoietin-1[181], bFGF[182], and SDF-1[181], augment endothelial progenitor cell mobilization and recruitment. Granulocyte–macrophage colony-stimulating factor (GM-CSF)[73, 154] and granulocyte CSF (G-CSF) also increase the number of endothelial progenitors[183]. Matrix metalloproteinase-9 (MMP-9) releases stem cell factor that enables bone marrow repopulating cells to translocate to a permissive vascular niche favoring differentiation and reconstitution of the stem/progenitor cell pool[184].

Previous studies indicate that the eNOS signal is very important for neovascularization. Dimmeler's group demonstrated that endothelial nitric oxide synthase (eNOS) and matrix metalloproteinase-9 (MMP-9) are essential to mobilize endothelial progenitor cells which accelerate neovascularization in ischemic tissues[185], and enhance reendothelialization after arterial injury[186]. Other groups also demonstrated that eNOS-mediated activation of MMP-9 is involved in estradiol enhanced recovery after myocardial infarction, by augmenting incorporation of bone marrow-derived endothelial progenitor cell into sites of ischaemia-induced neovascularization[187], and increased eNOS availability is required for statin-induced improvement of endothelial progenitor cell mobilization, myocardial neovascularization, LV dysfunction, interstitial fibrosis, and survival after MI[137]. Stromal cell-derived factor-1α (SDF-1α) is implicated as a chemokine for endothelial progenitor cell, which might be involved in endothelial progenitor cell recruitment under physiological and pathological circumstances. Previous studies revealed that SDF-1a promotes endothelial progenitor cell migration and attenuates endothelial progenitor cell apoptosis in vitro, and locally delivered SDF-1 augments vasculogenesis and subsequently contributes to ischaemic neovascularization in vivo by augmenting endothelial progenitor cell recruitment in ischaemic tissues[182].

Evidence provided by Hiasa and colleagues confirmed this point[188]. The unilateral hindlimb ischaemia mouse model with bone marrow transplantation (donor marrow taken from ROS mice) was applied, with plasmid DNA encoding SDF-1α injected into the ischaemic muscles. They observed that SDF-1α gene transfer mobilized endothelial progenitor cells into the peripheral blood, augmented recovery of blood perfusion to the ischemic limb, and increased capillary density associated with partial incorporation of LacZ-positive cells into the capillaries of the ischaemic limb. Their findings suggested that SDF-1α induced vasculogenesis and angiogenesis in ischaemic tissue. SDF-1α gene transfer did not affect ischaemia-induced expression of vascular endothelial growth factor (VEGF) but did enhance Akt and eNOS activity. Blockade of VEGF or NOS prevented all such SDF-1α-induced effects. Their study indicated that SDF-1α gene transfer enhanced ischaemia-induced vasculogenesis and angiogenesis in vivo through a VEGF/eNOS-related pathway.

Further evidence has demonstrated the critical role of caveolin in SDF-1-mediated mobilization and peripheral homing of progenitor cells in response to ischaemia[189]. Once mobilized, the stem/progenitor cells must home at the site of neovascularization or endothelialization. SDF-1 augments endothelial progenitor cell recruitment to ischaemic tissues and subsequently contributes to ischaemic neovascularization in vivo[181]. Similarly, it was reported that bone marrow monocytic lineage cells adhere to injured endothelium in a MCP-1-dependent manner, accelerating re-endothelialization by endothelial progenitor cells[127].

Angiogenic growth factors or cytokines are potent chemotactic factors for stem/progenitor cell mobilization and homing. However, key biological issues remain to be elucidated. Furthermore, the molecular phenotype of the putative stem/progenitor cells and the processes leading to their mobilization from the bone marrow and homing to sites of angiogenesis are not fully clarified. The relative contribution of these cells to postnatal physiological and pathological neovascularization has not been fully characterized.

MECHANISM OF STEM/PROGENITOR CELL DIFFERENTIATION INTO VASCULAR CELLS

Mature vascular cells isolated from adult artery or vein were used for engineering vascular tissues in the past decade. However, these mature vascular cells, especially EC, divide a finite number of times before undergoing growth arrest in a state known as senescence[190, 191].

The limited lifespan of adult vascular cells may, therefore, be the rate-limiting step in constructing autologous human vessels in vitro to replace diseased or injured vasculature. Hence, finding a new cell source to obtain large amounts of vascular cells is important to allow vascular tissue engineering to develop. In the last several years, an exciting achievement has been obtained in the field of cardiovascular research, in which stem/progenitor cells were reported to differentiate into vascular cells and cardiomyocytes, representing a potential cell source for cardiovascular tissue repair. The differentiated cells were positively identified by various specific cell markers. Concerning the mechanism underlying this kind of specific differentiation, efforts have been made and some progress has been achieved in the last few years. For instance, it has been found that mechanical forces exert their effects on embryonic stem cell differentiation. Yamamoto studied the effect of the shear stress on the differentiation of embryonic stem cells and reported that the mechanical forces generated by fluid flow, could induce endothelial cell differentiation[192]. Accordingly, Wang reported that shear stress significantly upregulated angiogenic growth factors while down-regulating growth factors associated with smooth muscle cell differentiation[193]. These results indicate that mechanical stress induces the differentiation to endothelial cells and promotes angiogenic factots that down-regulate differentation to smooth muscle cells. A number of growth factors and cytokines have been reported to be involved in stem cell differentiation. More specifically, it was recently reported that the expression levels of cytokines and growth factors are altered during the differentiation of mesenchymal stem cells[194]. Supporting the role of cytokines in stem cell differentiation is the fact that co-culture of mouse neural stem cells with human endothelial cells result in neural stem cells converting to endothelial like cells that have the capacity to form capillary networks[195]. These findings indicate that the use of different cytokines can direct differentiation down specific pathways. Thus, the differentiation of stem cells into a specific cell lineage, e.g. vascular cells will depend on its microenviroment, including cytokines or growth factors, extracellular matrix, mechanical forces and communication with adjacent cells.

Smooth Muscle Cells Differentiation

There is an excellent review providing an overview of the current state of knowledge of molecular mechanisms/processes that control differentiation of vascular smooth muscle cells during normal development and maturation of the vasculature, as well as how these mechanisms/processes are altered in vascular injury or disease[196]. In this chapter, we will just add some new interesting insights into the knowledge of mechanisms involved in smooth muscle cell differentiation from ES cells from work in our laboratory. We have isoalated Sca-1^+ progenitor cells from pre-differentiated ES cells and differentiated them into smooth muscle cells. We have developed a method for producing a large number of smooth muscle cells with high purity (>95% of cells were smooth muscle cell specific markers positive cells) from stem cells, and demonstrated for the first time that collagen IV has a crucial role in the initiation of smooth muscle cell differentiation from stem cells. We also demonstrated that the collagen IV-integrin (α1,β1 and αv)-FAK/paxillin-PI3K-MEK -ERK/JNK signaling pathway is involved in such smooth muscle cell differentiation and PDGF receptor-β-mediated signalling pathways are important for Sca-1[+] progenitor cell differentiation into smooth muscle cells[197]. Accompanying this finding is a most important observation, that stem cell-derived smooth muscle cells are more sensitive to apoptosis than arterial smooth muscle cells in vitro. First of all, we observed that many cells were detached and undergo apoptosis, then death, during the smooth muscle cell differentiation process. In response to 100 µM of H_2O_2 and serum-starvation, the cell viability of ES cell-derived smooth muscle cells (esSMC) is much lower than that of arterial smooth muscle cells. To further examine whether esSMCs are sensitive to apoptosis in vitro, or whether H_2O_2 or serum-starvation stimulates esSMCs apoptosis or death, flow cytometry analysis of double-stained smooth muscle cells with annexin V-FITC and propidium iodide (PI) was performed. Our data indicate that the higher number of spontaneous dead and apoptotic cells occurred in esSMCs, but not arterial smooth muscle cells, when cultured in basic DM. The main population of dying cells underwent apoptosis in esSMCs after treatment with H_2O_2 or serum-starvation. In other words, esSMCs had a higher rate of both spontaneous and H_2O_2 or serum-starvation-stimulated apoptosis and necrosis. A possible explanation for this phenomenon is that the apoptotic signals which exist in stem cells have been switched on or up-regulated during differentiation toward smooth muscle cells. Concomitantly, Dietrich et al[48] provide evidence that sustained exposure of smooth muscle cells to a hypercholesterolaemic environment alters the cell phenotype and promotes cell dedifferentiation, and the phenotype-altered smooth muscle cells are more sensitive to apoptotic stimuli in vitro or in vivo. Furthermore, during repopulation and differentiation, certain numbers of newly produced cells may die by apoptosis during neocardiovascular tissue remodeling and morphogenesis[198]. Accordingly to this finding, the mechanisms involved in esSMC apoptosis should be further clarified for clinical use of these differentiated smooth muscle cells. In our study, we found that p53 was not detectable and involved in such apoptosis processes. However, expression levels of Bax, a proapoptotic protein serving downstream of p53 and caspase-2, were much higher in the differentiated smooth muscle cells. Interestingly, caspase-2 protein levels and active subunits (indicated by caspase-2 fragment) were significantly different between differentiated and arterial smooth muscle cells. To further investigate the role of caspase-2 in the apoptosis of differentiated smooth muscle cells, we examined caspase-2 and Bax's target proteins, such as cytochrome c, Bad and caspase-3. We observed that cytochrome c and caspase-3 in differentiated smooth muscle cells were markedly elevated, compared to that in adult smooth muscle cells. In addition, Bad protein was detectable in both types of smooth muscle cells, but the level was higher in differentiated smooth muscle cells. Furthermore, caspase-2 activity in the differentiated smooth muscle cells had approximately a two-fold increase compared to normal smooth muscle cells. These results demonstrate that caspase-2 acts as a key protein in the regulation of apoptosis in esSMCs. Since the results of above experiments demonstrated Sca-1[+] progenitors underwent apoptosis during differentiation through the caspase-2 pathway, one can postulate that progenitor cells will direct toward differentiation, not apoptosis, if caspase-2 is inhibited. To test this hypothesis, the effect of the different concentrations of caspase-2 inhibitor (Z-VDVAD-fmk) on Sca-1[+] cells was determined. Our data revealed that the proliferation of Sca-1[+] cells reached a plateau when cells were treated with 5 to 20 µM of Z-VDVAD-fmk, and the inhibition of caspase-2 activity was dose-dependent. Sca-1$^+$ cells and arterial smooth muscle cells were cultured in the presence of Z-VDVAD-fmk at 37°C for 3 days. This resulted in a 2-fold reduction of caspase-2 activity in esSMCs, but no significant decrease in arterial smooth muscle cells. Furthermore, the active fragment of caspase-2 was not detected or very weak in Z-VDVAD-fmk-treated cell. Concomitantly, apoptotic cells were decreased compared to vehicle control (7.96% vs 32.12%, p<0.001), but no significant difference was seen in arterial smooth muscle cells (4.72% vs 6.3%, p>0.1). However, the proportion of dead cells was not significantly changed in the two types of smooth muscle cells (figure 3A and 3C). Importantly, the percentage of SMA$^+$ cells from Sca-1+ progenitors was significantly increased, when cells were treated with Z-VDVAD-fmk for 2 days (65.92% vs 75.43%, p<0.05; figure 3B and 3D). These data indicate that caspase-2 inhibitor can block the apoptotic pathway, and promote progenitor cell differentiation toward smooth muscle cells. These findings observed in our study implied that at least some of progenitor cells tending towards apoptosis can switch direction towards differentiation by blocking the apoptotic pathway. Support for this notion is the fact that SMA$^+$ cells were significantly increased when cells were treated with caspase-2 inhibitor. A possible explanation for this observation is that there are two kinds of fates in stem cells, i.e. differentiation and apoptosis, which can be triggered during development in vivo or by LIF withdrawal in vitro (figure 4). This phenomenon could be also observed during neural differentiation from stem cells induced by retinoic acid[199], p38 inhibitor or small heat shock protein (HSP27)[200, 201]. Thus, it could be interesting to further study the molecular mechanisms for regulating the balance between apoptosis and differentiation in stem cells.

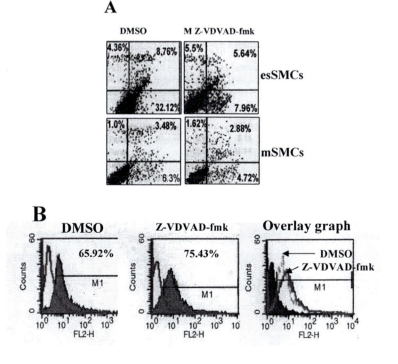

Figure 3 continued

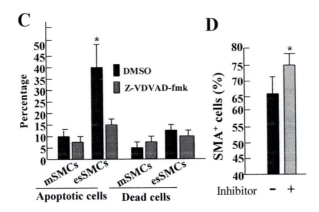

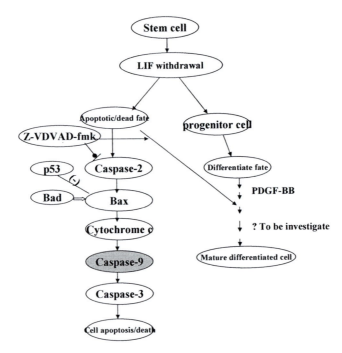

Figure 3. Caspase-2 inhibitor Z-VDVAD-fmk inhibited apoptosis and increased smooth muscle cell differentiation from Sca-1[+] cells. Arterial smooth muscle cells (mSMCs; A and C) and Sca-1[+] cells (designated as esSMCs, A to D) were incubated in DM medium supplemented with 10 ng/ml PDGF-BB with 0.2%DMSO (as vehicle control) or 20 µM/L Z-VDVAD-fmk for 3 days. Cells were harvested and analysed by FACS after labeling with annexin/PI (A) and SMA[+] cells (B). Data are representative FACS graphs from three independent experiments. Panel C shows quantitative analysis of apoptotic cells and dead cells in mSMCs and esSMCs. Panel D shows quantitative analysis of SMA[+] cells in esSMCs. Data are means±SEM of three independent experiments. *Significant difference between controls and Z-VDVAD-fmk-treated cells (p<0.05).

Figure 4. Balance between differentiation and apoptosis during smooth muscle cells differentiation from ES cells. There are two kinds of fates in stem cells leading to differentiation or apoptosis, which can be triggered during the spontaneous differentiation by LIF withdrawal or differentiation with other methods in vitro. During smooth muscle cells differentiation, stem cells will undergo differentiation and apoptosis through Caspase-2-Bax-Cytochrome c-Caspase-9-Caspase-3 apoptotic pathway. Strikingly, some of proapoptotic cells will be rescued and switch to differentiation after the apoptotic pathway is blocked.

Endothelial Cells Differentiation

Endothelial cells are critical cellular components of blood vessels, functioning as selectively permeable barriers between blood and tissues. The denudation or dysfunction of the intact endothelial monolayer causes lipid accumulation, monocyte adhension and inflammatory reactions that initiate atherosclerotic lesion development[202, 203]. Recently, accumulating evidence indicates that stem/progenitor cells play an important role in endothelial repair[45, 132, 135, 139, 204] due to their abilities to self-renew and differentiate into mature functional endothelial cells. Under specific stimulation, e.g. growth factors[205], extracellular matrix[206], mechanical forces[205, 207] and coculture with other cell types[195, 208], stem/progenitor cells will undergo specific lineage differentiation. In this review, we will briefly summarize recent progress in the understanding of how stem/progenitor cells differentiate into endothelial cells and related mechanisms.

Mechanical Stress

Generally, there are two types of mechanical stress, laminar flow stress (shear stress) and disturbed flow (stretch stress). It is believed that shear stress, a mechanical force generated from blood flow, can induce stem/progenitor cells to differentiate into endothelial cells, and stretch stress, a mechanical stress generated from sudden change of blood flow direction, may stimulate stem/progenitor cells develop into smooth muscle cell under physiological conditions in vivo. Data from in vitro experiments suggest that endothelial progenitor cells can differentiate into endothelial phenotypes when shear stress is applied to the cells[209, 210]. Several groups first investigated the effects of shear stress on embryonic mesenchymal progenitor cells[193], endothelial progenitor cells[210] and ES cells[192] derived endothelial cell differentiation. When endothelial progenitor cells from human blood and Flk-1+ cells derived from mouse ES cells were subjected to shear stress, their cell density increased markedly, and a larger percentage of the cells were in the S and G(2)-M phases of the cell cycle than endothelial progenitor cells and Flk-1(+) ES cells cultured under static conditions. Shear stress significantly increased the expression of the vascular endothelial cell-specific markers Flk-1, Flt-1, vascular endothelial cadherin, and PECAM-1 at both the protein level and the mRNA level, but it had no effect on expression of the mural cell marker smooth muscle alpha-actin, blood cell marker CD3, or the epithelial cell marker keratin. They also found that shear stress induced tyrosine phosphorylation of Flk-1 in Flk-1(+) ES cells that was blocked by a Flk-1 kinase inhibitor, SU1498, but not by a neutralizing antibody against VEGF. SU1498 also abolished the shear stress-induced proliferation and differentiation of Flk-1(+) ES cells, indicating that ligand-independent activation of Flk-1 plays an important role in shear stress-mediated proliferation and differentiation by Flk-1(+) ES cells[192].

Illi and colleagues further investigated the molecular basis for the effects of shear stress on endothelial cell differentiation from ES cells[209]. Their data revealed that shear stress enhanced lysine acetylation of histone H3 at position 14 (K14), as well as serine phosphorylation at position 10 (S10) and lysine methylation at position 79 (K79), and cooperated with HDAC inhibitor TSA, inducing acetylation of histone H4 and phosphoacetylation of S10 and K14 of histone H3.

Rossig and colleagues provided firm evidence that histone deacetylase (HDAC) activity is essential for Hox9A expression and endothelial cell differentiation from progenitor cells. They demonstrated that Hox9A is regulated by HDACs and is critical for postnatal neovascularization.

Our recently study further clarified which HDAC is involved in endothelial cell differentiation and the related molecular mechanisms about shear stress-induced endothelial cell differentiation from ES cells[126]. In this study, we demonstrated for first time that HDAC3 is essential for shear stress-induced endothelial cell differentiation, and that laminar flow enhanced ES cell-derived progenitor cells to functionally differentiate into endothelial cells. During the endothelial lineage differentiation, p53 was up-regulated and deacetylated by HDAC1and HDAC3, which in turn activated p21. p21 activation promoted the differentiation of progenitor cells into mature endothelial cells. This data may provide some understanding of the mechanisms involved in the re-endothelialization of injured blood vessels and atherosclerosis-prone arteries by stem/progenitor cells, and provides basic information on targeting proteins that promote endothelial differentiation.

Growth Factors

Many angiogenic growth factors and cytokines are released from stem/progenitor cells, which in turn stimulate stem/progenitor cells to differentiate into endothelial cells and exert their therapeutic function in various vascular diseases.

Kim and colleagues[194] examined the gene expression profile of cytokines and growth factors during differentiation of bone marrow-derived mesenchymal stem cells (MSC). They observed that cytokine and growth factor genes, including IL-6, IL-8, IL-11, IL-12, IL-14, IL-15, LIF, G-CSF, GM-CSF, M-SCF, FL and SCF, were found to be expressed in the MSCs. In contrast, there was no IL-1alpha, IL-1beta, or IL-7 expression observed. The IL-12, IL-14, G-CSF, and GM-CSF mRNA expression levels either disappeared or decreased after the MSCs differentiated into osteoblasts, adipocytes, and endothelial cells. Among the differentiated cells derived from MSCs; osteoblasts, adipocytes, and endothelial cells expressed osteopontin, aP2, and the VEGFR-2 gene, respectively, which indicated that VEGF has a unique role in mediating endothelial cell differentiation from stem/progenitor cells. VEGF is a major angiogenic growth factor, which promotes stem/progenitor cells to differentiate into endothelial cells[211, 212]. Little is known about the implication of the VEGF-receptor tyrosine kinases and about the implication of the VEGF-R co-receptor, neuropilin-1, in this process. For this purpose, an in vitro model of differentiation of human bone marrow AC133+ (BM-AC133+) cells into vascular precursors was used[213]. In this work, authors have demonstrated that the effect of VEGF-A on BM-AC133+ cells relies on an early action of VEGF-A on the expression of its tyrosine kinase receptors followed by an activation of a VEGF-R2/neuropilin-1-dependent signaling pathway. This signaling promotes the differentiation of BM-AC133+ cells into endothelial precursor cells, followed by the proliferation of these differentiated cells. Using wild-type and SH2 domain mutated (R522K) Shb overexpression system, Rolny et al. demonstrated that Shb may play a crucial role during early ES cell differentiation to vascular structures by transducing VEGFR-2 and PDGFR-beta signals[214]. Our group recently demonstrated that HDAC3 is essential for VEGF-induced endothelial cell differentiation from mouse ES cells[4], but little is known about the down- or up-stream signaling pathway. To resolve this problem, one excellent study had been performed by Wang and colleagues[215]. They have used global gene expression analysis to establish a comprehensive list of candidate genes in the developing vasculature during ES cell differentiation in vitro. A large set of genes, including growth factors, cell surface molecules, transcriptional factors, and members of several signal transduction pathways that are known to be involved in vasculogenesis or angiogenesis, were found to have expression patterns as expected. Some unknown or functionally uncharacterized genes were differentially regulated in flk1+ cells compared with flk1- cells, suggesting possible roles for these genes in vascular commitment. Particularly, multiple components of the Wnt signaling pathway were differentially regulated in flk1+ cells, including Wnt proteins, their receptors, downstream transcriptional factors, and other components belonging to this pathway. Activation of the Wnt signal was able to expand vascular progenitor populations whereas suppression of Wnt activity reduced flk1+ populations. Suppression of Wnt signaling also inhibited the formation of matured vascular capillary-like structures during late stages of embryoid body differentiation. This data indicates a requisite and ongoing role for Wnt activity during vascular development, and the gene expression profiles identify candidate components of this pathway that participate in vascular cell differentiation. It will be interesting to investigate the relationship between Wnt signal pathway and HDAC or Shb.

Extracellular Matrix

The extracellular matrix (ECM) is a complex structural entity surrounding and supporting cells that are found within mammalian tissues. Previous studies demonstrated that ECM is an important factor affecting cell adherence[216], growth[216], migration[216], apoptosis[217], and differentiation[218]. ECM is composed of 3 major classes of biomolecules including structural proteins (collagen and elastin), specialized proteins (fibrillin, fibronectin, and laminin), and proteoglycans. Collagens are the most abundant proteins found in the animal kingdom and are the major proteins comprising the ECM. There are at least 12 types of collagen. Types I, II and III are the most abundant and form fibrils of similar structure. Type IV collagen forms a two-dimensional reticulum and is a major component of the basal lamina. Previous studies have shown that collagen type IV has a crucial role in the early stage of differentiation of F9 stem cells[219].

Yamashita et al[220] and Sone et al[221] demonstrated that VEGFR2+ progenitor cells can differentiate into endothelial cells with addition of VEGF. Both soluble factors and the type of extracellular matrix seem to be critical in directing differentiation of ES cells and the formation of tissue-like structures. In the course of normal embryogenesis, ES cells differentiate along different lineages in the context of complex three-dimensional (3D) tissue structures. A 3D collagen matrix (collagen gels and porous collagen sponges) mimicked such 3D tissue structure in vitro, and induced rhesus monkey ES cells to differentiate into various cell linages[222]. In particular, in collagen gels ES cells formed gland-like circular structures, whereas in collagen sponges ES cells were scattered through the matrix or formed aggregates. Soluble factors produced by feeder cells or added to the culture medium facilitated ES cell differentiation into particular lineages. In collagen sponges, keratinocytes facilitated ES cell differentiation into cells of an endothelial lineage expressing factor VIII. Exogenous granulocyte-macrophage colony-stimulating factor further enhanced endothelial differentiation. It is possible that growth factors produced by feeder cells or cocultured cells, ECM molecules and cell-surface receptors expressed by ES Cells are critical in setting up the appropriate micro-environment to drive stem cell differentiation towards particular lineages. The type of ECM molecules, cell-surface receptors for ECM, cell–cell adhesion molecules and glycoconjugates (that is structural mucopolysaccharides, glycans or highly glycosylated proteins) present in the ESCs' micro-environment were analyzed by the same group.

ESCs were cultured under three different conditions: (1) control culture with ESCs on a 3D collagen gel in a culture insert; (2) ESCs on a 3D collagen gel with a feeder layer of HPI.1 cells separated by the membrane of the insert; or (3) ESCs in a 3D collagen gel with HPI.1 cells embedded in the collagen gel[223]. They found ECM molecules such as laminins and fibronectins were synthesized and formed a ring-like matrix surrounding the gland-like structures. Differentiated ES cells were positive for many kinds of lectin receptors including SBA, BSA-1, BSA-1-B4, HPA, DBA, RCA-1, and UEA-1, but negative for SJA. Cell-surface receptors such as integrins β1, α5β1, N-cadherin, and β-catenin were upregulated during differentiation. These findings suggest that such ECM molecules and related receptors possibly mediate ES cell differentiation into endothelial cells.

Vijelath's findings supported the possibility that fibronectin and integrin α5β1 are involved in endothelial cells differentiation[224]. They found that fibronectin significantly promotes CD34+ cells to develop more endothelial colonies in vitro culture than collagen I, IV and vitronectin, and enhanced VEGF-mediated CD34+ cell migration. Blockade of α5β1, but not αvβ3 or αvβ5, inhibited both VEGF-mediated CD34+ cell differentiation and migration. These observations indicate that VEGF and fibronectin together could significantly promote the migration and differentiation of CD34+ cells. This synergism is specific to fibronectin and α5β1 integrin. Combinations of VEGF and FN may be useful in promoting differentiation of circulating endothelial progenitors into endothelial cells for tissue engineering. Another study further extended the molecular pathway that integrin α5β1 participates in the activation of both VEGFR-3 and its downstream PI3 kinase/Akt signaling pathway[225], which is essential for FN-mediated lymphatic endothelial cell survival and proliferation. However, there is a need to better understand the more detailed molecular pathways involved in the proliferation and differentiation of stem/progenitor cells to take full advantage of their clinical potential.

Co-Culture with other Cell Lines

Cell to cell communication is very important for cell survival, growth, and differentiation. After infusion, stem/progenitor cells will home to specific sites, have contact with resident cells, communicate with host cells, and differentiate into specific adult somatic cells. This indicates that cocultured cells will provide a microenvironment which guide stem/progenitor cell differentiation into related cell linage through growth factors secretion and other signal transduction pathways occurring in membrane proteins, for instance, growth factor or integrin signaling. Cocultured CD34+ cell with human microvascular endothelial cells stimulate CD34+ cells to differentiate into endothelial cells. Moreover, cell-cell direct contact between CD34+ and CD34- cells facilitated the endothelial differentiation of CD34+ cells, and coculture with CD34- cells led to 68% enhancement of neovascularization of CD34+ cells[226]. This data suggests that administration of CD34+-enriched cell populations may significantly improve neovascularization and point at an important supportive role for (endogenous or exogenous) CD34- cells.

Human bone marrow stromal cells (HBMSC) were cultured alone or cocultured with human umbilical vein endothelial cells (HUVEC) in different models (co-culture with or without direct contact, conditioned medium) to determine the influence of VEGF on these cells and on their relationship[227]. The data shows that HBMSC express and synthesize VEGF, HUVEC conditioned medium has a proliferative effect on them, and early osteoblastic marker (Alkaline phosphatase activity) levels increase when these cells are co-cultured with HUVEC only in direct contact. However, VEGF had no effect on these processes. These results suggest that the intercommunication between endothelial cells and osteoblastic-like cells requires not only diffusible factors, but also involves cell membrane proteins. However, which membrane protein and signal pathway mediates such cell differentiation is still unknown and continues to be investigated. It is worth exploring the potential target protein and signal pathways which can provide basic information on cell differentiation. Knowledge of these pathways may enable us to direct cell differentation when stem cells are used in cellular therapy, and help us prevent pluripotent cells differentiating into unwanted or dangerous lineage cells.

CLINICAL APPLICATIONS OF STEM/PROGENITOR CELLS IN VASCULAR DISEASES

As mentioned already, vascular disease causing stroke or myocardial infacrtion is the leading killer in the developed world. Animal models have demonstrated that stem/progenitor cells may play a role in both the development of atherosclerosis and in the response to endothelial damage and tissue ischaemia. As such, they provide huge potential to revolutionise the treatment and prevention of cardiovascular disease if only their complex interactions in the human could be fully understood.

The role of progenitor cells in human vascular disease will now be discussed, the argument for their involvement in the development of atherosclerosis is predominantly from animal models and has already been described, this next section will discuss the clinical roles of progenitor cells; as a prognostic indicator, and in the treatment of acute and chronic ischaemia.

Endothelial Progenitor Cell Number and Cardiovascular Disease in Humans

The mechanism of endothelial progenitor cell involvement in endothelial repair may be two fold: are they depleted in vascular disease by means of consumption, or are their number increased in response to a continued requirement? Endothelial progenitor cells have been studied in a variety of patients including those with established vascular disease and those with risk factors for vascular disease. Initially Vasa documented an inverse correlation between the number of endothelial progenitor cells and the number of cardiovascular risk factors in patients with established coronary artery disease [130]. This concept was developed by Hill who demonstrated a reduced number of endothelial progenitor cells in healthy individuals with risk factors for cardiovascular disease[129], correlating endothelial progenitor cell colony forming units to Framingham risk score. Importantly, Hill also noted that reduced endothelial progenitor cell number was predictive of reduced brachial artery flow mediated vasodilatation (FMD), a clinical study of endothelial function. This was the first time a functional clinical endpoint had been correlated to endothelial progenitor cell number in humans, and this clinical endpoint in itself is a predictor of cardiovascular events and restenosis[228]. This leads to speculation that endothelial progenitor cell number may be predictive of cardiovascular events.

Other investigators have shown reduced endothelial progenitor cell number in patients with risk factors for cardiovascular disease such as diabetes[229, 230] and smoking[231], with cessation of smoking resulting in a return of endothelial progenitor cell numbers to normal. Endothelial progenitor cell number is also reduced in groups of patients known to be at higher risk of cardiovascular disease such as those with rheumatoid arthritis[232] or chronic renal failure[233].

Endothelial progenitor cell number is also known to be reduced in established non-coronary cardiovascular disorders such as in patients with strokes[234], peripheral vascular disease[229] and patients with erectile dysfunction[235].

It follows that exposure to cardiovascular risk factors consumes endothelial progenitor cells and atherosclerosis subsequently develops as a result of deficient endothelial repair capacity. This theory is supported by work by Simper and colleagues who described the reduction of endothelial progenitor cell outgrowth colonies in the blood of cardiac allograft patients with documented transplant vasculopathy as opposed to transplant patients without transplant atherosclerosis[53]. He went on to show that endothelial cells seeded at the sites of atherosclerosis in patients who had received sex mismatched transplants were from recipient origin and not from the donor, further confirming the presence of circulating cells contributing to endothelial repair.

As described above, endothelial progenitor cell number is inversely correlated to risk factors for cardiovascular disease in healthy individuals and in those with established ischaemia[129, 130]. Endothelial progenitor cell number was also correlated to brachial FMD[129, 236], a measure of endothelial function, which itself is identified as a predictor of cardiovascular events[228, 237] and restenosis[238].

Endothelial progenitor cell functional impairment has been described in patients with restenosis following percutaneous coronary intervention[24], but until recently endothelial progenitor cell number has been indicative only of the potential presence of cardiovascular dysfunction rather than predictive of its outcome.

In late 2005, Werner published a large study of endothelial progenitor cell levels in patients attending for coronary angiography and then followed the patients for 12 months. Initial endothelial progenitor cell level was predictive of cardiovascular events and death from cardiovascular causes over the follow up period. This suggests that as well as being implicated in the development of cardiovascular disease, endothelial progenitor cells may play a role in the progression from stable disease to unstable events and as such, measurement of endothelial progenitor cell level may be a useful test in the clinic to identify patients at high risk of acute events and hence those in need of urgent intervention[239]. Importantly this correlation between endothelial progenitor cells and outcome was positive across a variety of laboratory methods the authors used for endothelial progenitor cell measurement.

Endothelial Progenitor Cells and Established Ischaemia – Clinical Trials

The clinical studies of cellular therapy are numerous and have followed the animal studies, using a variety of cell types and delivery methods. Below are detailed the published clinical trials.

Peripheral Vascular Disease

Bone marrow mononuclear cells were shown to improve ankle-brachial index when injected autologously into the gastrocnemius of patients with peripheral vascular disease[240], whilst peripheral blood mononuclear cells were not as effective. A recent study of 6 patients has shown that peripheral blood mononuclear cells were effective in improving limb perfusion when injected into the calf muscle of patients with severe peripheral vascular disease, however, the patients were all pre-treated with G-CSF as an attempt to mobilize stem cells from the bone marrow prior to cell harvest [241].

Myocardial Ischaemia

In clinical trials of myocardial ischaemia many studies have now reported. Some have shown significant benefit, whilst others have demonstrated only modest effects or no effect at all. It is important to note that many of these trials started with little understanding of the mechanisms by which cell transplantation would have its effects. Equally, as demonstrated by the animal studies detailed earlier, there is no consensus on the optimal cell type to use or the optimal mode of delivery. Hence the published literature contains heterogeneous evidence that should be interpreted carefully.

Despite success in animal models, use of cell transplantation in humans first had to be demonstrated as safe as there were concerns that the technique may provoke arrhythmias as was seen when skeletal muscle cells were used[242]. Several small feasibility studies reported that intramyocardial injection of mononuclear cells did not cause the type of ventricular arrhythmias seen with skeletal cell use[243-245].

Trials Following Acute Myocardial Infarction

Strauer transplanted autologous bone marrow mononuclear cells via the intracoronary route 5-9 days after myocardial infarction and demonstrated a reduced infarct size with improved stroke volume index and myocardial perfusion in the cell therapy group[246]. The TOPCARE-AMI trial isolated endothelial progenitor cells from peripheral blood and compared them to bone marrow mononuclear cells for intracoronary reinfusion following acute myocardial infarction[3]. Both groups were seen to have improved regional wall motion and reduced end systolic volume when compared to nonrandomized controls. These improvements were still present after one year of follow-up[171]. Subsequently the BOOST study, the first randomized control trial of intracoronary injection of bone marrow mononuclear cells following AMI, reported improved global left ventricular function in the cell treated group at six months[247] but this did not continue to improve in the following 12 months[248]. Recently other larger trials have reported mixed results. The REPAIR-AMI trial, the largest trial of this nature to date, used a multi-centre setting to randomize patients to intracoronary culture expanded bone marrow cells or placebo. Cell treated patients demonstrated a small overall improvement in LV function (5.5% vs. 3.0%) and a reduction in adverse events during 1 year follow up[249]. In the same journal issue however, the ASTAMI trial reported no improvement in LV function in the patients treated with bone marrow mononuclear cells as compared to controls at 6 months[250].

The majority of trials using cell therapy following AMI provide the suggestion that improvement may just reach statistical significance, however, the jury is still out on whether there is any real evidence of clinically significant improvement. Importantly the safety profile of such therapy has been encouraging except in the MAGIC trial[251]. This trial reported enhanced stent restenosis in the cell treated group and was stopped prematurely. However, the design of this trial, which utilized G-CSF mobilisation of stem cells prior to the initial PCI has been criticized and postulated as the cause of the restenosis. In later studies, Kang addressed the issue of restenosis after G-SCF mobilization in the drug eluting stent era and shown that G-CSF based stem cell therapy is safe and does not influence restenosis[252], it should be noted that the timing of G-CSF therapy was modified as well as the change to drug eluting stent use.

Chronic Myocardial Ischaemia

The setting of chronic myocardial ischaemia is somewhat different from that of AMI. In acute ischaemia, ongoing inflammation and cell damage may act as a homing signal for mobilized or injected stem or progenitor cells. Also the cell therapy has the possibility of modulating the deleterious effects of the remodelling process. In patients with chronic ischaemia this is not the case and hence the potential benefits of cell therapy are arguably not as high in the short term.

The initial small, safety and feasibility studies took place in this setting, with Hamano and Stamm demonstrating improved perfusion in viable target areas[244, 245] and Galinanes demonstrating improved regional wall motion in non-viable target areas but only when these territories received a concomitant bypass graft[243]. All these studies used the intramyocardial route for cell delivery as compared to the more common use of intracoronary infusion following acute ischaemia.

Recently three trials have reported on autologous bone marrow transplantation into chronically ischaemic myocardium.

The ICAT study used a non randomized protocol and the intracoronary route of delivery for cultured bone marrow mononuclear cells which were harvested 1 day prior to reinfusion, with the control patients those who refused entry into the trial. Cell treated patients showed improved global and segmental ventricular function[253].

In the first randomized trial of its type, Patel and colleagues randomized patients to OPCAB or OPCAB plus intramyocardial cell therapy. The cells were bone marrow cells harvested prior to sternotomy and then processed during surgery to achieve a mononuclear cell suspension. Patients who received OPCAB plus cell therapy had improved global LV function over the 6 month follow up period[254].

Finally TOPCARE-CHD investigated the intracoronary delivery of bone marrow or circulating progenitor cells in patients on average 6 years following myocardial infarction. The study was performed in a randomized crossover fashion, demonstrating a small benefit of bone marrow derived cells on global LV function irrespective of the order the cells were given[255].

The findings of improvement of ventricular function following cellular therapy in the chronically ischaemic patients suggests that cell therapy offers more than just enhancement of the healing process or attenuation of harmful remodelling after the acute event, however the biological process by which this occurs is poorly understood.

Mechanism of Benefit in Ischaemia?

Despite the numerous studies mentioned above which have detailed beneficial effects of bone marrow derived progenitor cells in acute and chronic myocardial ischaemia, the mechanism by which such effects occur is still elusive. Do these cells differentiate into myocardial cells and couple into the existing ventricular geometry to enhance contractile function? Do they differentiate into endothelial cells to facilitate angiogenesis and thereby provide perfusion to hibernating areas of myocardium? Do they merely secrete cytokines which attract as yet undefined stem cells from another location to facilitate myocardial regeneration?

Despite initial promise of myocardial differentiation of bone marrow derived cells in-vitro[117] and in vivo[75], this mechanism is now severely questioned due to the laboratory techniques used in the in vivo work[106, 107]. It is now thought that bone marrow derived cells can not differentiate into cardiac myocytes in ischaemic myocardium[107].

It has also been shown that the majority of cells infused during cellular therapy do not stay in the injected heart[256], if cells are injected intravenously none home to infarcted myocardium, whereas between 2% and 39% of unselected bone marrow cells or CD34 selected bone marrow cells stayed in the heart after intracoronary infusion.

In summary, early trials of cellular therapy have encouraging results, however, we still do not fully understand the biology of the cells currently being used for therapy, nor do we have enough data to define which cell type should be used, when they should be collected and by which route they should be reinfused. The fact remains that clinical trials are surging ahead without robust basic science and animal data about the cells in use.

Clinical Potential of Endothelial Progenitor Cell Transfusion after Arterial Intervention

Despite much animal work on the benefit of endothelial progenitor cells following vascular intervention a therapeutic role for endothelial progenitor cell has not emerged. The major issues limiting this progression into the clinical arena are the low numbers of circulating endothelial progenitor cells in patients with vascular disease and the difficulty in culture expanding them in a timely fashion without the use of animal serum.

Also the real worry following vascular intervention is the development of neointimal hyperplasia and restenosis, and, in the era of the drug eluting coronary stent, data would have to be extremely convincing to allow clinical trials of endothelial progenitor cells versus drug eluting stents following angioplasty. There is already data to suggest that drug eluting stents inhibit endothelialisation of the stent via their action on endothelial progenitor cells as well as inhibiting smooth muscle proliferation and the development of restenosis[257]. Therefore, attempts to use endothelial progenitor cells in this setting would be unsuccessful. However, there is potential for their clinical use in the absence of drug eluting stents.

One setting in which the use of endothelial progenitor cells has potential is that of preserving vascular access for treatments such as renal replacement therapy. Often long term vascular access is achieved via a surgically created PTFE expanded arterio-venous fistula which are frequently troubled by neointimal formation and stenosis. Rotmans attempted to enhance endothelial progenitor cell adhesion to the site of the PTFE grafts by coating the grafts with anti-CD34 antibodies prior to placement in pigs. As endothelial progenitor cells are a subpopulation of the CD34 mononuclear fragment, progenitor cells should show enhanced adherence to the graft, promote re-endothelialisation and reduce neointimal formation. Although the CD34 coated grafts did show improved reendothelialisation compared to uncoated grafts by 72 hours, they in fact went on to develop a profound increase in neointimal hyperplasia and stenosis[258]. Hence, this study demonstrated that an attempt to harness endothelial progenitor cells via a non-specific marker although resulting in increased endothelial coverage had a deleterious effect on stenosis. This acts as a warning of potential surprises when attempts are made to manipulate progenitor cells whose biology we do not yet completely understand.

At present, despite initial encouraging animal data, the use of endothelial progenitor cells following vascular procedures has not yet emerged as a viable option. However, once the real biology of endothelial progenitor cells is understood, they have the potential to be utilized to prolong graft longevity.

PROSPECTIVE/CONCLUSIONS

In conclusion, stem/progenitor cells isolated from embryonic or adult species have the capacity to proliferate, migrate, and differentiate into vascular lineage cells but have not yet acquired mature endothelial markers. Stem/progenitor cells are mobilized from bone marrow and other harboring sites including adipose tissue and vessel adventitia into the circulation and then home to sites of neovascularization in response to physiological and pathological stimuli, thereby contributing to postnatal neovascularization. Since animal experiments on stem/progenitor cells transplantation proved the therapeutic potential of cell-based strategy, the application of stem/progenitor cells for regenerative medicine has been expected with keen interest. Although early clinical trials showed optimistic results, larger randomized control trials have shown only modest benefit of cellular therapy. A number of issues remain to be addressed in this research field, and when the answers are available, hopefully stem cell therapy can fulfill its potential and revolutionise the treatment of vascular disease. Some of the future perspectives are as follows:

1　identification of a specific marker for stem/progenitor cells which is not shared by other lineage cells. Specific markers ideally would identify different stem/progenitor subsets with different mechanisms of action.

2　evaluation of stem/progenitor cell transdifferentiation in vitro and in physiological and pathological regeneration of tissues and organs. There is still debate on the role of transdifferentiation in cardiac tissues.

3　methodological optimization of stem/progenitor cells differentiation, purification, expansion, gene transfer, and administration to improve the efficacy of cell transplantation.

4　comparison of the therapeutic impact between purified stem/progenitor subpopulations and total bone marrow MNCs, as well as different stem/progenitor cells. We frankly do not know for sure what cell(s) is responsible for the arterial wall repair, which cellular subset is most active in neovascularisation or which cell type acts predominantly via angiogenic cytokine secretion. It is indeed quite possible that several progenitor cell types contribute to each function, meaning that attempts to isolate a single cell type for therapy may be unsuccessful, for example cells incorporating into neo vessels may only act in the presence of helper cells. It is also equally possible that endothelial progenitor cells are sufficient to provide adequate repair of the arterial wall, with required plasticity to provide not only mature endothelial cells but also other cells for the arterial wall such as smooth muscle cells.

5　investigation of related mechanisms controlling stem/progenitor cell differentiation into vascular cells, and mediating their therapeutic effects when transplanted by streamlined differentiation control.

6　optimization of methodologies to generate a large number of vascular cells from stem/progenitor cells with high purity for use in tissue engineering.

7　large multicentre clinical trials with strict guidelines for stem/progenitor cell treatments in vascular diseases to define the optimal cell type, mode of delivery and timing of delivery.

Although new therapeutic opportunities in clinical medicine are created by stem/progenitor cell research, we should also point out the following limitations in such research. Most of the cells charged with the repair mission have been tagged as vascular or endothelial progenitor cells in the current literature, not as "stem cells." We have to define well whether stem and progenitor are two kinds of cells, or the same cell population but just two different terms. It is believed that the term stem cell should be reserved to cells that satisfy certain criteria: (a) it must be capable of unlimited self-renewal by symmetric division; (b) it must be able to divide asymmetrically with one daughter cell resembling the mother cell and the other a more differentiated type of cell; and (c) it must originate from an embryonic or adult stem cell reservoir. However, the criteria to define and identify progenitor cells are less well defined. We anticipate that with the substantial body of research currently applied to this topic, most of these questions will be answered in the near future.

ACKNOWLEDGEMENTS

This work was supported by Grants from British Heart Foundation and the Oak Foundation. None of the authors have a financial interest related to this work.

REFERENCES

[1] Asahara, T., et al., Isolation of putative progenitor endothelial cells for angiogenesis. *Science,* 1997. 275(5302): p. 964-7.

[2] Kalka, C., et al., Transplantation of ex vivo expanded endothelial progenitor cells for therapeutic neovascularization. *Proc. Natl. Acad. Sci. U S A,* 2000. 97(7): p. 3422-7.

[3] Assmus, B., et al., Transplantation of Progenitor Cells and Regeneration Enhancement in Acute Myocardial Infarction (TOPCARE-AMI). *Circulation,* 2002. 106(24): p. 3009-17.

[4] Xiao, Q., et al., Sca-1+ progenitors derived from embryonic stem cells differentiate into endothelial cells capable of vascular repair after arterial injury. *Arterioscler. Thromb. Vasc. Biol,* 2006. 26(10): p. 2244-51.

[5] Xu, Q., The impact of progenitor cells in atherosclerosis. *Nat. Clin. Pract. Cardiovasc. Med,* 2006. 3(2): p. 94-101.

[6] Knowles, J.W. and N. Maeda, Genetic modifiers of atherosclerosis in mice. *Arterioscler. Thromb. Vasc. Biol,* 2000. 20(11): p. 2336-45.

[7] Mohler, E.R., 3rd, et al., Identification and characterization of calcifying valve cells from human and canine aortic valves. *J. Heart Valve Dis,* 1999. 8(3): p. 254-60.

[8] Tintut, Y., et al., Multilineage potential of cells from the artery wall. *Circulation,* 2003. 108(20): p. 2505-10.

[9] Sata, M., et al., Hematopoietic stem cells differentiate into vascular cells that participate in the pathogenesis of atherosclerosis. *Nat. Med,* 2002. 8(4): p. 403-9.

[10] Bentzon, J.F., et al., Smooth muscle cells in atherosclerosis originate from the local vessel wall and not circulating progenitor cells in ApoE knockout mice. *Arterioscler. Thromb. Vasc. Biol,* 2006. 26(12): p. 2696-702.

[11] Rauscher, F.M., et al., Aging, progenitor cell exhaustion, and atherosclerosis. *Circulation,* 2003. 108(4): p. 457-63.

[12] Zulli, A., et al., CD34 Class III positive cells are present in atherosclerotic plaques of the rabbit model of atherosclerosis. *Histochem. Cell Biol,* 2005. 124(6): p. 517-22.

[13] Torsney, E., et al., Characterisation of progenitor cells in human atherosclerotic vessels. *Atherosclerosis,* 2006.

[14] Wilcox, J.N., et al., Perivascular responses after angioplasty which may contribute to postangioplasty restenosis: a role for circulating myofibroblast precursors? *Ann. N. Y. Acad. Sci,* 2001. 947: p. 68-90; dicussion 90-2.

[15] Clowes, A.W., M.A. Reidy, and M.M. Clowes, Kinetics of cellular proliferation after arterial injury. I. Smooth muscle growth in the absence of endothelium. *Lab. Invest,* 1983. 49(3): p. 327-33.

[16] Clowes, A.W., M.A. Reidy, and M.M. Clowes, Mechanisms of stenosis after arterial injury. *Lab. Invest,* 1983. 49(2): p. 208-15.

[17] Reidy, M.A., J. Fingerle, and V. Lindner, Factors controlling the development of arterial lesions after injury. *Circulation,* 1992. 86(6 Suppl): p. III43-6.

[18] Kakuta, T., et al., Differences in compensatory vessel enlargement, not intimal formation, account for restenosis after angioplasty in the hypercholesterolemic rabbit model. *Circulation,* 1994. 89(6): p. 2809-15.

[19] Post, M.J., C. Borst, and R.E. Kuntz, The relative importance of arterial remodeling compared with intimal hyperplasia in lumen renarrowing after balloon angioplasty. A study in the normal rabbit and the hypercholesterolemic Yucatan micropig. *Circulation,* 1994. 89(6): p. 2816-21.

[20] Mintz, G.S., et al., Arterial remodeling after coronary angioplasty: a serial intravascular ultrasound study. *Circulation,* 1996. 94(1): p. 35-43.

[21] Shoji, M., et al., Temporal and spatial characterization of cellular constituents during neointimal hyperplasia after vascular injury: Potential contribution of bone-marrow-derived progenitors to arterial remodeling. *Cardiovasc. Pathol,* 2004. 13(6): p. 306-12.

[22] Hibbert, B., Y.X. Chen, and E.R. O'Brien, c-kit-immunopositive vascular progenitor cells populate human coronary in-stent restenosis but not primary atherosclerotic lesions. *Am. J. Physiol. Heart Circ. Physiol,* 2004. 287(2): p. H518-24.

[23] Skowasch, D., et al., Presence of bone-marrow- and neural-crest-derived cells in intimal hyperplasia at the time of clinical in-stent restenosis. Cardiovasc Res, 2003. 60(3): p. 684-91.

[24] George, J., et al., Number and adhesive properties of circulating endothelial progenitor cells in patients with in-stent restenosis. *Arterioscler. Thromb. Vasc. Biol,* 2003. 23(12): p. e57-60.

[25] Matsuo, Y., et al., The effect of senescence of endothelial progenitor cells on in-stent restenosis in patients undergoing coronary stenting. *Intern. Med,* 2006. 45(9): p. 581-7.

[26] Schober, A., et al., Peripheral CD34+ cells and the risk of in-stent restenosis in patients with coronary heart disease. *Am. J. Cardiol,* 2005. 96(8): p. 1116-22.

[27] Xu, Q., Mouse models of arteriosclerosis: from arterial injuries to vascular grafts. *Am. J. Pathol,* 2004. 165(1): p. 1-10.

[28] Zou, Y., et al., Mouse model of venous bypass graft arteriosclerosis. *Am. J. Pathol,* 1998. 153(4): p. 1301-10.

[29] Mayr, M., et al., Biomechanical stress-induced apoptosis in vein grafts involves p38 mitogen-activated protein kinases. *Faseb. J,* 2000. 14(2): p. 261-70.

[30] Han, C.I., G.R. Campbell, and J.H. Campbell, Circulating bone marrow cells can contribute to neointimal formation. *J. Vasc. Res,* 2001. 38(2): p. 113-9.

[31] Hillebrands, J.L., et al., Origin of neointimal endothelium and alpha-actin-positive smooth muscle cells in transplant arteriosclerosis. *J. Clin. Invest,* 2001. 107(11): p. 1411-22.

[32] Hu, Y., et al., Smooth muscle cells in transplant atherosclerotic lesions are originated from recipients, but not bone marrow progenitor cells. *Circulation,* 2002. 106(14): p. 1834-9.

[33] Li, J., et al., Vascular smooth muscle cells of recipient origin mediate intimal expansion after aortic allotransplantation in mice. *Am. J. Pathol,* 2001. 158(6): p. 1943-7.

[34] Saiura, A., et al., Circulating smooth muscle progenitor cells contribute to atherosclerosis. *Nat. Med,* 2001. 7(4): p. 382-3.

[35] Shimizu, K., et al., Host bone-marrow cells are a source of donor intimal smooth-muscle-like cells in murine aortic transplant arteriopathy. *Nat. Med,* 2001. 7(6): p. 738-41.

[36] Owens, G.K., Regulation of differentiation of vascular smooth muscle cells. *Physiol. Rev,* 1995. 75(3): p. 487-517.

[37] Schwartz, S.M., The intima : A new soil. *Circ. Res,* 1999. 85(10): p. 877-9.

[38] Simper, D., et al., Smooth muscle progenitor cells in human blood. *Circulation,* 2002. 106(10): p. 1199-204.

[39] Le Ricousse-Roussanne, S., et al., Ex vivo differentiated endothelial and smooth muscle cells from human cord blood progenitors home to the angiogenic tumor vasculature. *Cardiovasc. Res,* 2004. 62(1): p. 176-84.

[40] Hu, Y., et al., Both donor and recipient origins of smooth muscle cells in vein graft atherosclerotic lesions. *Circ. Res,* 2002. 91(7): p. e13-20.

[41] Caplice, N.M., et al., Smooth muscle cells in human coronary atherosclerosis can originate from cells administered at marrow transplantation. *Proc. Natl. Acad. Sci. U S A,* 2003. 100(8): p. 4754-9.

[42] Hu, Y., et al., Abundant progenitor cells in the adventitia contribute to atherosclerosis of vein grafts in ApoE-deficient mice. *J. Clin. Invest,* 2004. 113(9): p. 1258-65.

[43] Margariti, A., L. Zeng, and Q. Xu, Stem cells, vascular smooth muscle cells and atherosclerosis. *Histol. Histopathol,* 2006. 21(9): p. 979-85.

[44] Torsney, E., Y. Hu, and Q. Xu, Adventitial progenitor cells contribute to arteriosclerosis. *Trends Cardiovasc. Med,* 2005. 15(2): p. 64-8.

[45] Xu, Q., et al., Circulating progenitor cells regenerate endothelium of vein graft atherosclerosis, which is diminished in ApoE-deficient mice. *Circ. Res,* 2003. 93(8): p. e76-86.

[46] Mayr, U., et al., Accelerated arteriosclerosis of vein grafts in inducible NO synthase(-/-) mice is related to decreased endothelial progenitor cell repair. *Circ. Res,* 2006. 98(3): p. 412-20.

[47] Torsney, E., et al., Thrombosis and neointima formation in vein grafts are inhibited by locally applied aspirin through endothelial protection. *Circ. Res,* 2004. 94(11): p. 1466-73.

[48] Dietrich, H., et al., Rapid development of vein graft atheroma in ApoE-deficient mice. *Am. J. Pathol,* 2000. 157(2): p. 659-69.

[49] Johnson, P., et al., Recipient cells form the intimal proliferative lesion in the rat aortic model of allograft arteriosclerosis. *Am. J. Transplant,* 2002. 2(3): p. 207-14.

[50] Hu, Y., et al., Endothelial replacement and angiogenesis in arteriosclerotic lesions of allografts are contributed by circulating progenitor cells. *Circulation,* 2003. 108(25): p. 3122-7.

[51] Glaser, R., et al., Smooth muscle cells, but not myocytes, of host origin in transplanted human hearts. *Circulation,* 2002. 106(1): p. 17-9.

[52] Hillebrands, J., et al., Recipient origin of neointimal vascular smooth muscle cells in cardiac allografts with transplant arteriosclerosis. *J. Heart Lung Transplant,* 2000. 19(12): p. 1183-92.

[53] Simper, D., et al., Endothelial progenitor cells are decreased in blood of cardiac allograft patients with vasculopathy and endothelial cells of noncardiac origin are enriched in transplant atherosclerosis. *Circulation,* 2003. 108(2): p. 143-9.

[54] Feraud, O. and D. Vittet, Murine embryonic stem cell in vitro differentiation: applications to the study of vascular development. *Histol. Histopathol,* 2003. 18(1): p. 191-9.

[55] Vittet, D., et al., Embryonic stem cells differentiate in vitro to endothelial cells through successive maturation steps. *Blood,* 1996. 88(9): p. 3424-31.

[56] Levenberg, S., et al., Endothelial cells derived from human embryonic stem cells. *Proc. Natl. Acad. Sci. U S A,* 2002. 99(7): p. 4391-6.

[57] Fisher, K.A. and R.S. Summer, 4. Stem and progenitor cells in the formation of the pulmonary vasculature. *Curr. Top Dev. Biol,* 2006. 74: p. 117-31.

[58] Doetschman, T.C., et al., The in vitro development of blastocyst-derived embryonic stem cell lines: formation of visceral yolk sac, blood islands and myocardium. *J. Embryol. Exp. Morphol,* 1985. 87: p. 27-45.

[59] Risau, W., et al., Vasculogenesis and angiogenesis in embryonic-stem-cell-derived embryoid bodies. *Development,* 1988. 102(3): p. 471-8.

[60] Wang, R., R. Clark, and V.L. Bautch, Embryonic stem cell-derived cystic embryoid bodies form vascular channels: an in vitro model of blood vessel development. *Development,* 1992. 114(2): p. 303-16.

[61] Young, P.E., S. Baumhueter, and L.A. Lasky, The sialomucin CD34 is expressed on hematopoietic cells and blood vessels during murine development. *Blood,* 1995. 85(1): p. 96-105.

[62] Wartenberg, M., et al., The embryoid body as a novel in vitro assay system for antiangiogenic agents. *Lab. Invest,* 1998. 78(10): p. 1301-14.

[63] Nakagami, H., et al., Model of vasculogenesis from embryonic stem cells for vascular research and regenerative medicine. *Hypertension,* 2006. 48(1): p. 112-9.

[64] Li, Z.J., et al., [In vitro vasculogenesis and angiogenesis of mouse embryonic stem cells]. Zhongguo Yi Xue Ke Xue Yuan Xue Bao, 2005. 27(1): p. 62-6.

[65] Feraud, O., Y. Cao, and D. Vittet, Embryonic stem cell-derived embryoid bodies development in collagen gels recapitulates sprouting angiogenesis. *Lab. Invest,* 2001. 81(12): p. 1669-81.

[66] Asahara, T. and A. Kawamoto, Endothelial progenitor cells for postnatal vasculogenesis. *Am. J. Physiol. Cell Physiol,* 2004. 287(3): p. C572-9.

[67] Asahara, T., et al., Bone marrow origin of endothelial progenitor cells responsible for postnatal vasculogenesis in physiological and pathological neovascularization. *Circ. Res,* 1999. 85(3): p. 221-8.

[68] Asahara, T., et al., VEGF contributes to postnatal neovascularization by mobilizing bone marrow-derived endothelial progenitor cells. *Embo J,* 1999. 18(14): p. 3964-72.

[69] Majka, S.M., et al., Distinct progenitor populations in skeletal muscle are bone marrow derived and exhibit different cell fates during vascular regeneration. *J. Clin. Invest,* 2003. 111(1): p. 71-9.

[70] Iwaguro, H., et al., Endothelial progenitor cell vascular endothelial growth factor gene transfer for vascular regeneration. *Circulation,* 2002. 105(6): p. 732-8.

[71] Schatteman, G.C., et al., Blood-derived angioblasts accelerate blood-flow restoration in diabetic mice. *J. Clin. Invest,* 2000. 106(4): p. 571-8.

[72] Crosby, J.R., et al., Endothelial cells of hematopoietic origin make a significant contribution to adult blood vessel formation. *Circ. Res,* 2000. 87(9): p. 728-30.

[73] Takahashi, T., et al., Ischemia- and cytokine-induced mobilization of bone marrow-derived endothelial progenitor cells for neovascularization. *Nat. Med,* 1999. 5(4): p. 434-8.

[74] Rafii, S., Circulating endothelial precursors: mystery, reality, and promise. *J. Clin. Invest,* 2000. 105(1): p. 17-9.

[75] Orlic, D., et al., Bone marrow cells regenerate infarcted myocardium. *Nature,* 2001. 410(6829): p. 701-5.

[76] Orlic, D., et al., Mobilized bone marrow cells repair the infarcted heart, improving function and survival. *Proc. Natl. Acad. Sci. U S A,* 2001. 98(18): p. 10344-9.

[77] Kocher, A.A., et al., Neovascularization of ischemic myocardium by human bone-marrow-derived angioblasts prevents cardiomyocyte apoptosis, reduces remodeling and improves cardiac function. *Nat. Med,* 2001. 7(4): p. 430-6.

[78] Jackson, K.A., et al., Regeneration of ischemic cardiac muscle and vascular endothelium by adult stem cells. *J. Clin. Invest,* 2001. 107(11): p. 1395-402.

[79] Edelberg, J.M., et al., Young adult bone marrow-derived endothelial precursor cells restore aging-impaired cardiac angiogenic function. Circ Res, 2002. 90(10): p. E89-93.

[80] Shi, Q., et al., Evidence for circulating bone marrow-derived endothelial cells. *Blood,* 1998. 92(2): p. 362-7.

[81] Bhattacharya, V., et al., Enhanced endothelialization and microvessel formation in polyester grafts seeded with CD34(+) bone marrow cells. *Blood,* 2000. 95(2): p. 581-5.

[82] Kaushal, S., et al., Functional small-diameter neovessels created using endothelial progenitor cells expanded ex vivo. *Nat. Med,* 2001. 7(9): p. 1035-40.

[83] Noishiki, Y., et al., Autocrine angiogenic vascular prosthesis with bone marrow transplantation. *Nat. Med,* 1996. 2(1): p. 90-3.

[84] Otani, A., et al., Bone marrow-derived stem cells target retinal astrocytes and can promote or inhibit retinal angiogenesis. *Nat. Med,* 2002. 8(9): p. 1004-10.

[85] Grant, M.B., et al., Adult hematopoietic stem cells provide functional hemangioblast activity during retinal neovascularization. *Nat. Med,* 2002. 8(6): p. 607-12.

[86] Crisa, L., et al., Human cord blood progenitors sustain thymic T-cell development and a novel form of angiogenesis. *Blood,* 1999. 94(11): p. 3928-40.

[87] Young, P.P., A.A. Hofling, and M.S. Sands, VEGF increases engraftment of bone marrow-derived endothelial progenitor cells (EPCs) into vasculature of newborn murine recipients. *Proc. Natl. Acad. Sci. U S A,* 2002. 99(18): p. 11951-6.

[88] Lyden, D., et al., Impaired recruitment of bone-marrow-derived endothelial and hematopoietic precursor cells blocks tumor angiogenesis and growth. *Nat. Med,* 2001. 7(11): p. 1194-201.

[89] Reyes, M., et al., Origin of endothelial progenitors in human postnatal bone marrow. *J. Clin. Invest,* 2002. 109(3): p. 337-46.

[90] Gehling, U.M., et al., In vitro differentiation of endothelial cells from AC133-positive progenitor cells. *Blood,* 2000. 95(10): p. 3106-12.

[91] Marchetti, S., et al., Endothelial cells genetically selected from differentiating mouse embryonic stem cells incorporate at sites of neovascularization in vivo. *J. Cell Sci,* 2002. 115(Pt 10): p. 2075-85.

[92] Davidoff, A.M., et al., Bone marrow-derived cells contribute to tumor neovasculature and, when modified to express an angiogenesis inhibitor, can restrict tumor growth in mice. *Clin. Cancer Res,* 2001. 7(9): p. 2870-9.

[93] Shi, Q., et al., Utilizing granulocyte colony-stimulating factor to enhance vascular graft endothelialization from circulating blood cells. *Ann. Vasc. Surg,* 2002. 16(3): p. 314-20.

[94] Montesinos, M.C., et al., Adenosine A(2A) receptor activation promotes wound neovascularization by stimulating angiogenesis and vasculogenesis. *Am. J. Pathol,* 2004. 164(6): p. 1887-92.

[95] Galiano, R.D., et al., Topical vascular endothelial growth factor accelerates diabetic wound healing through increased angiogenesis and by mobilizing and recruiting bone marrow-derived cells. *Am. J. Pathol,* 2004. 164(6): p. 1935-47.

[96] Suh, W., et al., Transplantation of endothelial progenitor cells accelerates dermal wound healing with increased recruitment of monocytes/macrophages and neovascularization. *Stem Cells,* 2005. 23(10): p. 1571-8.

[97] Madeddu, P., et al., Transplantation of low dose CD34+KDR+ cells promotes vascular and muscular regeneration in ischemic limbs. *Faseb. J,* 2004. 18(14): p. 1737-9.

[98] Botta, R., et al., Heart infarct in NOD-SCID mice: therapeutic vasculogenesis by transplantation of human CD34+ cells and low dose CD34+KDR+ cells. *Faseb J,* 2004. 18(12): p. 1392-4.

[99] Friedrich, E.B., et al., CD34-/CD133+/VEGFR-2+ endothelial progenitor cell subpopulation with potent vasoregenerative capacities. *Circ. Res,* 2006. 98(3): p. e20-5.

[100] Iwase, T., et al., Comparison of angiogenic potency between mesenchymal stem cells and mononuclear cells in a rat model of hindlimb ischemia. *Cardiovasc. Res,* 2005. 66(3): p. 543-51.

[101] McFarlin, K., et al., Bone marrow-derived mesenchymal stromal cells accelerate wound healing in the rat. *Wound Repair Regen,* 2006. 14(4): p. 471-8.

[102] Nakagawa, H., et al., Human mesenchymal stem cells successfully improve skin-substitute wound healing. *Br. J. Dermatol,* 2005. 153(1): p. 29-36.

[103] Satoh, H., et al., Transplanted mesenchymal stem cells are effective for skin regeneration in acute cutaneous wounds. *Cell Transplant,* 2004. 13(4): p. 405-12.

[104] Kim, S.W., et al., Successful stem cell therapy using umbilical cord blood-derived multipotent stem cells for Buerger's disease and ischemic limb disease animal model. *Stem Cells,* 2006. 24(6): p. 1620-6.

[105] Moon, M.H., et al., Human adipose tissue-derived mesenchymal stem cells improve postnatal neovascularization in a mouse model of hindlimb ischemia. *Cell Physiol. Biochem*, 2006. 17(5-6): p. 279-90.

[106] Balsam, L.B., et al., Haematopoietic stem cells adopt mature haematopoietic fates in ischaemic myocardium. *Nature*, 2004. 428(6983): p. 668-73.

[107] Murry, C.E., et al., Haematopoietic stem cells do not transdifferentiate into cardiac myocytes in myocardial infarcts. *Nature*, 2004. 428(6983): p. 664-8.

[108] Nygren, J.M., et al., Bone marrow-derived hematopoietic cells generate cardiomyocytes at a low frequency through cell fusion, but not transdifferentiation. *Nat. Med*, 2004. 10(5): p. 494-501.

[109] Reinecke, H., et al., Evidence for fusion between cardiac and skeletal muscle cells. *Circ. Res*, 2004. 94(6): p. e56-60.

[110] Shi, D., et al., Myogenic fusion of human bone marrow stromal cells, but not hematopoietic cells. *Blood*, 2004. 104(1): p. 290-4.

[111] Kajstura, J., et al., Bone marrow cells differentiate in cardiac cell lineages after infarction independently of cell fusion. *Circ. Res*, 2005. 96(1): p. 127-37.

[112] Kawada, H., et al., Nonhematopoietic mesenchymal stem cells can be mobilized and differentiate into cardiomyocytes after myocardial infarction. *Blood*, 2004. 104(12): p. 3581-7.

[113] Fukuda, K. and J. Fujita, Mesenchymal, but not hematopoietic, stem cells can be mobilized and differentiate into cardiomyocytes after myocardial infarction in mice. *Kidney Int*, 2005. 68(5): p. 1940-3.

[114] Hattan, N., et al., Purified cardiomyocytes from bone marrow mesenchymal stem cells produce stable intracardiac grafts in mice. *Cardiovasc. Res*, 2005. 65(2): p. 334-44.

[115] Barbash, I.M., et al., Systemic delivery of bone marrow-derived mesenchymal stem cells to the infarcted myocardium: feasibility, cell migration, and body distribution. *Circulation*, 2003. 108(7): p. 863-8.

[116] Aicher, A., et al., Assessment of the tissue distribution of transplanted human endothelial progenitor cells by radioactive labeling. *Circulation*, 2003. 107(16): p. 2134-9.

[117] Badorff, C., et al., Transdifferentiation of blood-derived human adult endothelial progenitor cells into functionally active cardiomyocytes. *Circulation*, 2003. 107(7): p. 1024-32.

[118] Kawamoto, A., et al., Therapeutic potential of ex vivo expanded endothelial progenitor cells for myocardial ischemia. *Circulation*, 2001. 103(5): p. 634-7.

[119] Kawamoto, A., et al., Intramyocardial transplantation of autologous endothelial progenitor cells for therapeutic neovascularization of myocardial ischemia. *Circulation*, 2003. 107(3): p. 461-8.

[120] Iwasaki, H., et al., Dose-dependent contribution of CD34-positive cell transplantation to concurrent vasculogenesis and cardiomyogenesis for functional regenerative recovery after myocardial infarction. *Circulation*, 2006. 113(10): p. 1311-25.

[121] Werner, L., et al., Transfer of endothelial progenitor cells improves myocardial performance in rats with dilated cardiomyopathy induced following experimental myocarditis. *J. Mol. Cell Cardiol*, 2005. 39(4): p. 691-7.

[122] Jiang, Y., et al., Pluripotency of mesenchymal stem cells derived from adult marrow. *Nature,* 2002. 418(6893): p. 41-9.

[123] Rafii, S. and D. Lyden, Therapeutic stem and progenitor cell transplantation for organ vascularization and regeneration. *Nat. Med,* 2003. 9(6): p. 702-12.

[124] Rafii, S., et al., Characterization of hematopoietic cells arising on the textured surface of left ventricular assist devices. *Ann. Thorac. Surg,* 1995. 60(6): p. 1627-32.

[125] Urbich, C. and S. Dimmeler, Endothelial progenitor cells functional characterization. *Trends Cardiovasc. Med,* 2004. 14(8): p. 318-22.

[126] Zeng, L., et al., HDAC3 is crucial in shear- and VEGF-induced stem cell differentiation toward endothelial cells. *J. Cell Biol,* 2006. 174(7): p. 1059-69.

[127] Fujiyama, S., et al., Bone marrow monocyte lineage cells adhere on injured endothelium in a monocyte chemoattractant protein-1-dependent manner and accelerate reendothelialization as endothelial progenitor cells. *Circ. Res,* 2003. 93(10): p. 980-9.

[128] Wassmann, S., et al., Improvement of endothelial function by systemic transfusion of vascular progenitor cells. *Circ. Res,* 2006. 99(8): p. e74-83.

[129] Hill, J.M., et al., Circulating endothelial progenitor cells, vascular function, and cardiovascular risk. *N. Engl. J. Med,* 2003. 348(7): p. 593-600.

[130] Vasa, M., et al., Number and migratory activity of circulating endothelial progenitor cells inversely correlate with risk factors for coronary artery disease. *Circ. Res,* 2001. 89(1): p. E1-7.

[131] Werner, N. and G. Nickenig, Clinical and therapeutical implications of EPC biology in atherosclerosis. *J. Cell Mol. Med,* 2006. 10(2): p. 318-32.

[132] Werner, N., et al., Intravenous transfusion of endothelial progenitor cells reduces neointima formation after vascular injury. *Circ. Res,* 2003. 93(2): p. e17-24.

[133] Takamiya, M., et al., Granulocyte colony-stimulating factor-mobilized circulating c-Kit+/Flk-1+ progenitor cells regenerate endothelium and inhibit neointimal hyperplasia after vascular injury. *Arterioscler. Thromb. Vasc. Biol,* 2006. 26(4): p. 751-7.

[134] Urao, N., et al., Erythropoietin-mobilized endothelial progenitors enhance reendothelialization via Akt-endothelial nitric oxide synthase activation and prevent neointimal hyperplasia. *Circ. Res,* 2006. 98(11): p. 1405-13.

[135] Werner, N., et al., Bone marrow-derived progenitor cells modulate vascular reendothelialization and neointimal formation: effect of 3-hydroxy-3-methylglutaryl coenzyme a reductase inhibition. *Arterioscler. Thromb. Vasc. Biol,* 2002. 22(10): p. 1567-72.

[136] Spyridopoulos, I., et al., Statins enhance migratory capacity by upregulation of the telomere repeat-binding factor TRF2 in endothelial progenitor cells. *Circulation,* 2004. 110(19): p. 3136-42.

[137] Landmesser, U., et al., Statin-induced improvement of endothelial progenitor cell mobilization, myocardial neovascularization, left ventricular function, and survival after experimental myocardial infarction requires endothelial nitric oxide synthase. *Circulation,* 2004. 110(14): p. 1933-9.

[138] Assmus, B., et al., HMG-CoA reductase inhibitors reduce senescence and increase proliferation of endothelial progenitor cells via regulation of cell cycle regulatory genes. *Circ. Res,* 2003. 92(9): p. 1049-55.

[139] Walter, D.H., et al., Statin therapy accelerates reendothelialization: a novel effect involving mobilization and incorporation of bone marrow-derived endothelial progenitor cells. *Circulation*, 2002. 105(25): p. 3017-24.

[140] Llevadot, J., et al., HMG-CoA reductase inhibitor mobilizes bone marrow--derived endothelial progenitor cells. *J. Clin. Invest*, 2001. 108(3): p. 399-405.

[141] Dimmeler, S., et al., HMG-CoA reductase inhibitors (statins) increase endothelial progenitor cells via the PI 3-kinase/Akt pathway. *J. Clin. Invest*, 2001. 108(3): p. 391-7.

[142] Vasa, M., et al., Increase in circulating endothelial progenitor cells by statin therapy in patients with stable coronary artery disease. *Circulation*, 2001. 103(24): p. 2885-90.

[143] Hill, W.D., et al., SDF-1 (CXCL12) is upregulated in the ischemic penumbra following stroke: association with bone marrow cell homing to injury. *J. Neuropathol. Exp. Neurol*, 2004. 63(1): p. 84-96.

[144] Newman, M.B., et al., Stroke-induced migration of human umbilical cord blood cells: time course and cytokines. *Stem Cells Dev*, 2005. 14(5): p. 576-86.

[145] Shen, L.H., et al., Therapeutic benefit of bone marrow stromal cells administered 1 month after stroke. *J. Cereb. Blood Flow Metab*, 2006.

[146] Li, Y., et al., Human marrow stromal cell therapy for stroke in rat: neurotrophins and functional recovery. *Neurology*, 2002. 59(4): p. 514-23.

[147] Borlongan, C.V., et al., Central nervous system entry of peripherally injected umbilical cord blood cells is not required for neuroprotection in stroke. *Stroke*, 2004. 35(10): p. 2385-9.

[148] Chen, J., et al., Intravenous bone marrow stromal cell therapy reduces apoptosis and promotes endogenous cell proliferation after stroke in female rat. *J. Neurosci. Res*, 2003. 73(6): p. 778-86.

[149] Chen, J., et al., Intravenous administration of human bone marrow stromal cells induces angiogenesis in the ischemic boundary zone after stroke in rats. *Circ. Res*, 2003. 92(6): p. 692-9.

[150] Willing, A.E., et al., Mobilized peripheral blood cells administered intravenously produce functional recovery in stroke. *Cell Transplant*, 2003. 12(4): p. 449-54.

[151] Kang, S.K., et al., Improvement of neurological deficits by intracerebral transplantation of human adipose tissue-derived stromal cells after cerebral ischemia in rats. *Exp. Neurol*, 2003. 183(2): p. 355-66.

[152] Roybon, L., et al., Failure of transdifferentiation of adult hematopoietic stem cells into neurons. *Stem Cells*, 2006. 24(6): p. 1594-604.

[153] Castro, R.F., et al., Failure of bone marrow cells to transdifferentiate into neural cells in vivo. *Science*, 2002. 297(5585): p. 1299.

[154] Cho, H.J., et al., Mobilized endothelial progenitor cells by granulocyte-macrophage colony-stimulating factor accelerate reendothelialization and reduce vascular inflammation after intravascular radiation. *Circulation*, 2003. 108(23): p. 2918-25.

[155] Ohtaki, H., et al., Progressive expression of vascular endothelial growth factor (VEGF) and angiogenesis after chronic ischemic hypoperfusion in rat. *Acta Neurochir. Suppl*, 2006. 96: p. 283-7.

[156] Hai, J., et al., Vascular endothelial growth factor expression and angiogenesis induced by chronic cerebral hypoperfusion in rat brain. *Neurosurgery*, 2003. 53(4): p. 963-70; discussion 970-2.

[157] Marti, H.J., et al., Hypoxia-induced vascular endothelial growth factor expression precedes neovascularization after cerebral ischemia. *Am. J. Pathol*, 2000. 156(3): p. 965-76.

[158] Nakagami, H., et al., Novel autologous cell therapy in ischemic limb disease through growth factor secretion by cultured adipose tissue-derived stromal cells. *Arterioscler. Thromb. Vasc. Biol*, 2005. 25(12): p. 2542-7.

[159] Rehman, J., et al., *Secretion of angiogenic and antiapoptotic factors by human adipose stromal cells. Circulation*, 2004. 109(10): p. 1292-8.

[160] Urbich, C., et al., Soluble factors released by endothelial progenitor cells promote migration of endothelial cells and cardiac resident progenitor cells. *J. Mol. Cell Cardiol*, 2005. 39(5): p. 733-42.

[161] Kupatt, C., et al., Embryonic endothelial progenitor cells expressing a broad range of proangiogenic and remodeling factors enhance vascularization and tissue recovery in acute and chronic ischemia. *Faseb. J*, 2005. 19(11): p. 1576-8.

[162] Rehman, J., et al., Peripheral blood "endothelial progenitor cells" are derived from monocyte/macrophages and secrete angiogenic growth factors. *Circulation*, 2003. 107(8): p. 1164-9.

[163] Murohara, T., et al., Transplanted cord blood-derived endothelial precursor cells augment postnatal neovascularization. *J. Clin. Invest*, 2000. 105(11): p. 1527-36.

[164] Takagi, Y., et al., Survival and differentiation of neural progenitor cells derived from embryonic stem cells and transplanted into ischemic brain. *J. Neurosurg*, 2005. 103(2): p. 304-10.

[165] Orlic, D., et al., Transplanted adult bone marrow cells repair myocardial infarcts in mice. *Ann. N Y Acad. Sci*, 2001. 938: p. 221-9; discussion 229-30.

[166] Miranville, A., et al., Improvement of postnatal neovascularization by human adipose tissue-derived stem cells. *Circulation*, 2004. 110(3): p. 349-55.

[167] Yang, C., et al., Enhancement of neovascularization with cord blood CD133+ cell-derived endothelial progenitor cell transplantation. *Thromb. Haemost*, 2004. 91(6): p. 1202-12.

[168] Aoki, M., M. Yasutake, and T. Murohara, Derivation of functional endothelial progenitor cells from human umbilical cord blood mononuclear cells isolated by a novel cell filtration device. *Stem Cells*, 2004. 22(6): p. 994-1002.

[169] Matsumoto, T., et al., Therapeutic potential of vasculogenesis and osteogenesis promoted by peripheral blood CD34-positive cells for functional bone healing. *Am. J. Pathol*, 2006. 169(4): p. 1440-57.

[170] Suuronen, E.J., et al., Tissue-engineered injectable collagen-based matrices for improved cell delivery and vascularization of ischemic tissue using CD133+ progenitors expanded from the peripheral blood. *Circulation*, 2006. 114(1 Suppl): p. I138-44.

[171] Schachinger, V., et al., Transplantation of progenitor cells and regeneration enhancement in acute myocardial infarction: final one-year results of the TOPCARE-AMI Trial. *J. Am. Coll. Cardiol,* 2004. 44(8): p. 1690-9.

[172] Wu, X.J., et al., Effects of endothelial cell growth states on the proliferation and migration of vascular smooth muscle cells in vitro. Sheng Li Xue Bao, 2003. 55(5): p. 554-9.

[173] Vendrame, M., et al., Anti-inflammatory effects of human cord blood cells in a rat model of stroke. *Stem Cells Dev,* 2005. 14(5): p. 595-604.

[174] Goldschmidt-Clermont, P.J., Loss of bone marrow-derived vascular progenitor cells leads to inflammation and atherosclerosis. *Am. Heart J,* 2003. 146(4 Suppl): p. S5-12.

[175] Tse, W.T., et al., Suppression of allogeneic T-cell proliferation by human marrow stromal cells: implications in transplantation. *Transplantation,* 2003. 75(3): p. 389-97.

[176] Pluchino, S., et al., Neurosphere-derived multipotent precursors promote neuroprotection by an immunomodulatory mechanism. *Nature,* 2005. 436(7048): p. 266-71.

[177] Tepper, O.M., et al., Newly emerging concepts in blood vessel growth: recent discovery of endothelial progenitor cells and their function in tissue regeneration. *J. Investig. Med,* 2003. 51(6): p. 353-9.

[178] Kalka, C., et al., Vascular endothelial growth factor(165) gene transfer augments circulating endothelial progenitor cells in human subjects. *Circ. Res,* 2000. 86(12): p. 1198-202.

[179] Luttun, A., M. Tjwa, and P. Carmeliet, Placental growth factor (PlGF) and its receptor Flt-1 (VEGFR-1): novel therapeutic targets for angiogenic disorders. *Ann. N Y Acad. Sci,* 2002. 979: p. 80-93.

[180] Hattori, K., et al., Placental growth factor reconstitutes hematopoiesis by recruiting VEGFR1(+) stem cells from bone-marrow microenvironment. *Nat. Med,* 2002. 8(8): p. 841-9.

[181] Yamaguchi, J., et al., Stromal cell-derived factor-1 effects on ex vivo expanded endothelial progenitor cell recruitment for ischemic neovascularization. *Circulation,* 2003. 107(9): p. 1322-8.

[182] Wang, C., et al., Mechanical, cellular, and molecular factors interact to modulate circulating endothelial cell progenitors. *Am. J. Physiol. Heart Circ. Physiol,* 2004. 286(5): p. H1985-93.

[183] Mohle, R., et al., Transendothelial migration of CD34+ and mature hematopoietic cells: an in vitro study using a human bone marrow endothelial cell line. *Blood,* 1997. 89(1): p. 72-80.

[184] Heissig, B., et al., Recruitment of stem and progenitor cells from the bone marrow niche requires MMP-9 mediated release of kit-ligand. *Cell,* 2002. 109(5): p. 625-37.

[185] Aicher, A., et al., Essential role of endothelial nitric oxide synthase for mobilization of stem and progenitor cells. *Nat. Med,* 2003. 9(11): p. 1370-6.

[186] Iwakura, A., et al., Estrogen-mediated, endothelial nitric oxide synthase-dependent mobilization of bone marrow-derived endothelial progenitor cells contributes to reendothelialization after arterial injury. *Circulation,* 2003. 108(25): p. 3115-21.

[187] Iwakura, A., et al., Estradiol enhances recovery after myocardial infarction by augmenting incorporation of bone marrow-derived endothelial progenitor cells into sites of ischemia-induced neovascularization via endothelial nitric oxide synthase-mediated activation of matrix metalloproteinase-9. *Circulation*, 2006. 113(12): p. 1605-14.

[188] Hiasa, K., et al., Gene transfer of stromal cell-derived factor-1alpha enhances ischemic vasculogenesis and angiogenesis via vascular endothelial growth factor/endothelial nitric oxide synthase-related pathway: next-generation chemokine therapy for therapeutic neovascularization. *Circulation*, 2004. 109(20): p. 2454-61.

[189] Sbaa, E., et al., Caveolin plays a central role in endothelial progenitor cell mobilization and homing in SDF-1-driven postischemic vasculogenesis. *Circ. Res*, 2006. 98(9): p. 1219-27.

[190] Liao, S., et al., Accelerated replicative senescence of medial smooth muscle cells derived from abdominal aortic aneurysms compared to the adjacent inferior mesenteric artery. *J. Surg. Res*, 2000. 92(1): p. 85-95.

[191] van der Loo, B., M.J. Fenton, and J.D. Erusalimsky, Cytochemical detection of a senescence-associated beta-galactosidase in endothelial and smooth muscle cells from human and rabbit blood vessels. *Exp. Cell Res*, 1998. 241(2): p. 309-15.

[192] Yamamoto, K., et al., Fluid shear stress induces differentiation of Flk-1-positive embryonic stem cells into vascular endothelial cells in vitro. *Am. J. Physiol. Heart Circ. Physiol*, 2005. 288(4): p. H1915-24.

[193] Wang, H., et al., Shear stress induces endothelial differentiation from a murine embryonic mesenchymal progenitor cell line. *Arterioscler. Thromb. Vasc. Biol*, 2005. 25(9): p. 1817-23.

[194] Kim, D.H., et al., Gene expression profile of cytokine and growth factor during differentiation of bone marrow-derived mesenchymal stem cell. *Cytokine*, 2005. 31(2): p. 119-26.

[195] Wurmser, A.E., et al., Cell fusion-independent differentiation of neural stem cells to the endothelial lineage. *Nature*, 2004. 430(6997): p. 350-6.

[196] Owens, G.K., M.S. Kumar, and B.R. Wamhoff, Molecular regulation of vascular smooth muscle cell differentiation in development and disease. *Physiol. Rev*, 2004. 84(3): p. 767-801.

[197] Xiao, Q., et al., Stem Cell-derived Sca-1+ Progenitors Differentiate into Smooth Muscle Cells, which is Mediated by Collagen IV-Integrin {alpha}1/{beta}1/{alpha}v and PDGF Receptor Pathways. *Am. J. Physiol. Cell Physiol*, 2006.

[198] Geng, Y.J., Molecular mechanisms for cardiovascular stem cell apoptosis and growth in the hearts with atherosclerotic coronary disease and ischemic heart failure. *Ann. N Y Acad. Sci*, 2003. 1010: p. 687-97.

[199] Okazawa, H., et al., Bcl-2 inhibits retinoic acid-induced apoptosis during the neural differentiation of embryonal stem cells. *J. Cell Biol*, 1996. 132(5): p. 955-68.

[200] Duval, D., et al., A p38 inhibitor allows to dissociate differentiation and apoptotic processes triggered upon LIF withdrawal in mouse embryonic stem cells. *Cell Death Differ*, 2004. 11(3): p. 331-41.

[201] Mehlen, P., et al., hsp27 as a switch between differentiation and apoptosis in murine embryonic stem cells. *J. Biol. Chem,* 1997. 272(50): p. 31657-65.

[202] Lusis, A.J., Atherosclerosis. *Nature,* 2000. 407(6801): p. 233-41.

[203] Shimokawa, H., Primary endothelial dysfunction: atherosclerosis. *J. Mol. Cell Cardiol,* 1999. 31(1): p. 23-37.

[204] Sata, M., Circulating vascular progenitor cells contribute to vascular repair, remodeling, and lesion formation. *Trends Cardiovasc. Med,* 2003. 13(6): p. 249-53.

[205] Schaper, W. and D. Scholz, Factors regulating arteriogenesis. *Arterioscler. Thromb. Vasc. Biol,* 2003. 23(7): p. 1143-51.

[206] Kleinman, H.K., D. Philp, and M.P. Hoffman, Role of the extracellular matrix in morphogenesis. *Curr. Opin. Biotechnol,* 2003. 14(5): p. 526-32.

[207] Ingber, D.E., Mechanical signaling and the cellular response to extracellular matrix in angiogenesis and cardiovascular physiology. *Circ. Res,* 2002. 91(10): p. 877-87.

[208] Shen, Q., et al., Endothelial cells stimulate self-renewal and expand neurogenesis of neural stem cells. *Science,* 2004. 304(5675): p. 1338-40.

[209] Illi, B., et al., Epigenetic histone modification and cardiovascular lineage programming in mouse embryonic stem cells exposed to laminar shear stress. *Circ. Res,* 2005. 96(5): p. 501-8.

[210] Yamamoto, K., et al., Proliferation, differentiation, and tube formation by endothelial progenitor cells in response to shear stress. *J. Appl. Physiol,* 2003. 95(5): p. 2081-8.

[211] Cerdan, C., A. Rouleau, and M. Bhatia, VEGF-A165 augments erythropoietic development from human embryonic stem cells. *Blood,* 2004. 103(7): p. 2504-12.

[212] Hirashima, M., et al., A chemically defined culture of VEGFR2+ cells derived from embryonic stem cells reveals the role of VEGFR1 in tuning the threshold for VEGF in developing endothelial cells. *Blood,* 2003. 101(6): p. 2261-7.

[213] Fons, P., et al., VEGF-R2 and neuropilin-1 are involved in VEGF-A-induced differentiation of human bone marrow progenitor cells. *J. Cell Physiol,* 2004. 200(3): p. 351-9.

[214] Rolny, C., et al., Shb promotes blood vessel formation in embryoid bodies by augmenting vascular endothelial growth factor receptor-2 and platelet-derived growth factor receptor-beta signaling. *Exp. Cell Res,* 2005. 308(2): p. 381-93.

[215] Wang, H., et al., Gene expression profile signatures indicate a role for Wnt signaling in endothelial commitment from embryonic stem cells. *Circ. Res,* 2006. 98(10): p. 1331-9.

[216] Hutchings, H., N. Ortega, and J. Plouet, Extracellular matrix-bound vascular endothelial growth factor promotes endothelial cell adhesion, migration, and survival through integrin ligation. *Faseb J,* 2003. 17(11): p. 1520-2.

[217] Choy, J.C., et al., Granzyme B induces smooth muscle cell apoptosis in the absence of perforin: involvement of extracellular matrix degradation. *Arterioscler. Thromb. Vasc. Biol,* 2004. 24(12): p. 2245-50.

[218] Flaim, C.J., S. Chien, and S.N. Bhatia, An extracellular matrix microarray for probing cellular differentiation. *Nat. Methods,* 2005. 2(2): p. 119-25.

[219] Kawasaki, H., et al., Generation of dopaminergic neurons and pigmented epithelia from primate ES cells by stromal cell-derived inducing activity. *Proc. Natl. Acad. Sci. U S A,* 2002. 99(3): p. 1580-5.

[220] Yamashita, J., et al., Flk1-positive cells derived from embryonic stem cells serve as vascular progenitors. *Nature,* 2000. 408(6808): p. 92-6.

[221] Sone, M., et al., Different differentiation kinetics of vascular progenitor cells in primate and mouse embryonic stem cells. *Circulation,* 2003. 107(16): p. 2085-8.

[222] Chen, S.S., et al., Multilineage differentiation of rhesus monkey embryonic stem cells in three-dimensional culture systems. *Stem Cells,* 2003. 21(3): p. 281-95.

[223] Michelini, M., et al., Primate embryonic stem cells create their own niche while differentiating in three-dimensional culture systems. *Cell Prolif,* 2006. 39(3): p. 217-29.

[224] Wijelath, E.S., et al., Fibronectin promotes VEGF-induced CD34 cell differentiation into endothelial cells. *J. Vasc. Surg,* 2004. 39(3): p. 655-60.

[225] Zhang, X., J.E. Groopman, and J.F. Wang, Extracellular matrix regulates endothelial functions through interaction of VEGFR-3 and integrin alpha5beta1. *J. Cell Physiol,* 2005. 202(1): p. 205-14.

[226] Rookmaaker, M.B., et al., CD34+ cells home, proliferate, and participate in capillary formation, and in combination with CD34- cells enhance tube formation in a 3-dimensional matrix. *Arterioscler. Thromb. Vasc. Biol,* 2005. 25(9): p. 1843-50.

[227] Villars, F., et al., Effect of human endothelial cells on human bone marrow stromal cell phenotype: role of VEGF? *J. Cell Biochem,* 2000. 79(4): p. 672-85.

[228] Brevetti, G., et al., Endothelial dysfunction and cardiovascular risk prediction in peripheral arterial disease: additive value of flow-mediated dilation to ankle-brachial pressure index. *Circulation,* 2003. 108(17): p. 2093-8.

[229] Fadini, G.P., et al., Circulating endothelial progenitor cells are reduced in peripheral vascular complications of type 2 diabetes mellitus. *J. Am. Coll. Cardiol,* 2005. 45(9): p. 1449-57.

[230] Tepper, O.M., et al., Human endothelial progenitor cells from type II diabetics exhibit impaired proliferation, adhesion, and incorporation into vascular structures. *Circulation,* 2002. 106(22): p. 2781-6.

[231] Kondo, T., et al., Smoking cessation rapidly increases circulating progenitor cells in peripheral blood in chronic smokers. *Arterioscler. Thromb. Vasc. Biol,* 2004. 24(8): p. 1442-7.

[232] Grisar, J., et al., Depletion of endothelial progenitor cells in the peripheral blood of patients with rheumatoid arthritis. *Circulation,* 2005. 111(2): p. 204-11.

[233] Choi, J.H., et al., Decreased number and impaired angiogenic function of endothelial progenitor cells in patients with chronic renal failure. *Arterioscler. Thromb. Vasc. Biol,* 2004. 24(7): p. 1246-52.

[234] Ghani, U., et al., Endothelial progenitor cells during cerebrovascular disease. *Stroke,* 2005. 36(1): p. 151-3.

[235] Foresta, C., et al., Circulating endothelial progenitor cells in subjects with erectile dysfunction. *Int. J. Impot. Res,* 2005. 17(3): p. 288-90.

[236] Heiss, C., et al., Impaired progenitor cell activity in age-related endothelial dysfunction. *J. Am. Coll. Cardiol,* 2005. 45(9): p. 1441-8.

[237] Gokce, N., et al., Risk stratification for postoperative cardiovascular events via noninvasive assessment of endothelial function: a prospective study. *Circulation,* 2002. 105(13): p. 1567-72.

[238] Patti, G., et al., Impaired flow-mediated dilation and risk of restenosis in patients undergoing coronary stent implantation. *Circulation,* 2005. 111(1): p. 70-5.

[239] Werner, N., et al., Circulating endothelial progenitor cells and cardiovascular outcomes. *N. Engl. J. Med,* 2005. 353(10): p. 999-1007.

[240] Tateishi-Yuyama, E., et al., Therapeutic angiogenesis for patients with limb ischaemia by autologous transplantation of bone-marrow cells: a pilot study and a randomised controlled trial. *Lancet,* 2002. 360(9331): p. 427-35.

[241] Ishida, A., et al., Autologous peripheral blood mononuclear cell implantation for patients with peripheral arterial disease improves limb ischemia. *Circ. J,* 2005. 69(10): p. 1260-5.

[242] Menasche, P., et al., Autologous skeletal myoblast transplantation for severe postinfarction left ventricular dysfunction. *J. Am. Coll. Cardiol,* 2003. 41(7): p. 1078-83.

[243] Galinanes, M., et al., Autotransplantation of unmanipulated bone marrow into scarred myocardium is safe and enhances cardiac function in humans. *Cell Transplant,* 2004. 13(1): p. 7-13.

[244] Hamano, K., et al., Local implantation of autologous bone marrow cells for therapeutic angiogenesis in patients with ischemic heart disease: clinical trial and preliminary results. *Jpn. Circ. J,* 2001. 65(9): p. 845-7.

[245] Stamm, C., et al., Autologous bone-marrow stem-cell transplantation for myocardial regeneration. *Lancet,* 2003. 361(9351): p. 45-6.

[246] Strauer, B.E., et al., Repair of infarcted myocardium by autologous intracoronary mononuclear bone marrow cell transplantation in humans. *Circulation,* 2002. 106(15): p. 1913-8.

[247] Wollert, K.C., et al., Intracoronary autologous bone-marrow cell transfer after myocardial infarction: the BOOST randomised controlled clinical trial. *Lancet,* 2004. 364(9429): p. 141-8.

[248] Meyer, G.P., et al., Intracoronary bone marrow cell transfer after myocardial infarction: eighteen months' follow-up data from the randomized, controlled BOOST (BOne marrOw transfer to enhance ST-elevation infarct regeneration) trial. *Circulation,* 2006. 113(10): p. 1287-94.

[249] Schachinger, V., et al., Intracoronary bone marrow-derived progenitor cells in acute myocardial infarction. *N. Engl. J. Med,* 2006. 355(12): p. 1210-21.

[250] Lunde, K., et al., Intracoronary injection of mononuclear bone marrow cells in acute myocardial infarction. *N. Engl. J. Med,* 2006. 355(12): p. 1199-209.

[251] Kang, H.J., et al., Effects of intracoronary infusion of peripheral blood stem-cells mobilised with granulocyte-colony stimulating factor on left ventricular systolic function and restenosis after coronary stenting in myocardial infarction: the MAGIC cell randomised clinical trial. *Lancet,* 2004. 363(9411): p. 751-6.

[252] Kang, H.J., et al., Differential effect of intracoronary infusion of mobilized peripheral blood stem cells by granulocyte colony-stimulating factor on left ventricular function and remodeling in patients with acute myocardial infarction versus old myocardial infarction: the MAGIC Cell-3-DES randomized, controlled trial. *Circulation,* 2006. 114(1 Suppl): p. I145-51.

[253] Strauer, B.E., et al., Regeneration of human infarcted heart muscle by intracoronary autologous bone marrow cell transplantation in chronic coronary artery disease: the IACT Study. *J. Am. Coll. Cardiol,* 2005. 46(9): p. 1651-8.

[254] Patel, A.N., et al., Surgical treatment for congestive heart failure with autologous adult stem cell transplantation: a prospective randomized study. *J. Thorac. Cardiovasc. Surg,* 2005. 130(6): p. 1631-8.

[255] Assmus, B., et al., Transcoronary transplantation of progenitor cells after myocardial infarction. *N. Engl. J. Med,* 2006. 355(12): p. 1222-32.

[256] Hofmann, M., et al., Monitoring of bone marrow cell homing into the infarcted human myocardium. *Circulation,* 2005. 111(17): p. 2198-202.

[257] Fukuda, D., et al., Potent inhibitory effect of sirolimus on circulating vascular progenitor cells. *Circulation,* 2005. 111(7): p. 926-31.

[258] Rotmans, J.I., et al., In vivo cell seeding with anti-CD34 antibodies successfully accelerates endothelialization but stimulates intimal hyperplasia in porcine arteriovenous expanded polytetrafluoroethylene grafts. *Circulation,* 2005. 112(1): p. 12-8.

In: Stem Cell Research Developments
Editor: Calvin A. Fong, pp. 65-106

ISBN: 978-1-60021-601-5
© 2007 Nova Science Publishers, Inc.

Chapter II

Gata Transcription Factors and T Cell Development from Hematopoietic Stem Cells

Kam-Wing Ling, Jan Piet van Hamburg and Rudi W. Hendriks[*]

Department of Immunology, Erasmus MC Rotterdam,
P.O.Box 1738, 3000 DR Rotterdam, The Netherlands

ABSTRACT

Various members of the Gata family transcription factors play a crucial role in the regulation of T lymphocyte development from hematopoietic stem cells (HSCs). In this review, we will summarize recent interesting findings on how multiple stages of the T cell developmental program are controlled by Gata family transcription factors. In the adult bone marrow Gata1, 2 and 3 transcripts are present in a subpopulation of HSCs that is commonly defined as LSK (Lin⁻Sca-1^{hi}c-kit^{hi}) cells. Both Gata2 and Gata3 are also expressed in the sub-aorta region in mid-gestation stage embryos. It has been shown that Gata2 gene dosage affects the expansion of HSCs in this intra-embryonic hematopoietic site. By contrast, the Gata3 expression pattern suggests that it might regulate embryonic HSC production through effects on the microenvironment. While Gata2 expression also regulates adult HSC function in the bone marrow, Gata3 positive cells mark a previously undescribed Lin⁻ subpopulation in the bone marrow and in early uncommitted thymocytes, suggesting a role for Gata3 in T lineage specification from hematopoietic multipotent progenitors. Although the findings that the generation of T-lineage cells is absolutely dependent on Gata3 and that Gata3 is expressed throughout thymic T cell development suggest a role of Gata3 in T-lineage commitment, direct evidence demonstrating Gata3 as a T-lineage commitment factor is still lacking. The analysis of overexpression and conditionally deficient mouse mutants showed that in the thymus Gata3 (i) is essential for β-selection upon successful T cell receptor (TCR) β chain gene

[*] Correspondence to: Rudi W. Hendriks, Department of Immunology, Erasmus MC Rotterdam, P. O. Box 1738, 3000 DR Rotterdam, The Netherlands, e-mail: r.hendriks@erasmusmc.nl, phone: +31 10 4087180, fax: +31 10 4089456.

rearrangement, (ii) can negatively regulate TCR signals via E2A and CD5, and (iii) is absolutely required for CD4 single positive T cell development. In the spleen, Gata3 is active in CD4[+] T helper-2 (Th2) T cells and is crucial for the induction of Th2 cytokine expression. The essential role of Gata factors in the regulation of cell division and differentiation is also underscored by various findings implicating Gata family members, including Gata2 and Gata3, in the etiology of specific leukemias. Knowledge on the control of T cell development by Gata factors facilitates improvement of clinical strategies for the generation of various T cell subtypes from HSCs, e.g. in the context of bone marrow or stem cell transplantation, or for the specific expansion of particular mature T cell subpopulations for immuno-based therapies.

Keywords: GATA-2; GATA-3; Transcription factors, Haematopoietic stem cells; T cells; transgenic models.

LIST OF ABBREVIATIONS

AGM	aorta-gonads-mesonephros
CFU-S	colony forming unit-spleen
CLP	common lymphoid progenitor
CM	common myeloid progenitor
DN	double negative
DP	double positive
E	erythrocyte
E10.5	embryonic day 10.5
FDG	fluorescein-di-β-D-galactopyranoside
GFP	green fluorescent protein
G	Granulocyte
IL	interleukin
LSK	Lin-Sca-1^{hi}c-kit^{hi}
LT-HSC	long term hematopoietic stem cell
HSC	hematopoietic stem cell
M	macrophage
Mk	megakaryocyte
P-Sp	para-aortic splanchnopleura
Rag	recombination activating gene
Sp	splanchnopleura
SP	single positive
ST-HSC	short term hematopoietic stem cell
TCR	T cell receptor
Th1	T helper-1
Th2	T helper-2
WT	wild type
YS	yolk sac

INTRODUCTION

T lymphocytes play a central role in the mammalian immune response against potentially hazardous pathogens, such as parasites, bacteria, viruses and fungi. These cells have the remarkable capacity to specifically recognize foreign substances, termed antigens, to which they respond by clonal amplification and cellular differentiation, conferring lifelong protective immunity to reinfection with the same pathogen. T lymphocytes express an antigen-specific receptor, called the T cell receptor (TCR), which recognizes peptide fragments derived from foreign proteins or pathogens that have entered into host cells. Defective T cell development and function can result in increased susceptibility to infections and even development of leukemias, allergies and autoimmune diseases. On the other hand, T lymphocytes can be manipulated to eradicate tumor and control graft rejection after organ transplantation. Therefore, in addition to biological interest, knowledge on T cell biology is important for understanding the etiology of a wide variety of diseases and potentially improves current therapies.

Virtually all T lymphocytes are produced in the thymus, a bi-lobed grayish organ in the upper chest above the heart. The thymus is seeded by precursor cells in the adult bone marrow, but the precise identity of these thymus-seeding cells is currently under debate (Bhandoola and Sambandam, 2006; Petrie and Kincade, 2005; Rothenberg and Taghon, 2005; Zuniga-Pflucker and Schmitt, 2005). While it is clear that adult T cells are derived from HSCs, which can differentiate into progenitors with a more restricted lineage potential and generate all the lympho/hematopoietic lineages via a cascade of commitment events (Spangrude et al., 1991). During embryonic development, when the immune system is first established, progenitors with lymphoid potential are detectable before the first HSCs (Cumano et al., 1996; Yokota et al., 2006). Therefore, T cells may arise independent of HSC. Moreover, several embryonic sites harbor HSC activity and could thus be the origin of the first cells that seed the thymus (Durand and Dzierzak, 2005; Godin and Cumano, 2005; Mikkola and Orkin, 2006). Taken together, it is presently unclear how and where the first embryonic thymus-seeding cell is produced.

During early stages of thymocyte development, the TCR gene segments, which are inherited as large arrays of variable (V), diversity (D) and joining (J) gene segments, are irreversibly joined by DNA recombination to form a stretch of DNA encoding a complete variable region. Developing thymocytes first rearrange the TCRβ and then the TCRα locus. After each TCR gene rearrangement, there is a stringent selection process to ensure that only cells expressing functional and functionally relevant TCRs can survive and receive signals for further development. Although various molecules have been shown to be crucial for thymic T cell development (Rothenberg and Taghon, 2005), the molecular mechanisms guiding these selection processes are still quite unclear. In the peripheral lymphoid organs, early immune responses instruct naive T cells to differentiate into distinctive effector T cell subsets with specialized function. In mature T cell differentiation, cytokines provide crucial instructive signal leading to the generation of various T cell subsets, whereby the intracellular molecular pathways mediating the differentiation into one subtype and suppressing the others are currently being unraveled (Ansel et al., 2006; Lee et al., 2006).

The differentiation of HSCs to T cells in the thymus, as well as the generation of effector T cells in the periphery, are tightly regulated processes involving interaction of several signaling molecules, which result in expression of lineage-specific transcription factors. Such transcription factors define and restrict the developmental potential and function of the cells in which they are expressed. Interesting, most of these transcription factors are critical at multiple stages during T cell development and their function can be very different depending on the developmental stage. The Gata family is one out of many multigene families that are essential for the development of the lympho/hematopoietic system at multiple stages.

While the function of Gata1 in the development of the hematopoietic system has recently been reviewed (Ferreira et al., 2005), we will focus in this chapter on Gata2 and Gata3. Gata2 is essential for the production of embryonic hematopoietic stem and progenitor cells in a cell-autonomous fashion (Ling et al., 2004; Tsai et al., 1994; Tsai and Orkin, 1997). In contrast, the role of Gata3 during in the lympho/hematopoietic system in the embryo is less clear. Expression of Gata3 has is associated with HSC, but this factor may regulate the microenvironment of the developing embryonic lympho/hematopoietic system (Bertrand et al., 2005; Manaia et al., 2000). In the adult, Gata2 activity is required for HSC function (Ling et al., 2004; Rodrigues et al., 2005). Functional data on the role of Gata3 in bone marrow HSC and progenitors with T lineage potential are still lacking. Our analyses in *Gata3-LacZ* knock-in mice (Hendriks et al., 1999), show that Gata3 expression marks a previously undescribed population that is present both in the bone marrow and the thymus, which may contain the potential thymus seeding cells. Within the thymus, Gata2 and Gata3 are required for the inhibition of the progenitor cells into the myeloid lineage while Gata3 is necessary for the generation of all thymic T cells (de Pooter et al., 2006; Hendriks et al., 1999; Laiosa et al., 2006; Ting et al., 1996). Gata3 is also required for the two developmental checkpoints after TCRβ and TCRα chain gene rearrangement (Pai et al., 2003). Interestingly, there is a specific requirement of Gata3 for CD4 T cell development within the thymus and the subsequent differentiation into Th2 cells in the peripheral lymphoid organs (Pai et al., 2003; Zhu et al., 2004). Recently identified upstream and downstream pathways linking these two Gata proteins to the other signal molecules and their targets will also be reviewed.

THE GATA PROTEIN FAMILY

All Gata family transcription regulators contain C4 zinc finger motifs with the characteristic Cys-X_2-Cys-X_{17-18}-Cys-X_2-Cys sequence, which bind to a six-nucleotide consensus sequence (A/T)GATA(A/G) (Evans et al., 1988; Martin and Orkin, 1990). Gata proteins are present in a wide range of organisms from slime molds to vertebrates (Lowry and Atchley, 2000). Although the overall homologies for individual members are high between species and between different members of the same species (Yamamoto et al., 1990; Zon et al., 1991), sequence homologies outside the zinc finger regions are low among species. Therefore, unlike other evolutionarily conserved protein families, Gata transcription factors represent a family of proteins that are solely related to each other by their homologous zinc finger DNA binding domains. The founding member of the Gata family, Gata1 (also known as Ery-1, NF-E1, NF-1, and GF-1) was originally cloned as an erythroid nuclear protein (Tsai et al., 1989). Gata2 and Gata3 were subsequently discovered through cross-hybridization in a chicken reticulocyte cDNA library (Yamamoto et al., 1990). In total, six mammalian Gata transcription factors have been isolated, all containing two zinc fingers. The Gata factors show overlapping, but distinctive expression patterns. GATA1, 2 and 3 are predominantly expressed in the hematopoietic system and are often collectively referred to as the hematopoietic subfamily. In contrast, Gata4, Gata5, and Gata6 have been implicated in the gene expression and cellular differentiation in a variety of embryonic tissues, including the heart, lung, gastro-intestical epithelium, testis and ovaries (Burch, 2005; Peterkin et al., 2005).

Gata1 and Gata2 expression patterns overlap substantially, because they are both expressed in erythroid cells, megakaryocytes and mast cells (Fujiwara et al., 1996; Leonard et al., 1993; Martin et al., 1990; Nagai et al., 1994; Zon et al., 1993). In addition, Gata1 is expressed in eosinophils (Zon et al., 1993), while Gata2 is expressed in immature hematopoietic multipotent cells (Nagai et al., 1994). Gata2 is also expressed in embryonic brain, inner ear, endothelial cells, urogenital organs, liver, adipose tissue and cardiac muscle.

Alternative promoters regulate transcription of the Gata2 gene: transcription initiates from two distinct first exons, both of which encode entirely untranslated regions, while the remaining five exons are shared by each of the two divergent mRNAs. The proximal first exon is utilized in general tissues, while in hematopoietic progenitor cells transcription is initiated at the distal first exon (Minegishi et al., 1998; Pan et al., 2000). Differential use of two exons, which was first described for the Gata1 gene, is also found for the Gata3 locus, which was shown to contain a brain-specific and a thymus-specific promoter in mouse and human (Asnagli et al., 2002). The Gata3 expression pattern is quite unique: it is abundantly expressed in the developing nervous system, including the inner ear and different parts of the auditory nervous system, in hair follicles, in the adrenal gland and in the kidney (George et al., 1994; Kaufman et al., 2003; Lillevali et al., 2004; Pandolfi et al., 1995; van der Wees et al., 2004), but within the hematopoietic system expression appears to be confined to the T and NK cell lineages (Hendriks et al., 1999; Oosterwegel et al., 1992; Samson et al., 2003; Vosshenrich et al., 2006; Yamamoto et al., 1990). Gata factors are essential for the early development of the lympho/hematopoietic system at the embryonic stage and all Gata null mutations cause embryonic lethality (Fujiwara et al., 1996; Pandolfi et al., 1995; Tsai and Orkin, 1997).

The biochemical properties of Gata2 and Gata3 are less well characterized than those of Gata1. Gata1 protein contains at least 3 functional domains: the N-terminal activation domain, the N-terminal zinc finger and the C-terminal zinc finger. Initial studies showed that the C-terminal zinc finger is essential for Gata1 function, because it recognizes the Gata consensus sequence and therefore is responsible for DNA binding; nevertheless, also the N-terminal zinc finger contributes to stable and specific DNA binding (Martin and Orkin, 1990; Trainor et al., 2000; Trainor et al., 1996; Whyatt et al., 1993; Yang and Evans, 1992). Later *in vivo* transgenic rescue experiment confirmed that all these 3 domains can function collaboratively as well as independently of each other (Shimizu et al., 2001). While similar *in vivo* analyses with respect to the functional domains of Gata2 and Gata3 are lacking, *in vitro* studies have revealed a comparable activation domain in the Gata3 N-terminus (Yang et al., 1994). Intriguingly, the N-terminal domain of Gata2 was shown to be inhibitory (Minegishi et al., 2003). The N-terminal zinc fingers of Gata2 and Gata3 are capable of strong independent binding with a preference for the GATC motif (Pedone et al., 1997). Minor differences within the three functional domains of the Gata proteins collectively distinguish their specific roles in the tissues in which they are expressed.

While it is clear that Gata1 activity is subject to various forms of regulation on the protein level by post-translational modifications and protein degradation (reviewed in (Ferreira et al., 2005)), knowledge on regulation of Gata2 and Gata3 activity are relatively limited. As in Gata1, acetylation of GATA2 and GATA3 affect both their DNA binding activities and physiological functions (Ferreira et al., 2005; Hayakawa et al., 2004; Yamagata et al., 2000). The stability of the Gata1 and Gata2 proteins is affected by caspase-mediated and ubiquitin-proteasome degradation pathways (De Maria et al., 1999; Minegishi et al., 2005). Likewise, it was very recently shown that stabilization of Gata3 is regulated by the polycomb group protein Bmi-1. Biochemical studies indicated that in effector T cells Bmi-1 binds to Gata3, whereby this interaction is dependent on the Ring finger of Bmi-1 (Hiroyuki Hosokawa, 2006). Overexpression of Bmi-1 resulted in decreased ubiquitination and increased Gata3 protein stability. In Bmi-1-deficient helper T cells, the levels of Th2 cell differentiation decreased as the degradation and ubiquitination on Gata3 increased. Yet, there is so far no report on the regulation of GATA3 turnover in developing thymocytes via similar mechanisms. Nevertheless, the identified co-expression of Gata2, Gata3 and Bmi-1 in HSCs (Ezoe et al., 2004) and below) would allow for a similar regulatory pathway in HSCs. In addition, the Fog1 (friend of Gata-1) multitype zinc finger protein, which was originally identified as a cofactor for transcription factor gata1 in erythroid and megakaryocytic differentiation (Tsang et al., 1997), can repress Gata3-dependent activation of the IL-4 and IL-5 promoters in activated T cells (Kurata et al., 2002; Zhou et al., 2001). Another Gata3 interacting protein, termed repressor of Gata(ROG) represses GATA-3-induced transactivation (Miaw et al., 2000). Recently, Gata1-containing complexes were identified by an *in vivo* biotinylation tagging, purification by streptavidin beads and subsequent mass spectrometry approach (Rodriguez et al., 2005). In addition to known Gata1 interacting factors, such as Fog1, Tal1 and Ldb1, new partners were identified including the essential hematopoietic factor Gfi-1b and the chromatin remodeling and modification complexes MeCP1 and ACF/WCRF. It was concluded that Gata1 forms several distinct complexes, whereby Fog1 serves as a bridging factor between Gata1 and the methyl-DNA binding protein MeCP1 complex. Interestingly, evidence was presented for the *in vivo* binding of the repressive Gata1/Fog1/MeCP1 complex to silenced hematopoietic genes in erythroid cells and of the activating Gata-1/Tal1 complex to erythroid-specific genes (Rodriguez et al., 2005). It is expected that similar approaches will be applied to identify Gata2 and Gata3 protein complexes.

The Gata target motif appears in a variety of regulatory contexts throughout the genome. Gata3 for example, binds to the promoter regions immediately upstream of the transcription start-point, as well as in enhancers of the Th2 cytokine locus (reviewed in (Lee et al., 2006). Therefore, Gata proteins can function as classical transcription factors, or by modifying chromatin structure and thereby facilitating interactions among enhancers, promoters and factors associated with the basal transcription machinery. The result can be activation or inhibition of the expression of target genes. Different Gata proteins can compete for their target sites, leading to a switching of associated DNA binding proteins and therefore different effects on their target genes. There is also accumulating evidence showing that Gata proteins have the capacity to regulate their own expression and cross-regulate the expression of each other (Grass et al., 2003; Grass et al., 2006; Kobayashi-Osaki et al., 2005; Philipsen et al., 1993). The presence of autoregulation and network regulation between the individual Gata family members appears to be essential and therefore, the outcome of Gata transcription factor regulation is highly complex, unpredictable and often cell-context and expression-level dependent.

EXPRESSION OF GATA FACTORS DURING EMBRYONIC LYMPHO/HEMATOPOIESIS

During embryonic development the lympho/hematopoietic system is generated from HSCs in the fetal liver. Shortly after birth, this function is replaced by the bone marrow. However, it is uncertain how the initial immune system is established before lympho/hematopoiesis begins in the fetal liver. Indeed, owing to the differences in functional requirements, the embryonic lympho/hematopoietic system is different from the adult. For example, HSCs in fetal liver have greater repopulating capacity than HSCs derived from adult bone marrow in irradiated recipients (Morrison et al., 1996). Primitive embryonic erythrocytes and macrophages are different from the definitive types found in the adult. Embryonic immunoglobulin and TCR repertoires are unique: only fetal liver HSCs can generate the innate-like $V\gamma5^+$ $\gamma\delta$ T cells (originally termed $V\gamma3^+$) in fetal thymuses, whereas adult bone marrow HSCs do not have this capacity. Likewise, $CD5^+$ B-1a B cells, which are predominantly localized in the peritoneum and pleural cavities, are readily generated from fetal/neonatal precursors, but inefficiently from precursors in the adult (Hardy, 2006). Furthermore, it has been shown that, whereas IL-7 is required for adult B cell development, it is dispensable during fetal hematopoiesis (Carvalho et al., 2001; Hardy and Hayakawa, 1991).

Also in the embryo the thymus is the main site of T cell production, but the first lympho/hematopoietic progenitors seeding the thymus may arise from various hematopoietic sites, including the extra-embryonic yolk sac (YS) and the intra-embryonic splanchnopleura (Sp), para-aortic splanchnopleura (P-Sp) or aorta-gonads-mesonephros (AGM) region (figure 1). Influx of lympho/hematopoietic progenitors to the thymus begins at about embryonic day 10.5 (E10.5) (Fontaine-Perus et al., 1981; Owen and Ritter, 1969). As early as E7, primitive erythroid cells can be observed in the YS blood islands (Russell ES, 1966). Until recently, it was believed that the blood islands of the YS produce the cells that are required to establish the adult lympho/hematopoietic system that seeds the liver and the thymus. However, it has now become clear that lymphoid potential in the YS is limited and is not detectable beyond E8 (Godin and Cumano, 2002). Rather, the intraembryonic Sp tissue has both erythro/myeloid and lymphoid potential before E8 (Cumano et al., 1996). Although cells with long-term multi-lineage potential can be detected in both YS and P-Sp when transplanted into conditioned newborn recipients (Yoder and Hiatt, 1997), adult HSCs that are able to provide long-term multi-lineage reconstitution in adult recipients are only detectable in the E10.5 P-

Sp /AGM region and only later in the YS at E11 (Muller et al., 1994). Progenitors with lymphoid potential detected before E10.5 in the AGM region and E11 in the YS could arise independent of HSC (Yokota et al., 2006). Thus, the developmental hierarchy of the embryonic lympho/hematopoietic system appears very different from that of the adult. The molecular pathways required for the maintenance of the embryonic lympho/hematopoietic system may therefore also differ from that of the adult. This would imply that the lympho/hematopoietic progenitors detected at E10.5 in the thymus could be either derived from the YS or from the AGM region. At the moment, the relative contribution of these two embryonic sites is still unknown.

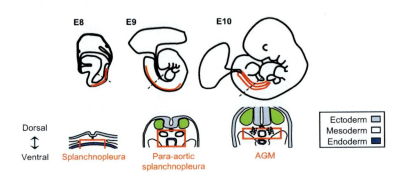

Figure 1. Location and development of the intra-embryonic sites with lympho/hemato-poietic potential in the mouse embryo. The top panel shows a schematic representation of whole mouse embryo at E8 (left), E9 (middle) and E10 (right). Cross sections marked by dotted lines of the corresponding stages are shown in the lower penal. Red boxes in the lower panel are the embryonic sites in which lympho/hematopoietic activity and progenitors can be detected. At E8, splanchnopleura (Sp) is defined as the mosoderm that is associated with the endoderm. The dorsal aortae will develop from this region. At E9, when the paired aortae have developed, this embryonic region is defined as the para-aortic splanchnopleura (P-Sp). At E10, the paired aortae fuse, forming a single aorta and the development of the gonads and mesonephros become apparent. Collectively, this region is referred to as the aorta, gonads and mesonephros (AGM) region.

The expression patterns of Gata2 and Gata3 in the P-Sp/AGM region suggest that these factors have distinctive roles in the control of the generation of the lympho/hematopoietic system in the developing embryo. Gata2 is expressed in E7.5 lateral plate mesoderm, in E8.5 dorsal aorta and the surrounding mesenchyme, and in the YS blood islands (Kobayashi-Osaki et al., 2005; Minegishi et al., 1998; Minegishi et al., 1999; Minegishi et al., 2003). In a Gata2-GFP transgenic mouse line, in which the GFP expression pattern recapitulates the early embryonic Gata2 expression pattern, the Gata2-GFP expressing cell population in E9 YS and P-Sp contains a high proportion of c-kit$^+$CD34$^+$ cells (Kobayashi-Osaki et al., 2005). The c-kit$^+$CD34$^+$ cells in these embryonic regions are enriched in neonatal repopulating HSCs (Yoder et al., 1997). Therefore, Gata2 possibly regulates the production of the cells that are required to generate the embryonic lympho/hematopoietic system. In contrast, Gata3 expression is undetectable in the YS (analyzed between E8 and E10) (Manaia et al., 2000), but is present in the P-Sp/AGM region from E8 through E11. Although Gata3-positive cells are closely associated with hematopoietic molecular marker expressing cells, such as AA4.1, Lmo2, and CD45, they do not overlap (Manaia et al., 2000). Gata3 may therefore play a role in the determination of the embryonic stromal microenvironment for generation of the embryonic lympho/hematopoietic system. Interestingly, cell clusters within the E10.5 splenic mesoderm, closely associated with the aorta epithelium in the AGM region, express both Gata2 and Gata3 (Bertrand et al., 2005). These sub-aortic clusters have been described in all vertebrates and are potentially involved in HSC generation. The overlapping expression patterns in these clusters suggest that Gata2 and Gata3 may cross-regulate or work coordinately with each other for the generation of HSCs in the E10.5 AGM region.

FUNCTION OF GATA FACTORS IN EMBRYONIC HSCs

GATA2$^{-/-}$ mutants die at E10.5 with severe anemia. E9.5 Gata2$^{-/-}$ embryos are pale and have lower numbers of circulating blood cells (Tsai et al., 1994). *In vitro*, clonogenic progenitor colonies obtained from Gata2$^{-/-}$ P-Sp, YS and ES cells are dramatically reduced but can be partially rescued by crossing into the p53$^{-/-}$ background (Tsai and Orkin, 1997). This suggests that these *in vitro* hematopoietic progenitors in the Gata2$^{-/-}$ mutants are generated, but that they failed to expand or survive. Consistently, when Gata2$^{-/-}$ ES cells were introduced into wild-type (WT) blastocysts, these cells contributed at a low level to the embryonic circulation in the chimeras, but not to the fetal liver hematopoietic compartment (Tsai et al., 1994). Therefore, it can be concluded that Gata2 plays a minor or redundant role in primitive hematopoiesis, whereas the development of the definitive hematopoietic system is highly dependent on Gata2. Hematopoietic progenitor cells arise in Gata2$^{-/-}$ embryos and can be derived from Gata$^{-/-}$ ES cells, but they fail to proliferate or survive. Thus, Gata2 function is dispensable for the generation of hematopoietic progenitors but is crucial for their maintenance and expansion (Tsai et al., 1994).

Since Gata2$^{-/-}$ mutants die before the first HSCs are detectable in the embryo at E10.5, the effect of Gata2 deletion in HSC production and function in the embryo cannot be analyzed *in vivo*. Heterozygous Gata2$^{+/-}$ mutant mice, which express reduced levels of Gata2 in hematopoietic cells, survive until adulthood without gross abnormalities. Studies on Gata2$^{+/-}$ mutant embryos have demonstrated that they are haploinsufficient and have revealed differential responses of YS and AGM to Gata2 gene dosage, thereby affecting the production, expansion and maintenance of HSCs in the developing embryo (Ling et al., 2004). Gata2$^{+/-}$ mutants have reduced number of CFU-S (colony forming units - spleen), both in the YS and in the AGM region. While this defect could be intrinsic to the expansion or survival of these erythro-myeloid progenitors, it could alternatively be due to the reduced HSCs production in both YS and AGM regions of the Gata2$^{+/-}$ mutants. Although HSCs are present in these embryonic sites in the Gata2$^{+/-}$ mutants, the detected HSC activities are reduced in both tissues. As the embryo develops, expansion of HSC activities in the Gata2$^{+/-}$ YS appears to be normal, both *in vivo* and *ex vivo*, while the Gata2$^{+/-}$ AGM region completely fails to maintain and expand the residual HSC activity present. Therefore, while Gata2 gene dosage affects HSCs production of both YS and AGM region, there is an intrinsic difference between YS and AGM region in the response to Gata2 levels in terms of HSC proliferation and survival. We concluded that HSC expansion and maintenance in the AGM region, but not in the YS, is dependent on Gata2 gene dosage (Ling et al., 2004).

GATA-3 AND EMBRYONIC HSC

Gata3[-/-] embryos die between E11 and E12 and display massive internal bleeding, marked growth retardation, severe malformation of the brain and spinal cord, and gross aberrations in fetal liver hematopoiesis. YS hematopoiesis appears to be normal, but fetal liver shows a mild reduction in hematopoietic progenitors obtained *in vitro*, suggesting that definitive hematopoiesis is Gata3-dependent (Pandolfi et al., 1995). Subsequent Rag2[-/-] complementation analyses showed the intrinsic requirement of Gata3 for T cell production (Hendriks et al., 1999; Ting et al., 1996), but the effects of Gata3 deficiency on the microenvironment of the embryonic hematopoietic system has remained unexplored. Also HSC production and lymphoid potential of the Gata3[-/-] AGM and P-Sp have not been analyzed to date.

Gata3[-/-] embryonic lethality is primarily due to noradrenalin deficiency of the sympathetic nervous system and secondarily due to heart failure (Lim et al., 2000). This discovery was based on a previous finding that a 625-kb Gata3 YAC transgene, mimicking endogenous Gata3 expression except in thymus and the sympatho-adrenal system, failed to overcome embryonic lethality. The hypothesis that a neuro-endocrine deficiency in the sympathetic nervous system might cause the embryonic lethality of Gata3 deficient mice was tested by feeding catechol intermediates to pregnant mice, which partially averted Gata3 mutation-induced lethality (Lim et al., 2000). This pharmacological rescue raised the possibility to further study the development of the lympho/hematopoietic system using rescued Gata3[-/-] embryos at a later developmental stage. The rescued Gata3[-/-] thymuses were small, which could be either due to an intrinsic role of Gata3 directly on the development of the thymic epithelium or to the lack of lympho/hematopoietic progenitors seeding the thymus. It is clear that more analyses on the Gata3[-/-] mutants have to be performed to have a better understanding of the role of Gata3 in the establishment of the embryonic lympho/hematopoietic system.

CONTROL OF GATA2 EXPRESSION IN EMBRYONIC HSCs

Given the network regulation between Gata factors, one possible downstream target of Gata3 could be the Gata2 gene. Six Gata factor binding sites are present upstream of the Gata2 locus, and both Gata1, -2 and -3 are able to bind to these Gata sites (Kobayashi-Osaki et al., 2005). Only five out of these six GATA binding sites are necessary for the expression of Gata2 in the YS and the major arteries, while only one is essential for the expression in the dorsal aorta. Thus, Gata2 expression in the embryonic hematopoietic sites is GATA factor-dependent and the expression in different sites is differentially regulated. However, Gata2-GFP expression is maintained in both Gata2 and Gata3 deletion mutants. Collectively, these data suggest that Gata2 expression in the P-Sp is Gata factor dependent and Gata2 and Gata3 may compensate each other, at least for the expression of Gata2 (Kobayashi-Osaki et al., 2005).

Gata2 expression in the P-Sp/AGM region is also regulated by the Notch signaling pathway (Robert-Moreno et al., 2005). Molecules necessary to transduce the Notch signal (the receptors Notch-1 and -4, the ligands Delta-like-1 (Dll-1, -3 and -4) and Jagged-1 and – 2) as well as Notch target genes, such as the Hes related proteins Hrt-1 and -2) and bone morphogenetic protein 4 (BMP4) are expressed in the endothelium of the P-Sp/AGM region. Expression of these genes was found in particular in the hematopoietic clusters on the ventral side of the dorsal aorta (Kumano et al., 2003; Robert-Moreno et al., 2005), which is the region where emerging HSCs are labeled in a recently developed transgenic mouse model (Ma et al., 2002) and the HSC-associated transcription factors Aml1/Runx1, Gata2, Scl/Tal1 are expressed (North et al., 2002; Porcher et al., 1996; Robb et al., 1996; Tsai et al., 1994; Tsai and Orkin, 1997).

Notch1 null mutants have reduced c-kit$^+$CD34$^+$ cell numbers and neonatal repopulating HSC activity (Kumano et al., 2003). In the Notch1$^{-/-}$ endothelium in the AGM region Gata2 and BMP4 expression are reduced. As Gata2 is under the control of BMP4 (Maeno et al., 1996), Notch1 could regulate Gata2 indirectly through BMP4 (Kumano et al., 2003). In addition, RBPjκ, a mediator of feedback regulation of Notch signals, binds to the promoter of GATA2. Moreover, Gata2 mRNA levels in the RBPjκ$^{-/-}$ P-Sp region are reduced (Robert-Moreno et al., 2005). Robert-Moreno et al. have also shown that (i) in WT embryos, Notch1 and Gata2 are co-expressed in cells lining the aorta endothelium at E9.5, (ii) Notch1 specifically associates with the Gata2 promoter in E9.5 WT embryos and 32D myeloid cells by chromatin immunoprecipitation, and (iii) the Notch1/Gata2 interaction is lost in RBPjκ$^{-/-}$ mutants. Taken together, these data strongly suggest that activation of Gata2 expression by Notch1/RBPjκ is a crucial event in the generation of HSC in the developing embryo.

GATA2 AND ADULT HSC FUNCTION

Long-term (LT) repopulation efficiency of adult HSC is directly related to their cell cycle status and is highest in the G0 phase (Passegue et al., 2005). It is estimated that about 75% of LT-HSCs are normally in G0 phase, but these quiescent HSCs do regularly enter the cell cycle. It has been estimated that almost all LT-HSCs are recruited into the cell cycle on average every 57 days (Passegue et al., 2005). It is clear that the regulation of the cell cycle of HSCs plays a central role in HSC function, but the molecular mechanisms regulating HSC cell cycle entry are not defined.

Adult HSCs express high levels of Gata2 and when they are induced to proliferate *in vitro*, the Gata2 expression levels are downregulated (Ezoe et al., 2002). These observations suggest that the Gata2 level plays a role in the maintenance of HSC quiescence, as high Gata2 levels may block HSC cell cycle entry. The early embryonic lethality of Gata2$^{-/-}$ mutants precludes the direct analysis of the role of this gene in adult HSC function. Early in vitro studies involving overexpression of ligand-inducible Gata2 chimeric proteins in hematopoietic cell lines were contradictory (Briegel et al., 1993) (Ezoe et al., 2002; Heyworth et al., 1999). Conditional activation of a Gata/estrogen receptor chimera produced essentially opposite effects to those observed with conditional, drug-inducible, Gata2 expression. Gata2 and Gata2/ER differ in their binding activities and transcriptional interactions (Kitajima et al., 2002). Recently, it is shown this discrepancy is due to the interaction between Gata2 and the Ets family member PU.1. While transcription of the PU.1

gene is regulated by Gata2, the function of Gata2 is modified in a context-dependent manner by expression of PU.1 (Kitajima et al., 2006). Nonetheless, overexpressing Gata2 in bone marrow cells blocks their engraftment to lethally irradiated recipients (Persons et al., 1999). Engrafted cells did not die, differentiate nor expand, thus Gata2 expression appears crucial for the function of HSC. Because enforced expression of Gata2 in pluripotent hematopoietic cells blocked both their amplification and differentiation, Persons *et al.* concluded that there is a critical dose-dependent effect of Gata2 on blood cell differentiation in that downregulation of Gata-2 expression is necessary for stem cells to contribute to hematopoiesis *in vivo*. On the other hand, it was demonstrated, using mouse ES cells co-cultured on the stromal cell line OP9, that Gata-2 increased the proliferation of immature hematopoietic cells (Kitajima et al., 2002). Recently, Gata2 function was analyzed by combining in vitro ES cell differentiation with tetracycline-based conditional gene expression (Kitajima et al., 2006). In this system, Gata2 expression inhibited macrophage differentiation and redirected the fate of hematopoietic differentiation to other lineages, including the megakaryocytic and erythroid lineages. In agreement with the previous finding that generation of mast cells requires co-operative functions of Gata2 and the transcription factor PU.1, also in these experiments, interaction between Gata2 and PU.1 appeared to play a critical role. The authors concluded that Gata2 function is modified in a context-dependent manner by expression of PU.1, which is in turn regulated by Gata2 (Kitajima et al., 2006).

Although Gata2$^{+/-}$ bone marrow cells express lower levels of Gata2 mRNA, the hematological profile of Gata2$^{+/-}$ mice, and the efficiency of engraftment of Gata2$^{+/-}$ bone marrow cells to the recipient's hematopoietic system, is comparable to the WT. Steady state hematopoiesis is normal in Gata2$^{+/-}$ mice, but phenotypically defined HSCs are under-represented in Gata2$^{+/-}$ mice. Gata2$^{+/-}$ HSC defects are only uncovered under a competitive transplantation scenario. When equal amounts of WT and Gata2$^{+/-}$ cells are transplanted into lethally irradiated recipients, a lower contribution of Gata2$^{+/-}$ cells to the hematopoietic system is observed (Rodrigues et al., 2005). This is not due to homing defects in the Gata2$^{+/-}$ HSCs, since a similar study, using sub-lethally irradiated Gata2$^{+/-}$ recipients, showed that lower dose of WT bone marrow cells are able to out-compete the residual Gata2$^{+/-}$ HSC (Ling et al., 2004). Reciprocal transplantation using Gata2$^{+/-}$ donor cells and WT recipients showed that a higher dose (about 10-fold) of donor cells is required to out-compete the endogenous HSCs (Ling et al., 2004). These data clearly show that proliferation of Gata2$^{+/-}$ HSCs is less advantageous, when compared with WT HSCs.

Interestingly, flow cytometric analysis showed that Gata2$^{+/-}$ bone marrow HSCs are phenotypically more quiescent (Rodrigues et al., 2005), which explains the proliferation defects in the competitive transplantation results, and would predict a delayed response to proliferation stress. When Gata2$^{+/-}$ mice were challenged by the cytotoxic drug 5-FU, which specifically targets cycling cells, regeneration of the hematopoietic system in the Gata2$^{+/-}$ mutants was found to be delayed (Ling et al., 2004). The recoveries of all progenitors studied in the Gata2$^{+/-}$ mutants were decreased at various time points after 5-FU treatment, but Gata2$^{+/-}$ bone marrow cells were able to fully recover when given sufficient time. Thus, Gata2$^{+/-}$ mutants are defective in proliferation when under stress (Ling et al., 2004). The Gata2 gene dosage affects HSC proliferation during regeneration of the lympho/hematopoietic system, most likely by regulating HSC cell cycle entry.

EARLY THYMIC PROGENITORS AND LYMPHOID LINEAGE COMMITMENT

Early thymic progenitors are short-lived and contain only lymphoid potential. The thymus is seeded via the blood, but the identity of thymus-seeding cells in the circulation of adult mice is unknown (Bhandoola and Sambandam, 2006; Petrie and Kincade, 2005; Rothenberg and Taghon, 2005; Zuniga-Pflucker and Schmitt, 2005). Likewise, there is no consensus on where and how lymphoid lineage commitment of these early thymic progenitors occurs. Because HSCs can be isolated from the circulation, they would have the capacity to seed the thymus directly (Schwarz and Bhandoola, 2004). In this case, T cell specification would be initiated shortly after HSCs enter the thymus. However, oligopotent progenitors with lymphoid developmental potential can be isolated from the bone marrow, suggesting lymphoid lineage specification can occur before they leave the bone marrow (Igarashi et al., 2002; Kondo et al., 1997; Lai and Kondo, 2006; Martin et al., 2003). Recent data show the presence of bone marrow progenitors with robust lymphoid and limited myeloid potential, but lacking erythroid potential (Lai and Kondo, 2006), suggesting that lymphoid commitment is not a simple single event but a gradual loss of developmental potential to other non-lymphoid lineages. Nonetheless, bone marrow HSC and various progenitors with different lineage developmental potential could seed the thymus and the significance of each individual population may depend on different physiological requirements.

HSC activities in the mouse bone marrow are restricted to the $Lin^-Sca-1^{hi}c-kit^{hi}$ population (Osawa et al., 1996b), which is commonly referred to as the LSK population, whereby Lin^- refers to the negative expression of a cocktail of hematopoietic lineage markers. In particular, a single $CD34^{-/lo}$ cell (and in some mouse strains $Thy-1.1^{lo}$) within the LSK population can engraft a lethally irradiated recipient and regenerate the whole lympho/hematopoietic system (Osawa et al., 1996a; Smith et al., 1991). LSK $CD34^{lo}Thy-1.1^{lo}$ cells are LT-HSCs with extensive self-renewal capacity, which can sustain lympho/hematopoiesis for at least the lifespan of an animal. Upon commitment to differentiation, LT-HSCs progressively lose their self-renewal capacity and become short-term (ST)-HSCs that are still multipotent but their self-renewal capacity is transient (Morrison and Weissman, 1994). The expression of the fms-like receptor kinase Flt3 (also known as Flk2), divides LSK cells into LT-HSC and ST-HSC with increasing expression of this receptor kinase, and so they are designated the $Flt3^-$ and $Flt3^{-/lo}$ subset of LSK cells, respectively (figure 2) (Christensen and Weissman, 2001). The first step of HSCs differentiation is therefore the progressive loss of self-renewal capacity, probably by changes in the responsiveness to the environment.

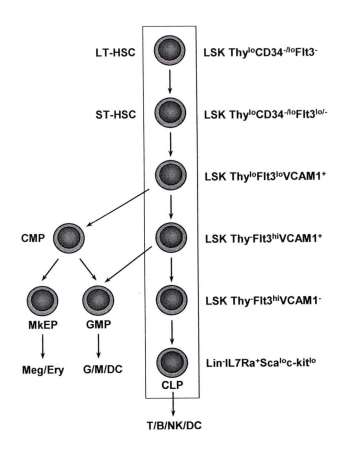

Figure 2. Proposed model of hierarchy in progenitor subset within the bone marrow. In this model, when HSCs differentiate into the lymphoid lineage, they progressively lose their self-renewal capacity and myeloid developmental potential. HSCs and progenitor cells that could possible seed the thymus are marked in the white box. Only phenotypic markers of HSC and progenitor cells with lymphoid potential, which are the potential source of T cells in the thymus are noted here. Adapted from Lai and Kondo (2006).

  The first lineage-committed progenitors isolated from the bone marrow are the common lymphoid progenitors (CLPs), which were defined as $Lin^{-} IL-7R\alpha^{+} Sca-1^{lo} c-kit^{lo}$ cells (Kondo et al., 1997; Manz et al., 2001). These cells have the potential to differentiate into B and dendritic cells *in vitro*, and also clonally into T and NK, cells but lack myeloid potential. Subsequently, an equivalent myeloid-lineage counterpart, the common myeloid progenitors (CMPs) were defined as $Lin^{-} IL7R\alpha^{-} Sca-1^{-} c-kit^{hi}$. These cells can give rise to granulocyte/macrophage (G/M) progenitors and megakaryocyte/erythroid (Mk/E) progenitors with exclusive G/M and Mk/E potential, respectively (Akashi et al., 2000) (figure 2). These early data suggest that the main branching of hematopoietic cell differentiation is the separation of lymphoid and myeloid lineages. Lacking all myeloid potential, CLP can possibly seed the thymus to produce all thymic T cells. Recently, an additional progenitor subset, defined as $Flt3^{lo}VCAM1^{+}$ LSK cells, which lack erythroid but has potent lymphoid and G/M developmental potential was isolated in the bone marrow. These cells can give rise to $Flt3^{hi}VCAM1^{+}$ LSK and subsequently $Flt3^{hi}VCAM1^{-}$ LSK cells, with increased lymphoid potential, and reduced G/M potential, but lacking Mk/E potential (Lai and Kondo, 2006) (figure 2). Therefore, bone marrow HSC may differentiate into the lymphoid lineage by sequentially and gradually losing the Mk/E and G/M differentiation potential, before commitment to the lymphoid lineage. Any of the intermediate progenitors with limited and biased developmental potential could also be the source for thymic T cell development.

While direct lineage relationships between these various different lymphoid progenitors and CLPs are lacking, thymopoiesis can carry on without detectable CLPs in the bone marrow of Ikaros-deficient mice (Allman et al., 2003). The presence of CLPs in the circulation is controversial, so they may not be physiological T lineage precursors (Schwarz and Bhandoola, 2006), but LSK cells are isolatable in the circulation and early immature thymic progenitors express markers more similar to LSK cells than to CLPs (Schwarz and Bhandoola, 2004). This would indicate that multipotent HSCs could also seed the thymus before lymphoid commitment initiates (figure 2).

GATA3 AND T CELL COMMITMENT

Flow cytometric and immunocytochemical analyses of fetal thymus cells in the mouse showed that Gata3 is already present in the most immature population of fetal thymus cells, which have the DN1 phenotype (CD44$^+$CD25$^-$ CD4$^-$CD8$^-$ double negative (DN) cells (Hattori et al., 1996). Antisense Gata3 oligonucleotides inhibited T cell development from fetal liver precursor cells in fetal thymic organ cultures, indicating the critical importance of Gata3 for T cell development (Hattori et al., 1996). Moreover, Rag2$^{-/-}$ complementation experiments *in vivo* demonstrated that the development of Gata3$^{-/-}$ embryonic stem cell-derived T cell precursors is arrested at or before the DN stage (Ting et al., 1996). Yet, in such Gata3$^{-/-}$ Rag-2$^{-/-}$ chimeric mice, the Gata3$^{-/-}$ cells did significantly contribute to non-hematopoietic tissues and to various hematopoietic lineages, including erythroid, myeloid en B cell lineages (Ting et al., 1996). In chimeric mice generated by injections of Gata3 deficient ES cells (harboring an allele in which the Gata3 gene was targeted by insertion of a *LacZ* reporter) in WT blastocysts, we showed that Gata3-deficient ES cells did not contribute to the T cell lineage, not even to the earliest subset of DN1 cells (Hendriks et al., 1999).

As (i) Gata3 is expressed within the hematopoietic system in a T cell specific fashion (Hendriks et al., 1999; Oosterwegel et al., 1992; Pandolfi et al., 1995), and (ii) GATA3 is essential for proper development of early thymocytes, it is attractive to propose that GATA3 acts as the decisive T cell commitment factor, equivalent to Pax-5 in the B cell lineage (Nutt et al., 1999; Rolink et al., 1999). However, forced expression of Gata3 in hematopoietic precursors does not appear to enhance T specification. On the contrary, it was found that overexpression of Gata3 in HSCs resulted in cessation of cell expansion, followed by selective induction of megakaryocytic and erythroid differentiation and inhibition of myeloid and lymphoid precursor development (Chen and Zhang, 2001; Rothenberg and Taghon, 2005). These findings indicate that in these experiments, Gata3 may mimic Gata1 function, suggesting functional redundancy among Gata proteins. Thus, induction of cell fate decisions by Gata proteins may well be regulated by their restricted expression patterns and not so much by the features of the individual Gata factors. Moreover, overexpression of Gata3 in developing thymocytes clearly has adverse effects and is associated with reduced cell survival (Anderson et al., 2002; Nawijn et al., 2001b; Taghon et al., 2001; K.W.L., unpublished).

Nevertheless, in support of a role for Gata3 as transcription factor important for T lineage identity, it was recently shown that Gata3 has the capacity to counteract C/EBPα-induced macrophage reprogramming of DN thymocytes cultured on OP9-Dll-1 stromal cells (Laiosa et al., 2006). The restriction of multipotent precursors in the thymus is normally accompanied by a downregulation of the transcription factors C/EBPα and PU.1. Retroviral transduction of C/EBPα in DN cells induced the formation of functional macrophages, but this reprogramming could be inhibited by expression of intracellular Notch1 or Gata3 (Laiosa et al., 2006). A similar antagonism for C/EBPαand Gata3 has been described in adipocyte differentiation, whereby both Gata2 and Gata3 form protein complexes with C/EBPα and C/EBPβ (Tong et al., 2005). In this context, it is intriguing that Gata3 was also shown to regulate the balance between hair follicle and epidermal cell fates by integrating various signaling networks including the WNT, Notch1 and BMP pathways (Kurek, 2006). Additional links with Gata3 and Notch1 include the finding that activation of the Notch1 pathway controls lineage commitment of early thymic precursors by altering the levels between Gata3 and Spi-B, which is an Ets family member transcription factor closely related to PU.1 that controls plasmacytoid dendritic cell development (Dontje et al., 2006).

Taken together, these findings indicate that Gata3 function is closely associated with T cell specification and development, and therefore we argued that Gata3 expression in the bone marrow progenitor cells might indicate their lymphoid lineage developmental potential. To be able to quantify Gata3 expression during T cell differentiation *in vivo* in the mouse, we had previously generated mutant mice in which the Gata3 gene was targeted by insertion of a *LacZ* reporter by homologous recombination in ES cells (Hendriks et al., 1999). In these mice, the expression of the *LacZ* reporter gene reflects transcription of the endogenous Gata3 gene and can be quantified by using fluorescein-di-β-D-galactopyranoside (FDG) as a fluorogenic substrate in conjunction with flow cytometry. We detected Gata3 gene transcription throughout T cell differentiation in the thymus, although the proportion of *LacZ*+ cells varied considerably between the distinct stages of differentiation (see below). In these experiments, ~20-25% of the DN1 population was *LacZ*+ (Hendriks et al., 1999).

Interestingly, we found that 2.5% of the Lin⁻ cells in the bone marrow of the *Gata3-LacZ* mice expressed the *LacZ* reporter gene (figure 3). These Lin⁻ FDG⁺ cells were all c-kit⁻, showing that they were neither LSK nor CLP cells, although they expressed a heterogeneous level of Sca-1 (figure 3). High proportions of Lin⁻ FDG⁺ cells expressed the lymphoid specific cytokine receptor IL-7Rα, suggesting that they could have lymphoid lineage potential and are not CMPs. It is not very likely that these cells represent Gata3⁺ IL-7Rα⁺ NK cells, as we would have excluded these cells using the Lin channel. Moreover, such Gata3⁺IL-7Rα⁺ NK cells were shown to be thymus-derived and not present in the bone marrow (Vosshenrich et al., 2006). While it is clear from previous RT-PCR data showing that HSCs express low levels of Gata3, and CMPs do not express Gata3 mRNA, it was also reported that CLPs (that are Sca-1^{lo}c-kit^{lo}) express low level Gata3 mRNA (Akashi et al., 2000). This discrepancy could be contributed to differences in (i) the sensitivity of the detection approach (one is PCR-based and the other is based on enzymatic reaction and flow cytometry), or (ii) the stability of the *LacZ* protein or the Gata3 transcripts. In any case, the lympho/hematopoietic lineage potential of our Gata3$^+$ IL-7Rα^+ Lin$^-$ cells is not clear, and needs further characterization.

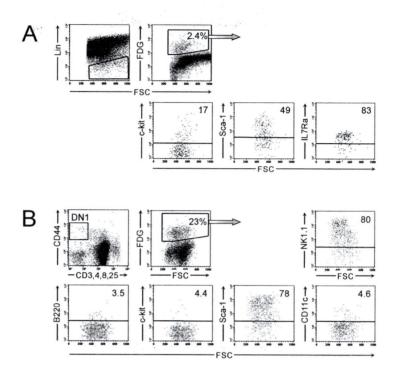

Figure 3. Flow cytometric analyses of Gata3 expressing cells in bone marrow and thymus of Gata3-LacZ knock-in mice. (A) Bone marrow Lin$^-$ FDG$^+$ cells were analyzed for developmental markers c-kit, Sca-1 and IL-7R . (B), Thymic DN1 FDG$^+$ cells were analyzed for expression of developmental markers (c-kit and Sca-1) and lineage markers (NK1.1, B220 and CD11c).

Obviously, the Gata3$^+$ IL-7Rα^+ Lin$^-$ cells may reflect intermediate progenitors in the bone marrow, which are on their way to becoming T cells, and would eventually leave the bone marrow and seed the thymus. Thus, we also investigated the *LacZ* expression pattern in the immature thymic T cell progenitor subset of DN1 cells in the *Gata3-LacZ* mice in more detail. Consistent with our previous report (Hendriks et al., 1999), we found that ~23% of the DN1 cells in the thymus are FDG$^+$ (figure 3). Further analysis of these DN1 FDG$^+$ cells showed that they are all c-kit$^-$ and express heterogeneous levels of Sca-1, an expression pattern similar to that of the bone marrow Lin$^-$ FDG$^+$ cells of these mice. However, about 80% of DN1 FDG$^+$ cells expressed the NK cell marker NK1.1, and were essentially negative for the DC and B cell markers CD11c and B220, respectively (figure 3). Therefore, it seems likely that they are the recently described Gata3$^+$IL-7Rα^+ NK cells present in the thymus (Vosshenrich et al.; 2006). In contrast to T cells, NK cells can be generated in the absence of Gata3, but Gata3is essential for NK cell function, as it promotes maturation, interferon-γ (IFNγ) production, and liver-specific homing of NK cells (Samson et al., 2003). The homeostasis of the thymus-derived Gata3$^+$IL-7Rα^+ NK cells, which repopulate peripheral lymphoid organs, is strictly dependent on Gata3 and IL-7 and have functional characteristics that are different from the bone marrow derived NK cells (Vosshenrich et al., 2006).

Nevertheless, a subpopulation of ~20% of the DN1 FDG$^+$ cells were NK$^-$B220$^-$CD11c$^-$ and possibly contained the lineage-uncommitted progenitors, which could be the cells that had recently migrated from the bone marrow to the thymus. A detailed characterization of the developmental potential of the bone marrow Lin$^-$ FDG$^+$ cells and the thymic NK1.1$^-$ DN1 FDG$^+$ cells (in particular with regards to their relationship to the other established bone marrow and thymic progenitors with lymphoid potential), would shed light on the cellular and molecular mechanisms of T cell commitment.

EXPRESSION OF GATA3 IN THYMOCYTES AND β-SELECTION

Early T lineage restricted precursors express neither CD4 nor CD8 co-receptor and are therefore referred to as DN cells (figure 4). Within the DN population, the CD44$^+$CD25$^-$ DN1 subset contains the most immature progenitors originating from the bone marrow (Allman et al., 2003; Porritt et al., 2004). DN1 cells develop into CD44$^+$CD25$^+$ DN2 thymocytes, in which specification is initiated and commitment is completed (Rothenberg, 2000). When cells have differentiated into CD44$^-$CD25$^+$ (DN3), the pro-T cells begin controlled locus-specific recombination of their TCR γ, δ or β genes, initiated by the Rag-1 and Rag-2 proteins (Rothenberg and Taghon, 2005). Pro-T cells that successfully rearrange TCRγ and TCRδ will express a γδ TCR and are eligible to develop further as γδ T cells (Burtrum et al., 1996). By contrast, cells that produce a functional TCR β chain, which associates with an invariant pTα chain to form a pre-TCR, are selected for further development, enter the cell cycle and differentiate into DN4 cells, a process referred to as β-selection (Godfrey and Zlotnik, 1993; Mallick et al., 1993; von Boehmer, 2005). Subsequently, they acquire both CD4 and CD8 co-receptors. In most mouse strains CD8 is expressed first, resulting in the generation of large cycling CD8$^+$ immature single positive (ISP) cells. In double positive (DP) thymocytes productive TCRα locus recombination results in the expression of the αβ TCR complex on the cell surface. After engagement of the αβ TCR by self-MHC peptide complexes, low- to intermediate-avidity interactions rescue DP thymocytes from death by neglect through a process termed positive selection (Bosselut, 2004; Germain, 2002; Kappes and He, 2005). By contrast, strong TCR signals resulting from interactions with endogenous peptides trigger apoptosis, which eliminates auto-reactive thymocytes, a process termed negative selection. Positive selection results in the differentiation of CD4 and CD8 single positive (SP) cells, which express an αβ TCR that recognizes peptide antigens presented by MHC class II and class I molecules, respectively. Mature SP cells exit the thymus to circulate to the periphery as naive CD4$^+$ T helper (Th) cells and CD8$^+$ cytotoxic T cells.

Using mice with the Gata3 *LacZ* reporter on one allele, we examined the proportion of *LacZ$^+$* cells as a function of T cell development (figure 4). Although Gata3 is expressed throughout T cell development, the fraction of *LacZ$^+$* cells was highly variable between different stages, indicating that expression levels of Gata3 may be crucial for regulation of T cell development (Hendriks et al., 1999; Nawijn et al., 2001b). High proportions of *LacZ$^+$* cells in the DN4, ISP and CD3$^+$ DP cell populations suggested a role for Gata3 in β-selection and in positive selection of CD4$^+$ T cells (Hendriks et al., 1999; Nawijn et al., 2001b). In particular, the finding of low Gata3 expression during the two waves of TCR gene recombination, separated by a stage of high Gata3 expression, suggested that Gata3 may function as a regulator of proliferation events associated with the essential coupling of V(D)J recombination activity to the cell cycle (Lee and Desiderio, 1999). In agreement with this, we find that transgenic overexpression of Gata3 is associated with thymic lymphoma (Nawijn et al., 2001b) and c-myc upregulation (J.P. v. H., unpublished).

Conditional deletion of the *Gata3* gene at the DN stage using the Cre-loxP system, whereby the *Cre* transgene was driven by the proximal *Lck* promoter, resulted in a developmental arrest at the DN3 stage, implicating Gata3 in β-selection (Pai et al., 2003). Gata3$^{-/-}$ DN3 cells can rearrange and express intracellular TCR β chain, but the DN3 TCRβ$^+$ cells fail to increase their cell size and do not downregulate CD25 surface expression. Interestingly, there is no evidence suggesting a survival defect in these arrested Gata3$^{-/-}$ DN3 cells. These findings indicate that β-selection is partially induced, because cells are rescued from apoptosis, but fail to expand or differentiate. Introduction of a pre-rearranged TCR transgene into these Gata3$^{-/-}$ thymocytes did not rescue the developmental block (Pai et al., 2003). On the other hand, expression of Gata3 alone is not sufficient to initiate β-selection: the developmental arrest at the DN3 stage in Rag2$^{-/-}$ mice (Mombaerts et al., 1992; Shinkai et al., 1992) could not be corrected by enforced transgenic expression of Gata3. In these Gata3 transgenic Rag2$^{-/-}$ mice cell size increase and CD25 downregulation in DN3 cells was negligible and no DN4 cells were detected (K.W.L, unpublished data). Taken together, these findings show that Gata3 functions as a key mediator for β-selection, but expression of Gata3 alone - in the absence of a functionally rearranged TCR β chain - is not sufficient to initiate β-selection.

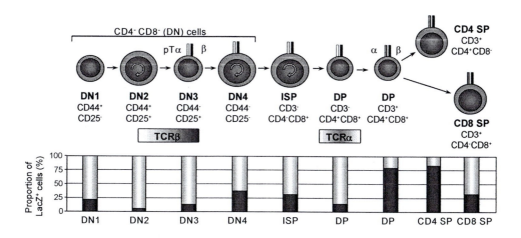

Figure 4. Schematic overview of T cell development and Gata3 expression. Developmental markers used to separate different developmental T cell subset are shown on the upper panel. Proportion of *LacZ*$^+$ cells (analyzed by flow cytometry using Gata3-*LacZ* knock-in mice and FDG substrate (Hendriks et al., 1999; Nawijn et al., 2001b) is shown in the lower panel.

ROLE OF GATA3 DURING POSITIVE SELECTION AND CD4 T CELL DEVELOPMENT

Conditional deletion of the *Gata3* gene after β-selection, using *CD4-Cre* transgenic mice, resulted in a profound specific deficiency of CD4 SP cells. This finding demonstrated the absolute requirement of Gata3 for survival or development of CD4 committed thymocytes *in vivo*. Together with the unique expression pattern of Gata3 – low in early immature DP cells and specifically upregulated when DP cells develop towards the CD4 lineage (figure 4), it is possible that Gata3 has a role in CD4 versus CD8 lineage commitment. Interestingly, TCR signal strength at the DP stage has been shown to affect CD4 versus CD8 lineage decision, i.e. strong TCR signals directs commitment towards the CD4 lineage (Bosselut, 2004; Germain, 2002; Kappes and He, 2005). Gata3 is upregulated by DP thymocytes in response to TCR stimulation, whereby its expression levels correlate with the strength of the TCR signal (Hernandez-Hoyos et al., 2003). To assess the stages at which the Gata3 expression levels diverge between cells taking the CD4 or CD8 pathway, quantitative real-time RT-PCR was used to analyze Gata3 transcripts from sorted thymocyte subpopulations from either MHC class I- or MHC class II-deficient mice to guarantee the CD4 or CD8 lineage of the sorted populations, respectively (Hernandez-Hoyos et al., 2003). In the MHC class II selected cells Gata3 mRNA levels increased to a maximum in CD69$^+$ CD4 lineage intermediates and then gradually decreased as the cells develop into CD4 SP mature cells, while in the MHC class I selected cells Gata3 was not induced (Hernandez-Hoyos et al., 2003). Taken together, these observations indicate that Gata3 could function to direct CD4 lineage commitment by translating the quantitative difference between TCR signals for CD4 versus CD8 lineage commitment.

However, in the absence of Gata3, while MHC class I-restricted T cell commitment was not affected, MHC class II-restricted T cells were not diverted into the CD8 lineage (Pai et al., 2003). Conversely, sustained over-expression of Gata3 in fetal thymic organ cultures favored selection of CD4 over CD8 SP cells, but did not divert MHC class I-restricted precursors into the CD4 lineage (Hernandez-Hoyos et al., 2003). On the basis of these findings it has been concluded that Gata3 is necessary for post-commitment CD4 generation, rather than for commitment to the CD4 lineage (Hernandez-Hoyos et al., 2003; Pai et al., 2003). Nevertheless, the possibility that Gata3 might promote CD4 lineage choice cannot be excluded, as it is still conceivable that MHC class II-restricted CD8$^+$ T cells or MHC class I-restricted CD4$^+$ T cells die as they fail to undergo MHC-TCR and CD4/CD8 co-engagement required for their survival (Bosselut, 2004).

To further investigate a possible role of Gata3 in CD4/CD8 lineage commitment, we have analyzed transgenic mice with enforced expression of Gata3, 5' tagged with 3 HA epitopes, driven by the human CD2 locus control region, which targets Gata3 expression to both the CD4 and the CD8 lineage. Two independent CD2-GATA3 Tg lines were established, and no differences were found between the two lines. These mice have a complex T cell phenotype, characterized by (i) impaired maturation of CD8 SP cells in the thymus, (ii) enhanced Th2 cell development of mature peripheral T cells, and (iii) thymic lymphoma in aging mice (Nawijn et al., 2001a; Nawijn et al., 2001b). We crossed the CD2-GATA3 Tg mice with mice in which the Gata3 gene is conditionally deleted in the T cell lineage using the CD4-Cre lox system. In this complex cross any differential expression of Gata3 between DP cells taking the CD4 or CD8 pathway was eliminated, because endogenous Gata3 was entirely substituted by transgenic Gata3, which is expressed at equal levels in developing CD4 and CD8 cells. In these mice both CD4 and CD8 cells were generated (K.W.L., manuscript submitted), we therefore conclude that Gata3 expression levels are not decisive for determination of CD4/CD8 lineage choice.

In Gata3-deficient DP cells, the proximal components of TCR signaling for positive selection, such as phosphorylation of Lck and ZAP70 appear to be unaffected (Pai et al., 2003). However, in the absence of Gata3 TCR signaling does not appear to induce cell size increase or CD69 and TCR upregulation (K.W.L., manuscript submitted). Conversely, in the CD2-GATA3 Tg mice we identified a small increase in DP cell size and in TCR$\alpha\beta$/CD3 expression levels in CD69$^+$ DP cells, suggesting that enforced Gata3 expression may influence the kinetics of positive selection (Nawijn et al., 2001b). Enforced expression of Gata3 is associated with decreased levels of CD5 at the DP stage, while in the absence of Gata3 CD5 levels are slightly elevated, when compared to WT mice (K.W.L., manuscript submitted). CD5 expression is first induced at the early DN stage, upregulated by pre-TCR signaling and increases progressively as T cells develop from the DN to the DP stage in a signal dose-dependent manner (Azzam et al., 1998). CD5 is a negative regulator of TCR signaling and thus participates in the fine-tuning of the TCR repertoire (Azzam et al., 2001). Taken together, Gata3 has the ability to downregulate CD5 and to upregulate TCR expression in developing CD4 T cell lineage cells (K.W.L., manuscript submitted). As Gata3 expression is induced by TCR signaling, these findings implicate Gata3 as a key regulator in a positive feedback loop. Induction of Gata3 by TCR signaling will increase TCR expression and thereby enhance the induction of Gata3. Moreover, Gata3 has the ability to increase TCR signal strength in an independent parallel pathway by downregulating CD5, leading to an efficient mode of signal amplification in this positive regulatory loop. As a result, during development of DP to CD4 SP cells the expression levels of the TCR and Gata3 will increase. It may be possible that Gata3 directly regulates TCR α and β transcription, as binding sites have been identified in these loci (Ho et al., 1991; Marine and Winoto, 1991). As Gata3 expression is not induced in the CD8 cell lineage (Hernandez-Hoyos et al., 2003), different nuclear factors should be responsible for the regulation of the expression level of CD5 and TCR molecules in the CD8 lineage.

GATA3 AS A MASTER REGULATOR OF TH2 DIFFERENTIATION

Upon antigenic stimulation naive CD4$^+$ T cells differentiate into effector T cells, which are classically divided into two functionally distinct subsets, termed Th1 and Th2 (See for review: Bottomly, 1988; Mosmann and Coffman, 1989; Murphy and Reiner, 2002; Kalinski and Moser, 2005). Th1 cells, which produce IFN-γ and lymphotoxin-α, are associated with the elimination of intracellular pathogens. Th2 cells, which produce IL-4, Il-5 and IL-13, are critically important for the eradication of parasitic worms, but are also implicated in allergic responses (Abbas et al., 1996; Szabo et al., 2003). Recently, new lineages of CD4$^+$ T cells have been identified, including CD25[+] regulatory T cells (Sakaguchi et al., 2006), and a helper T cell subset producing IL-17 and for this reason termed Th17. IL-17 is a pro-inflammatory cytokine, which has been linked to autoimmune diseases (such as systemic lupus erythematosus, experimental autoimmune encephalomyelitis and rheumatoid arthritis) and to allograft rejection (Batten et al., 2006; Harrington et al., 2005; Park et al., 2005; Veldhoen et al., 2006a; Veldhoen et al., 2006b). Differentiation towards individual T cell subsets and their maintenance is critically dependent on specific transcription factors, such as T-bet for Th1 (Szabo et al., 2000), Gata3 for Th2 (Zhang et al., 1997; Zheng and Flavell, 1997), RORγt for Th17 (Ivanov et al., 2006) and FoxP3 for regulatory T cells (Sakaguchi et al., 2006; Ziegler, 2006).

In response to chronic antigenic stimulation *in vivo*, progressive polarization of the cytokine responses ultimately leads to the commitment of naive CD4[+] precursors into mutually exclusive Th effector phenotypes, which are though to be maintained independent of extrinsic factors. Th1 development is facilitated by two major signaling pathways, one involving IL-12/Stat4 and the other involving IFNγ/Stat1/T-bet. Th2 differentiation is dependent on IL-4-induced activation of Stat6, leading to expression of Gata3 (Zhang et al., 1997; Zheng and Flavell, 1997). On its turn Gata3 auto-activates its own expression and increases the accessibility of the Th2 cytokine cluster containing the genes coding for IL-4, IL-5 and IL-13 (Agarwal and Rao, 1998; Lee et al., 2001; Ouyang et al., 2000). Furthermore, Gata3 suppresses Th1 development by downregulating the expression of Stat4 and the IL-12 receptor β2 chain (Ouyang et al., 1998; Usui et al., 2003; Usui et al., 2006). Only if T-bet is induced in naive cells at sufficient levels, such Gata3 suppression is counteracted, permitting Th1 differentiation to occur. This ability of T-bet to oppose the action of Gata3 now appears its most essential function in Th1 differentiation rather than any ability of T-bet to directly affect IFNγ gene transcription, as has been argued previously (Mullen et al., 2002). T-bet may act on Gata3 through multiple mechanisms, as it (i) inhibits Gata3 transcription and (ii) physically interacts with Gata3 and thereby prevents its binding to the IL-5 promoter (Hwang et al., 2005). Commitment of CD4[+] T cells to a particular Th phenotype is associated with the induction of epigenetic changes in the loci of effector cytokine genes, the Th2 cytokine locus (IL-4 / IL-13 / Rad50 / IL-5 locus) and the IFNγ locus (Agarwal and Rao, 1998; Lee et al., 2001). The mechanisms through which regulatory elements in these loci regulate cytokine expression by intra- and even inter-chromosomal interactions (Lee et al., 2005; Spilianakis and Flavell, 2004; Spilianakis et al., 2005), has recently been reviewed (Lee et al., 2006). Gata3 or chromatin remodeling using pharmacological histone deacetylase- and cytosine methylation-inhibitors can replace the essential role of Stat6 in Th2 differentiation (Bird et al., 1998; Grogan et al., 2001; Ouyang et al., 2000). The introduction of Gata3 into *in vitro*-cultured T cells was shown to generate Th2-specific DNAse I hypersensitive sites independently of Stat6, implicating Gata3 in the process of chromatin remodeling (Ouyang et al., 2000). These experiments also indicated that there is a positive auto-activation pathway, whereby Gata3, either directly or indirectly, activates its own expression. Interestingly, Th cell differentiation is controlled by the cell cycle and the instruction for the Th2 cytokines IL-4 and IL-10 requires progression into S phase (Bird et al., 1998; Richter et al., 1999). In conditional Gata3-deficient T cells, normal Th2 acetylation patterns in the IL-4, IL-5, and IL-13 genes are impaired (Yamashita et al., 2004). The effect is most prominent in the IL-5 gene, where there is a severe loss of Th2-associated hyperacetylation. The effect in the IL-4 and IL-13 genes is much less pronounced. The effect of Gata3 loss on Th2 cytokine production is more apparent in developing responses than in established Th2 cells. In a developing Th2 response, loss of Gata3 results in the inability to effectively mount a Th2 response, with a substantial reduction in the generation of IL-4-, IL-5-, and IL-13-producing cells (Pai et al., 2004; Yamashita et al., 2004; Zhu et al., 2004). In contrast, the loss of Gata3 in established Th2 cells causes a dramatic reduction in IL-5 production, a smaller effect on IL-13, but little effect on IL-4 (Pai et al., 2004; Zhu et al., 2004). Gata3 acts in part by maintaining hyperacetylation of promoter regions of the IL-5 gene. The maintenance of acetylation patterns and transcriptional activity of the IL-4 and IL-13 genes may be controlled by additional mechanisms.

To examine the functional capacities of Gata3 *in vivo*, we investigated Th cell differentiation in the CD2-GATA3 Tg mice with enforced expression of Gata3 in all T cells. These mice manifested increased serum levels of the IL-4/Th2-dependent isotype IgG1, when compared with non-transgenic littermates (Nawijn et al., 2001a). Upon immunisation with the TNP-KLH protein, antigen-specific IgG2a - which is an INFγ/Th1-dependent isotype – was significantly decreased and IgE – which is an IL-4/Th2-dependent isotype – was significantly increased (Nawijn et al., 2001a). We also found a severe reduction in the KLH-induced footpad swellings in *CD2-GATA3-Tg* mice, indicating that enforced Gata3 expression suppresses the Th1-dependent delayed type hypersensitivity response to KLH. The total population of CD4$^+$ T cells in spleen or mesenteric lymph node, manifested rapid secretion of the Th2 cytokines IL-4, IL-5, and IL-10, reminiscent of Th2 memory cells. At the same time, the ability to produce IL-2 and IFNγ was decreased (Nawijn et al., 2001a). We concluded that he increased functional capacity to secrete Th2 cytokines, along with the increased expression of surface markers for Ag-experienced Th2-committed cells, including T1/ST2, would argue for a role of Gata3 in Th2 memory formation (Nawijn et al., 2001a).

To analyze the effect of enforced Gata3 expression on the function of naive T cells, we isolated CD62L$^+$ naïve CD4$^+$ T cells from CD2-GATA3 Tg mice and wild-type littermates, and stimulated them with plate-bound anti-CD3 and anti-CD28 for 2 days under various polarizing conditions, and cultured them for another 5 days. As is clear from figure 5A, in the presence of the CD2-GATA3 transgene cellular expansion under Th1 and Th2 conditions was slightly impaired. In CD2-GATA3 Tg mice, the expression of Gata3, which is normally Th2-cell specific, was now quite similar in all CD4 conditions and in CD8 T cells (figure 5B). Gata3 overexpression did not affect the levels of T-bet transcription, not even in Th0 conditions that did not contain anti-IL-4 antibodies.

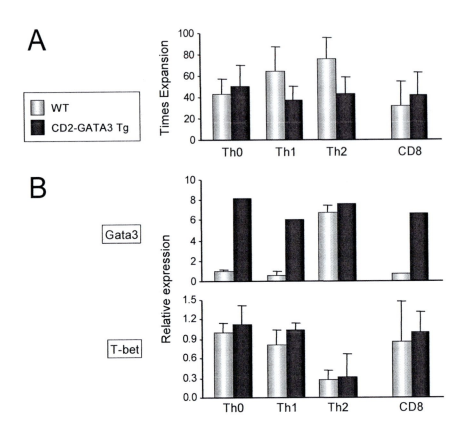

Figure 5. The effect of enforced Gata3 expression in T cell cultures. (A) Expansion rates of FACS-sorted CD62L[+] naïve CD4 or CD8 cells from the indicated WT or CD2-GATA3 Tg mice on the FVB background. (B) Expression of Gata3 and T-bet transcription factors at day 7, as determined by quantitative RT-PCR. Expression in WT Th0 cultures was set to one. Cells were stimulated with plate-bound anti-CD3 and anti-CD28 for 2 days and subsequently expanded in the presence of IL-2. For Th1 conditions IL-12 and anti-IL-4 was added, whereas for Th2 conditions IL-4, anti-IL-12 and anti-IFN . was added.

When we analyzed cytokine production at day 5 by intracellular flow cytometry, we found that CD2-GATA3 Tg T cell cultures contained large fractions of IL-4-expressing cells (~60%), irrespective of the culture conditions (figure 6). Under Th1 conditions, this resulted in cells co-expressing IL-4 and IFNγ. CD2-GATA3 Tg T cell cultures also contained fewer IL-2 producing cells and more IL-10 producing cells. Enforced Gata3 expression had only limited effect on IFNγ production by CD4 or CD8 cells, and even appeared to enhance Granzyme B expression by CD8 cells (figure 6B). Collectively, the findings from these experiments confirmed observations by various groups, that Gata3 supports Th2 development and inhibits Th1 development. In addition, we found that Gata3 expression is sufficient to induce IL-4 expression (figure 6A), IL-5 and IL-13 (data not shown), even under Th1 culture conditions when the cells express T-bet (and high levels of IL-12 and antibodies to IL-4 are present). Under these Th1 conditions T-bet is apparently unable to counteract Gata3, but nevertheless able to support Th1 differentiation in the presence of Gata3, as IFNγ is produced.

In summary, direct targets of Gata3 are mainly identified in the context of T helper cell development and include the Th2 cytokines IL-4, IL-5 and IL-13, Gata3 itself, and Stat4 (which is repressed). Our findings demonstrate that Gata3 expression is sufficient to activate transcription of the Th2 locus in activated and polarized INFγ-producing Th1 cells, but this does not imply that Gata3 has this ability in any cell. For example, expression of the Th2 cytokines in activated CD2-GATA3 CD8 T cells was usually lower (J.P.v.H., unpublished results). Furthermore, we did not detect enhanced IL-4, IL-5 or IL-13 expression in CD2-GATA3 Tg DP thymocytes, although expression of Gata3 was increased by a factor of ~5 to 10, when compared with WT DP cells. Also, in T cell lymphomas from CD2-GATA3 Tg mice, we found that cytokine production was variable and high-level expression was confined to particular areas of the tumors. Therefore, we conclude that the capacity of Gata3 to activate transcription of the Th2 locus is different between T cell differentiation stages, and thus context-dependent.

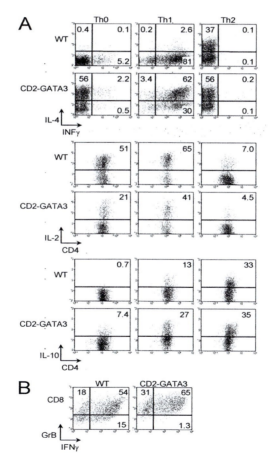

Figure 6. The effect of enforced Gata3 expression on cytokine production. Intracellular cytokine production in CD4 T cell (A) or CD8 T cell (B) cultures from the indicated WT or CD2-GATA3 Tg mice on the FVB background. FACS-sorted CD62L⁺ naïve CD4 or CD8 cells were stimulated with plate-bound anti-CD3 and anti-CD28 for 2 days and subsequently expanded in the presence of IL-2. For Th1 conditions IL-12 and anti-IL-4 was added, whereas for Th2 conditions IL-4, anti-IL-12 and anti-IFN , was added. GrB= Granzyme B.

GATA FACTORS AND HEMATOPOIETIC DISORDERS

As Gata factors are crucially involved in the regulation of self-renewal, cellular proliferation and differentiation, it is not surprising that there is evidence for a role of Gata factors in the etiology of specific tumors.

Acquired missense mutations in the Gata1 gene have been identified in almost all cases of Down's syndrome-related acute megakaryoblastic leukemia (AMKL) and transient myeoloproliferative disorder (Wechsler et al., 2002). Mutations are clustered and each mutation results in the introduction of a premature stop codon in the N-terminal activation domain region, preventing the synthesis of full-length Gata1. The mutations do not block the synthesis of a shorter Gata1 variant that is initiated downstream and lacks the N-terminal activation domain but can still bind to Fog1. T date, the molecular mechanism by which this short Gata1 variant induces AMKL remains unclear. Furthermore, a high incidence of leukemia was found in female mice heterozygous for the knock-down mutation allele Gata1.05, the expression of which is reduced to 5% of the WT level. Hemizygous male mice ($X^{Gata1.05}$/Y) die *in utero* due to severe anemia, but heterozygous females ($X^{Gata1.05}$/X) survive, although they show various degrees of anemia and thrombocytopenia. These $X^{Gata1.05}$/X female mice may be a valuable animal model for myelodysplastic syndrome, as they suffer from multilineage cytopenia which progresses to acute leukemia in aging mice (Pan et al., 2005; Shimizu et al., 2004).

An initial screening of more then 30 leukemias revealed a tight correlation of the expression of Gata2 and Gata3 in the leukemic cells comparable to their normal counterparts: Gata2 in leukemic cells with stem cell phenotypes and Gata3 in T lymphomas (Minegishi et al., 1997). The Gata2 gene is located near 3q21 breakpoints in acute myeloid leukaemia or myelodysplastic syndrome. The majority of 3q21 breakpoints are located telomeric to the transcribed portion of the Gata2 gene in a region that is necessary for proper promoter function in mice. Gata2 was found to be reproducibly overexpressed in 7 out of 9 patient samples with 3q21 abnormalities (Wieser et al., 2000). Gata2 can form a complex with the pro-myelocytic leukaemia protein (PML) and can potentiate its transactivation capacity (Tsuzuki et al., 2000). Gata2 can also physically interact with the PML-RARα (retinoic acid receptor α oncogenic fusion protein generated by the t(15;17) translocation characteristic of acute promyelocytic leukaemia. Functional experiments further showed that this interaction has the capacity to render a subset of Gata2 target genes subject to regulation by the retinoid acid signaling pathway (Tsuzuki et al., 2000). Although Gata2 can interact with these leukemic chimera proteins, it has not been demonstrated to date that Gata2 indeed functions in leukemogenesis.

It has been reported that Gata2 transcription is decreased in CD34$^+$ bone marrow-derived hematopoietic stem and progenitor cells in aplastic anemia (Tsuzuki et al., 2000). (Fujimaki et al., 2001) Aplastic anemia is a bone marrow failure syndrome due to impaired stem cell function, characterized by hypocellular bone marrow, reduced hematopoiesis and peripheral pancytopenia (Young, 1999). This appears to be inconsistent with our studies on the Gata2 haplo-insufficient mice showing that Gata2 expression level is crucial for HSC function (Ling et al., 2004), however, reduced Gata2 expression level only caused a delayed response to proliferative stress, which would not result in a long term hypocellular bone marrow. At the same time, it was postulated that the primary cause of aplastic anemia is not intrinsic to the HSC but due to a cytotoxic T lymphocyte-mediated attack on bone marrow CD34$^+$ cells (Young and Maciejewski, 1997). Recent DNA micro array analyses confirmed the reduced Gata2 expression in CD34$^+$ bone marrow cells from aplastic anemia patients. However, it also revealed an abnormal expression of genes involved in signal transduction pathways for apoptosis and terminal cytolytic enzyme generation and the reduced expression of anti-apoptotic genes in these cells. Furthermore, there is an increased expression level of immune response genes in aplastic anemia patients (Zeng et al., 2004). Taken together these data support the idea that the primary cause of aplastic anemia is an immune attack of bone marrow CD34$^+$ cells. The observed reduced Gata2 expression level is therefore not likely the primary cause of aplastic anemia.

Gata3, which is also highly expressed by the luminal epithelial cells in the breast, was found mutated in cases of human breast tumors (Usary et al., 2004). Recently, Gata3 has been identified as a prognostic marker in breast cancer (Mehra et al., 2005): patients whose tumors expressed low Gata3 had significantly shorter overall and disease-free survival when compared with those whose tumors had high Gata3 levels. Also Gata4, 5 and 6 have been implicated in various human tumors, including gastric and colon cancer, esophageal cancer, ovarian carcinoma and adrenocortical tumors (Akiyama et al., 2003; Guo et al., 2006; Kiiveri et al., 2004; Wakana et al., 2006).

Gata3 haplo-insufficiency is associated with HDR syndrome (hypopara-thyroidism, sensorineural deafness and renal anomalies) (Bilous et al., 1992; Van Esch et al., 2000). However, hematological disorders have not been reported so far in the HDR syndrome patients. Consistently, as Gata3 haplo-insufficiency can cause HDR syndrome, our Gata-LacZ knock-in heterozygous mice have a normal hematopoietic profile. In contrast to Gata2$^{+/-}$ mice (see above), regeneration of the hematopoietic system, including the T cell lineage, after cytotoxic drug treatment in the Gata3-LacZ heterozygous mice is comparable to that of the WT (K.W.L. unpublished observations).

Taken the oncogenic potential of Gata factors into account, we were wondering whether a link was present between the induction of DP thymic lymphomas in the CD2-GATA3 Tg mice (Nawijn et al., 2001b), the upregulation of Gata3 expression and the selection events that normally take place at the DP stage in the thymus. When the CD2-GATA3 Tg mice were followed up to 9 mo of age, ~50% developed thymic lymphomas, which were typically noticed as mice displayed respiratory distress. The thymic lymphomas often had a CD4$^+$CD8$^+$ phenotype and were generally positive for CD3ε and TCRαβ expression. Tumor frequencies were similar in two independent CD2-GATA3 Tg mouse lines and were not seen in non-transgenic littermates. Several animals with thymic lymphoma exhibited enlargement of spleen or lymph nodes. Lymphoma cells, were found in the spleen, liver, lymph nodes, and kidney, indicating that the thymic lymphomas metastasized to the periphery. This was confirmed by the presence of identical clonal TCRβ rearrangement patterns in Southern blotting analyses using probes specific for Jβ$_1$ or Jβ$_2$ gene segments (Nawijn et al., 2001b).

We crossed CD2-GATA3 Tg mice to various TCR transgenic mice that represent models for negative selection and positive selection towards CD4 or CD8. As we found tumors in all these models (J.P. v. H., unpublished results), it appears that thymic lymphoma formation is independent of the process of positive or negative selection. One possible mechanism by which the thymic lymphomas arise could be an aberrant expression of the Lmo2, E2A and Tal1 transcription factors, which are commonly found in human T-ALL. In particular, it has been shown that the gene for retinaldehyde dehydrogenase-2 is a direct target gene regulated by Tal1 and Lmo2 in T-ALL, whereby these two proteins act as cofactors for Gata3. Forced expression of Gata3 potentiated the induction of retinaldehyde dehydrogenase-2 by Tal1 and Lmo2, and these three factors formed a complex *in vivo* (Ono et al., 1997; Ono et al., 1998). However, expression analyses on cell lines obtained from CD2-GATA3 Tg mice showed no evidence for the involvement of these factors in tumor formation.

Several lines of evidence indicate that the transformation mechanism of CD2-GATA3 Tg DP thymocytes does not involves aberrant use of the V(D)J recombination machinery. Firstly, the CD2-GATA3 Tg lymphoma cells did not contain translocations involving TCR or Ig loci, as detected by spectral karyotyping (SKY) analysis. Secondly, the mRNA levels of Rag1 and Rag2 were very low in these cells. CD2-GATA3 Tg mice which were crossed onto a Rag-1$^{-/-}$ background (whereby thymic cellularity was restored by a pre-rearranged TCR transgene), still developed DP thymic lymphoma.

However, the SKY analyses revealed in four out of six cases a trisomy of chromosome 15 and in two of the cases this was the only chromosomal abnormality observed. Interestingly, chromosome 15 contains the gene encoding c-myc, the expression of which was also found to be increased in CD2-GATA3 Tg DP thymocytes, when compared with WT DP thymocytes (J.P. v. H., unpublished results). Together with the findings that CD2-GATA3 Tg DP thymocytes have an increased cell size and that Gata3-deficient TCRβ-expressing DN3 cells cannot increase their cell size during β-selection (Nawijn et al., 2001b; Pai et al., 2003; J.P. v. H., unpublished results), this may indicate an important role of deregulated c-myc expression in the induction of thymic lymphoma. It is attractive to hypothesize that c-myc is an important downstream target of Gata3, because (i) expression of c-myc, like Gata3, peaks in the largest DN cells and declines in DP cells, (ii) c-myc-deficient early thymocytes – just like Gata3-deficient cells - are blocked as small noncycling DN3 cells, and (iii) enforced expression of c-myc under the control of the human CD2 regulatory sequences is also associated with thymic lymphoma of CD3^{+} cells that are mostly DP (Douglas et al., 2001; Stewart et al., 1993). Intriguingly, it was recently reported that Notch1, which signaling pathway plays a critical role in T cell development and in the pathogenesis of human T cell lymphoblastic leukemia (Ellisen et al., 1991; Radtke et al., 2004; Weng et al., 2004; Weng et al., 2003), has the capacity to directly regulate c-myc gene expression. It appears that Notch1 and c-myc govern two directly interconnected transcriptional programs containing common target genes that together promote leukemic cell growth (Palomero et al., 2006; Weng et al., 2006). As expression of Gata3 is upregulated by Dl-1/Notch1 signaling (Dontje et al., 2006), it is very well conceivable that overexpression of Gata3 in the CD2-GATA3 Tg mice may induce part of the transcriptional program that is activated by Notch1 signaling in T cell leukemia, including the induction of c-myc gene transcription and various biosynthetic pathway genes associated with oncogenic transformation.

CONCLUSION

In this review, we have summarized recent progress related to the control of the T cell developmental program by Gata family transcription factors. Gata2 is essential for embryonic HSC production and adult HSC function. It also functions to limit the differentiation of thymocytes into non-T lineages. In contrast, Gata3 is implicated in nearly all major fate decisions during T cell development, starting from T cell specification, β-selection, positive selection and even up to the generation of mature effector Th2 cells. Gata factors are crucial regulators of the balance between cellular proliferation and differentiation. Interestingly, Gata3-mediated regulation of cell fate most likely involves the induction of proliferation at the stages of T cell commitment, β-selection or Th2 differentiation, but not during positive selection of CD4 SP cells in the thymus. Thus, the mechanism by which Gata3 regulates cell fate decisions during T cell differentiation may be very different between the individual developmental stages.

The various transgenic and (conditional) knock-out mouse models for Gata2 and Gata3 have evolved as invaluable tools to gain insight into the *in vivo* functions of these factors. In particular, since the functions of the Gata factors are context-dependent, with clear differences e.g. between fetal and adult hematopoiesis, or between T cell differentiation in the thymus and the activation of peripheral T cells. Moreover, expression levels of the Gata factors are decisive, as is obvious from the phenotypic consequences of reduced or enhanced expression of Gata2 or Gata3. The essential role of Gata factors in the regulation of cell division and differentiation is also underscored by their involvement in the pathogenesis of specific leukemias. Knowledge on the control of T cell development by Gata factors will facilitates improvement of clinical strategies for the generation of various T cell subtypes from HSCs, e.g. in the context of bone marrow or stem cell transplantation, or for the specific expansion of particular mature T cell subpopulations for immuno-based therapies.

ACKNOWLEDGEMENTS

We acknowledge M.J.W. de Bruijn, E. de Haas and the people from the EDC Animal Facility (Erasmus MC Rotterdam) for assistance at various stages of the project. We are also grateful to Dr. Pat Crowley for critical reading of the manuscript. This work was supported by the Association for International Cancer Research and the Dutch Cancer Society.

REFERENCES

Abbas, A. K., Murphy, K. M., and Sher, A. (1996). Functional diversity of helper T lymphocytes. *Nature.* 383, 787-793.

Agarwal, S., and Rao, A. (1998). Modulation of chromatin structure regulates cytokine gene expression during T cell differentiation. *Immunity.* 9, 765-775.

Akashi, K., Traver, D., Miyamoto, T., and Weissman, I. L. (2000). A clonogenic common myeloid progenitor that gives rise to all myeloid lineages. *Nature.* 404, 193-197.

Akiyama, Y., Watkins, N., Suzuki, H., Jair, K. W., van Engeland, M., Esteller, M., Sakai, H., Ren, C. Y., Yuasa, Y., Herman, J. G., and Baylin, S. B. (2003). GATA-4 and GATA-5 transcription factor genes and potential downstream antitumor target genes are epigenetically silenced in colorectal and gastric cancer. *Mol. Cell Biol.* 23, 8429-8439.

Allman, D., Sambandam, A., Kim, S., Miller, J. P., Pagan, A., Well, D., Meraz, A., and Bhandoola, A. (2003). Thymopoiesis independent of common lymphoid progenitors. *Nat. Immunol.* 4, 168-174.

Anderson, M. K., Hernandez-Hoyos, G., Dionne, C. J., Arias, A. M., Chen, D., and Rothenberg, E. V. (2002). Definition of regulatory network elements for T cell development by perturbation analysis with PU.1 and GATA-3. *Dev. Biol.* 246, 103-121.

Ansel, K. M., Djuretic, I., Tanasa, B., and Rao, A. (2006). Regulation of Th2 differentiation and Il4 locus accessibility. *Annu. Rev. Immunol.* 24, 607-656.

Asnagli, H., Afkarian, M., and Murphy, K. M. (2002). Cutting edge: Identification of an alternative GATA-3 promoter directing tissue-specific gene expression in mouse and human. *J. Immunol.* 168, 4268-4271.

Azzam, H. S., DeJarnette, J. B., Huang, K., Emmons, R., Park, C. S., Sommers, C. L., El-Khoury, D., Shores, E. W., and Love, P. E. (2001). Fine tuning of TCR signaling by CD5. *J. Immunol.* 166, 5464-5472.

Azzam, H. S., Grinberg, A., Lui, K., Shen, H., Shores, E. W., and Love, P. E. (1998). CD5 expression is developmentally regulated by T cell receptor (TCR) signals and TCR avidity. *J. Exp. Med.* 188, 2301-2311.

Batten, M., Li, J., Yi, S., Kljavin, N. M., Danilenko, D. M., Lucas, S., Lee, J., de Sauvage, F. J., and Ghilardi, N. (2006). Interleukin 27 limits autoimmune encephalomyelitis by suppressing the development of interleukin 17-producing T cells. *Nat. Immunol.* 7, 929-936.

Bertrand, J. Y., Giroux, S., Golub, R., Klaine, M., Jalil, A., Boucontet, L., Godin, I., and Cumano, A. (2005). Characterization of purified intraembryonic hematopoietic stem cells as a tool to define their site of origin. *Proc. Natl. Acad. Sci. U S A.* 102, 134-139.

Bhandoola, A., and Sambandam, A. (2006). From stem cell to T cell: one route or many? *Nat. Rev. Immunol.* 6, 117-126.

Bilous, R. W., Murty, G., Parkinson, D. B., Thakker, R. V., Coulthard, M. G., Burn, J., Mathias, D., and Kendall-Taylor, P. (1992). Brief report: autosomal dominant familial hypoparathyroidism, sensorineural deafness, and renal dysplasia. *N. Engl. J. Med.* 327, 1069-1074.

Bird, J. J., Brown, D. R., Mullen, A. C., Moskowitz, N. H., Mahowald, M. A., Sider, J. R., Gajewski, T. F., Wang, C. R., and Reiner, S. L. (1998). Helper T cell differentiation is controlled by the cell cycle. *Immunity.* 9, 229-237.

Bosselut, R. (2004). CD4/CD8-lineage differentiation in the thymus: from nuclear effectors to membrane signals. *Nat. Rev. Immunol.* 4, 529-540.

Bottomly, K. (1988). A functional dichotomy in CD4+ T lymphocytes. *Immunol. Today.* 9, 268-274.

Briegel, K., Lim, K. C., Plank, C., Beug, H., Engel, J. D., and Zenke, M. (1993). Ectopic expression of a conditional GATA-2/estrogen receptor chimera arrests erythroid differentiation in a hormone-dependent manner. *Genes Dev.* 7, 1097-1109.

Burch, J. B. (2005). Regulation of GATA gene expression during vertebrate development. *Semin. Cell Dev. Biol.* 16, 71-81.

Burtrum, D. B., Kim, S., Dudley, E. C., Hayday, A. C., and Petrie, H. T. (1996). TCR gene recombination and alpha beta-gamma delta lineage divergence: productive TCR-beta rearrangement is neither exclusive nor preclusive of gamma delta cell development. *J. Immunol.* 157, 4293-4296.

Carvalho, T. L., Mota-Santos, T., Cumano, A., Demengeot, J., and Vieira, P. (2001). Arrested B lymphopoiesis and persistence of activated B cells in adult interleukin 7(-/)- mice. *J. Exp. Med.* 194, 1141-1150.

Chen, D., and Zhang, G. (2001). Enforced expression of the GATA-3 transcription factor affects cell fate decisions in hematopoiesis. *Exp. Hematol.* 29, 971-980.

Christensen, J. L., and Weissman, I. L. (2001). Flk-2 is a marker in hematopoietic stem cell differentiation: a simple method to isolate long-term stem cells. *Proc. Natl. Acad. Sci. U S A.* 98, 14541-14546.

Cumano, A., Dieterlen-Lievre, F., and Godin, I. (1996). Lymphoid potential, probed before circulation in mouse, is restricted to caudal intraembryonic splanchnopleura. *Cell.* 86, 907-916.

De Maria, R., Zeuner, A., Eramo, A., Domenichelli, C., Bonci, D., Grignani, F., Srinivasula, S. M., Alnemri, E. S., Testa, U., and Peschle, C. (1999). Negative regulation of erythropoiesis by caspase-mediated cleavage of GATA-1. *Nature.* 401, 489-493.

de Pooter, R. F., Schmitt, T. M., de la Pompa, J. L., Fujiwara, Y., Orkin, S. H., and Zuniga-Pflucker, J. C. (2006). Notch signaling requires GATA-2 to inhibit myelopoiesis from embryonic stem cells and primary hemopoietic progenitors. *J. Immunol.* 176, 5267-5275.

Dontje, W., Schotte, R., Cupedo, T., Nagasawa, M., Scheeren, F., Gimeno, R., Spits, H., and Blom, B. (2006). Delta-like1-induced Notch1 signaling regulates the human plasmacytoid dendritic cell versus T-cell lineage decision through control of GATA-3 and Spi-B. *Blood.* 107, 2446-2452.

Douglas, N. C., Jacobs, H., Bothwell, A. L., and Hayday, A. C. (2001). Defining the specific physiological requirements for c-Myc in T cell development. *Nat. Immunol.* 2, 307-315.

Durand, C., and Dzierzak, E. (2005). Embryonic beginnings of adult hematopoietic stem cells. *Haematologica.* 90, 100-108.

Ellisen, L. W., Bird, J., West, D. C., Soreng, A. L., Reynolds, T. C., Smith, S. D., and Sklar, J. (1991). TAN-1, the human homolog of the Drosophila notch gene, is broken by chromosomal translocations in T lymphoblastic neoplasms. *Cell.* 66, 649-661.

Evans, T., Reitman, M., and Felsenfeld, G. (1988). An erythrocyte-specific DNA-binding factor recognizes a regulatory sequence common to all chicken globin genes. *Proc. Natl. Acad. Sci. U S A.* 85, 5976-5980.

Ezoe, S., Matsumura, I., Nakata, S., Gale, K., Ishihara, K., Minegishi, N., Machii, T., Kitamura, T., Yamamoto, M., Enver, T., and Kanakura, Y. (2002). GATA-2/estrogen receptor chimera regulates cytokine-dependent growth of hematopoietic cells through accumulation of p21(WAF1) and p27(Kip1) proteins. *Blood.* 100, 3512-3520.

Ezoe, S., Matsumura, I., Satoh, Y., Tanaka, H., and Kanakura, Y. (2004). Cell cycle regulation in hematopoietic stem/progenitor cells. *Cell Cycle.* 3, 314-318.

Ferreira, R., Ohneda, K., Yamamoto, M., and Philipsen, S. (2005). GATA1 function, a paradigm for transcription factors in hematopoiesis. *Mol. Cell Biol.* 25, 1215-1227.

Fontaine-Perus, J. C., Calman, F. M., Kaplan, C., and Le Douarin, N. M. (1981). Seeding of the 10-day mouse embryo thymic rudiment by lymphocyte precursors in vitro. *J. Immunol.* 126, 2310-2316.

Fujimaki, S., Harigae, H., Sugawara, T., Takasawa, N., Sasaki, T., and Kaku, M. (2001). Decreased expression of transcription factor GATA-2 in haematopoietic stem cells in patients with aplastic anaemia. *Br. J. Haematol.* 113, 52-57.

Fujiwara, Y., Browne, C. P., Cunniff, K., Goff, S. C., and Orkin, S. H. (1996). Arrested development of embryonic red cell precursors in mouse embryos lacking transcription factor GATA-1. *Proc. Natl. Acad. Sci. U S A.* 93, 12355-12358.

George, K. M., Leonard, M. W., Roth, M. E., Lieuw, K. H., Kioussis, D., Grosveld, F., and Engel, J. D. (1994). Embryonic expression and cloning of the murine GATA-3 gene. *Development.* 120, 2673-2686.

Germain, R. N. (2002). T-cell development and the CD4-CD8 lineage decision. *Nat. Rev. Immunol.* 2, 309-322.

Godfrey, D. I., and Zlotnik, A. (1993). Control points in early T-cell development. *Immunol. Today.* 14, 547-553.

Godin, I., and Cumano, A. (2002). The hare and the tortoise: an embryonic haematopoietic race. *Nat. Rev. Immunol.* 2, 593-604.

Godin, I., and Cumano, A. (2005). Of birds and mice: hematopoietic stem cell development. *Int. J. Dev. Biol.* 49, 251-257.

Grass, J. A., Boyer, M. E., Pal, S., Wu, J., Weiss, M. J., and Bresnick, E. H. (2003). GATA-1-dependent transcriptional repression of GATA-2 via disruption of positive autoregulation and domain-wide chromatin remodeling. *Proc. Natl. Acad. Sci. U S A.* 100, 8811-8816.

Grass, J. A., Jing, H., Kim, S. I., Martowicz, M. L., Pal, S., Blobel, G. A., and Bresnick, E. H. (2006). Distinct functions of dispersed GATA factor complexes at an endogenous gene locus. *Mol. Cell Biol.* 26, 7056-7067.

Grogan, J. L., Mohrs, M., Harmon, B., Lacy, D. A., Sedat, J. W., and Locksley, R. M. (2001). Early transcription and silencing of cytokine genes underlie polarization of T helper cell subsets. *Immunity.* 14, 205-215.

Guo, M., House, M. G., Akiyama, Y., Qi, Y., Capagna, D., Harmon, J., Baylin, S. B., Brock, M. V., and Herman, J. G. (2006). Hypermethylation of the GATA gene family in esophageal cancer. *Int. J. Cancer.* 119, 2078-2083.

Hardy, R. R. (2006). B-1 B cell development. *J Immunol.* 177, 2749-2754.

Hardy, R. R., and Hayakawa, K. (1991). A developmental switch in B lymphopoiesis. *Proc. Natl. Acad. Sci. U S A.* 88, 11550-11554.

Harrington, L. E., Hatton, R. D., Mangan, P. R., Turner, H., Murphy, T. L., Murphy, K. M., and Weaver, C. T. (2005). Interleukin 17-producing CD4+ effector T cells develop via a lineage distinct from the T helper type 1 and 2 lineages. *Nat. Immunol.* 6, 1123-1132.

Hattori, N., Kawamoto, H., Fujimoto, S., Kuno, K., and Katsura, Y. (1996). Involvement of transcription factors TCF-1 and GATA-3 in the initiation of the earliest step of T cell development in the thymus. *J. Exp. Med.* 184, 1137-1147.

Hayakawa, F., Towatari, M., Ozawa, Y., Tomita, A., Privalsky, M. L., and Saito, H. (2004). Functional regulation of GATA-2 by acetylation. *J. Leukoc. Biol.* 75, 529-540.

Hendriks, R. W., Nawijn, M. C., Engel, J. D., van Doorninck, H., Grosveld, F., and Karis, A. (1999). Expression of the transcription factor GATA-3 is required for the development of the earliest T cell progenitors and correlates with stages of cellular proliferation in the thymus. *Eur. J. Immunol.* 29, 1912-1918.

Hernandez-Hoyos, G., Anderson, M. K., Wang, C., Rothenberg, E. V., and Alberola-Ila, J. (2003). GATA-3 expression is controlled by TCR signals and regulates CD4/CD8 differentiation. *Immunity.* 19, 83-94.

Hosokawa, H., Kimura, M., Y., Shinnakasu, R., Suzuki, A., Miki, T., Koseki, H., van Lohuizen, M., Yamashita, M., and Nakayama, T (2006). Regulation of Th2 Cell Development by Polycomb Group Gene bmi-1 through the Stabilization of GATA3. *J. Immunol.* 177, 7656-7664.

Ho, I. C., Vorhees, P., Marin, N., Oakley, B. K., Tsai, S. F., Orkin, S. H., and Leiden, J. M. (1991). Human GATA-3: a lineage-restricted transcription factor that regulates the expression of the T cell receptor alpha gene. *Embo J.* 10, 1187-1192.

Hwang, E. S., Szabo, S. J., Schwartzberg, P. L., and Glimcher, L. H. (2005). T helper cell fate specified by kinase-mediated interaction of T-bet with GATA-3. *Science.* 307, 430-433.

Igarashi, H., Gregory, S. C., Yokota, T., Sakaguchi, N., and Kincade, P. W. (2002). Transcription from the RAG1 locus marks the earliest lymphocyte progenitors in bone marrow. *Immunity.* 17, 117-130.

Ivanov, II, McKenzie, B. S., Zhou, L., Tadokoro, C. E., Lepelley, A., Lafaille, J. J., Cua, D. J., and Littman, D. R. (2006). The orphan nuclear receptor RORgammat directs the differentiation program of proinflammatory IL-17+ T helper cells. *Cell.* 126, 1121-1133.

Kalinski, P., and Moser, M. (2005). Consensual immunity: success-driven development of T-helper-1 and T-helper-2 responses. *Nat. Rev. Immunol.* 5, 251-260.

Kappes, D. J., and He, X. (2005). CD4-CD8 lineage commitment: an inside view. *Nat. Immunol.* 6, 761-766.

Kaufman, C. K., Zhou, P., Pasolli, H. A., Rendl, M., Bolotin, D., Lim, K. C., Dai, X., Alegre, M. L., and Fuchs, E. (2003). GATA-3: an unexpected regulator of cell lineage determination in skin. *Genes Dev.* 17, 2108-2122.

Kiiveri, S., Liu, J., Heikkila, P., Arola, J., Lehtonen, E., Voutilainen, R., and Heikinheimo, M. (2004). Transcription factors GATA-4 and GATA-6 in human adrenocortical tumors. *Endocr. Res.* 30, 919-923.

Kitajima, K., Masuhara, M., Era, T., Enver, T., and Nakano, T. (2002). GATA-2 and GATA-2/ER display opposing activities in the development and differentiation of blood progenitors. *Embo J.* 21, 3060-3069.

Kitajima, K., Tanaka, M., Zheng, J., Yen, H., Sato, A., Sugiyama, D., Umehara, H., Sakai, E., and Nakano, T. (2006). Redirecting differentiation of hematopoietic progenitors by a transcription factor, GATA-2. *Blood.* 107, 1857-1863.

Kobayashi-Osaki, M., Ohneda, O., Suzuki, N., Minegishi, N., Yokomizo, T., Takahashi, S., Lim, K. C., Engel, J. D., and Yamamoto, M. (2005). GATA motifs regulate early hematopoietic lineage-specific expression of the Gata2 gene. *Mol. Cell Biol.* 25, 7005-7020.

Kondo, M., Weissman, I. L., and Akashi, K. (1997). Identification of clonogenic common lymphoid progenitors in mouse bone marrow. *Cell.* 91, 661-672.

Kumano, K., Chiba, S., Kunisato, A., Sata, M., Saito, T., Nakagami-Yamaguchi, E., Yamaguchi, T., Masuda, S., Shimizu, K., Takahashi, T., et al. (2003). Notch1 but not Notch2 is essential for generating hematopoietic stem cells from endothelial cells. *Immunity.* 18, 699-711.

Kurata, H., Lee, H. J., McClanahan, T., Coffman, R. L., O'Garra, A., and Arai, N. (2002). Friend of GATA is expressed in naive Th cells and functions as a repressor of GATA-3-mediated Th2 cell development. *J. Immunol.* 168, 4538-4545.

Kurek, D., Garinis, G.A., Van Doorninck, J.H., Van der Wees, J. and Grosveld, F. (2006). Transcriptome analysis reveals GATA3-dependent signalling pathways in murine hair follicles. *Development.* (in press).

Lai, A. Y., and Kondo, M. (2006). Asymmetrical lymphoid and myeloid lineage commitment in multipotent hematopoietic progenitors. *J. Exp. Med.* 203, 1867-1873.

Laiosa, C. V., Stadtfeld, M., Xie, H., de Andres-Aguayo, L., and Graf, T. (2006). Reprogramming of Committed T Cell Progenitors to Macrophages and Dendritic Cells by C/EBPalpha and PU.1 Transcription Factors. *Immunity.* 25, 731-744.

Lee, G. R., Fields, P. E., and Flavell, R. A. (2001). Regulation of IL-4 gene expression by distal regulatory elements and GATA-3 at the chromatin level. *Immunity.* 14, 447-459.

Lee, G. R., Kim, S. T., Spilianakis, C. G., Fields, P. E., and Flavell, R. A. (2006). T helper cell differentiation: regulation by cis elements and epigenetics. *Immunity.* 24, 369-379.

Lee, G. R., Spilianakis, C. G., and Flavell, R. A. (2005). Hypersensitive site 7 of the TH2 locus control region is essential for expressing TH2 cytokine genes and for long-range intrachromosomal interactions. *Nat. Immunol.* 6, 42-48.

Lee, J., and Desiderio, S. (1999). Cyclin A/CDK2 regulates V(D)J recombination by coordinating RAG-2 accumulation and DNA repair. *Immunity.* 11, 771-781.

Leonard, M., Brice, M., Engel, J. D., and Papayannopoulou, T. (1993). Dynamics of GATA transcription factor expression during erythroid differentiation. *Blood.* 82, 1071-1079.

Lillevali, K., Matilainen, T., Karis, A., and Salminen, M. (2004). Partially overlapping expression of Gata2 and Gata3 during inner ear development. *Dev. Dyn.* 231, 775-781.

Lim, K. C., Lakshmanan, G., Crawford, S. E., Gu, Y., Grosveld, F., and Engel, J. D. (2000). Gata3 loss leads to embryonic lethality due to noradrenaline deficiency of the sympathetic nervous system. *Nat. Genet.* 25, 209-212.

Ling, K. W., Ottersbach, K., van Hamburg, J. P., Oziemlak, A., Tsai, F. Y., Orkin, S. H., Ploemacher, R., Hendriks, R. W., and Dzierzak, E. (2004). GATA-2 plays two functionally distinct roles during the ontogeny of hematopoietic stem cells. *J. Exp. Med.* 200, 871-882.

Lowry, J. A., and Atchley, W. R. (2000). Molecular evolution of the GATA family of transcription factors: conservation within the DNA-binding domain. *J. Mol. Evol.* 50, 103-115.

Ma, X., de Bruijn, M., Robin, C., Peeters, M., Kong, A. S. J., de Wit, T., Snoijs, C., and Dzierzak, E. (2002). Expression of the Ly-6A (Sca-1) lacZ transgene in mouse haematopoietic stem cells and embryos. *Br. J. Haematol.* 116, 401-408.

Maeno, M., Mead, P. E., Kelley, C., Xu, R. H., Kung, H. F., Suzuki, A., Ueno, N., and Zon, L. I. (1996). The role of BMP-4 and GATA-2 in the induction and differentiation of hematopoietic mesoderm in Xenopus laevis. *Blood.* 88, 1965-1972.

Mallick, C. A., Dudley, E. C., Viney, J. L., Owen, M. J., and Hayday, A. C. (1993). Rearrangement and diversity of T cell receptor beta chain genes in thymocytes: a critical role for the beta chain in development. *Cell.* 73, 513-519.

Manaia, A., Lemarchandel, V., Klaine, M., Max-Audit, I., Romeo, P., Dieterlen-Lievre, F., and Godin, I. (2000). Lmo2 and GATA-3 associated expression in intraembryonic hemogenic sites. *Development.* 127, 643-653.

Manz, M. G., Traver, D., Miyamoto, T., Weissman, I. L., and Akashi, K. (2001). Dendritic cell potentials of early lymphoid and myeloid progenitors. *Blood.* 97, 3333-3341.

Marine, J., and Winoto, A. (1991). The human enhancer-binding protein Gata3 binds to several T-cell receptor regulatory elements. *Proc. Natl. Acad. Sci. U S A.* 88, 7284-7288.

Martin, C. H., Aifantis, I., Scimone, M. L., von Andrian, U. H., Reizis, B., von Boehmer, H., and Gounari, F. (2003). Efficient thymic immigration of B220+ lymphoid-restricted bone marrow cells with T precursor potential. *Nat. Immunol.* 4, 866-873.

Martin, D. I., and Orkin, S. H. (1990). Transcriptional activation and DNA binding by the erythroid factor GF-1/NF-E1/Eryf 1. *Genes Dev.* 4, 1886-1898.

Martin, D. I., Zon, L. I., Mutter, G., and Orkin, S. H. (1990). Expression of an erythroid transcription factor in megakaryocytic and mast cell lineages. *Nature.* 344, 444-447.

Mehra, R., Varambally, S., Ding, L., Shen, R., Sabel, M. S., Ghosh, D., Chinnaiyan, A. M., and Kleer, C. G. (2005). Identification of GATA3 as a breast cancer prognostic marker by global gene expression meta-analysis. *Cancer Res.* 65, 11259-11264.

Miaw, S. C., Choi, A., Yu, E., Kishikawa, H., and Ho, I. C. (2000). ROG, repressor of GATA, regulates the expression of cytokine genes. *Immunity.* 12, 323-333.

Mikkola, H. K., and Orkin, S. H. (2006). The journey of developing hematopoietic stem cells. *Development.* 133, 3733-3744.

Minegishi, N., Morita, S., Minegishi, M., Tsuchiya, S., Konno, T., Hayashi, N., and Yamamoto, M. (1997). Expression of GATA transcription factors in myelogenous and lymphoblastic leukemia cells. *Int. J. Hematol.* 65, 239-249.

Minegishi, N., Ohta, J., Suwabe, N., Nakauchi, H., Ishihara, H., Hayashi, N., and Yamamoto, M. (1998). Alternative promoters regulate transcription of the mouse GATA-2 gene. *J. Biol. Chem.* 273, 3625-3634.

Minegishi, N., Ohta, J., Yamagiwa, H., Suzuki, N., Kawauchi, S., Zhou, Y., Takahashi, S., Hayashi, N., Engel, J. D., and Yamamoto, M. (1999). The mouse GATA-2 gene is expressed in the para-aortic splanchnopleura and aorta-gonads and mesonephros region. *Blood.* 93, 4196-4207.

Minegishi, N., Suzuki, N., Kawatani, Y., Shimizu, R., and Yamamoto, M. (2005). Rapid turnover of GATA-2 via ubiquitin-proteasome protein degradation pathway. *Genes Cells.* 10, 693-704.

Minegishi, N., Suzuki, N., Yokomizo, T., Pan, X., Fujimoto, T., Takahashi, S., Hara, T., Miyajima, A., Nishikawa, S., and Yamamoto, M. (2003). Expression and domain-specific function of GATA-2 during differentiation of the hematopoietic precursor cells in midgestation mouse embryos. *Blood.* 102, 896-905.

Mombaerts, P., Iacomini, J., Johnson, R. S., Herrup, K., Tonegawa, S., and Papaioannou, V. E. (1992). RAG-1-deficient mice have no mature B and T lymphocytes. *Cell.* 68, 869-877.

Morrison, S. J., Wandycz, A. M., Akashi, K., Globerson, A., and Weissman, I. L. (1996). The aging of hematopoietic stem cells. *Nat. Med.* 2, 1011-1016.

Morrison, S. J., and Weissman, I. L. (1994). The long-term repopulating subset of hematopoietic stem cells is deterministic and isolatable by phenotype. *Immunity.* 1, 661-673.

Mosmann, T. R., and Coffman, R. L. (1989). TH1 and TH2 cells: different patterns of lymphokine secretion lead to different functional properties. *Annu. Rev. Immunol.* 7, 145-173.

Mullen, A. C., Hutchins, A. S., High, F. A., Lee, H. W., Sykes, K. J., Chodosh, L. A., and Reiner, S. L. (2002). Hlx is induced by and genetically interacts with T-bet to promote heritable T(H)1 gene induction. *Nat. Immunol.* 3, 652-658.

Muller, A. M., Medvinsky, A., Strouboulis, J., Grosveld, F., and Dzierzak, E. (1994). Development of hematopoietic stem cell activity in the mouse embryo. *Immunity.* 1, 291-301.

Murphy, K. M., and Reiner, S. L. (2002). The lineage decisions of helper T cells. *Nat. Rev. Immunol.* 2, 933-944.

Nagai, T., Harigae, H., Ishihara, H., Motohashi, H., Minegishi, N., Tsuchiya, S., Hayashi, N., Gu, L., Andres, B., Engel, J. D., and et al. (1994). Transcription factor GATA-2 is expressed in erythroid, early myeloid, and CD34+ human leukemia-derived cell lines. *Blood.* 84, 1074-1084.

Nawijn, M. C., Dingjan, G. M., Ferreira, R., Lambrecht, B. N., Karis, A., Grosveld, F., Savelkoul, H., and Hendriks, R. W. (2001a). Enforced expression of GATA-3 in transgenic mice inhibits Th1 differentiation and induces the formation of a T1/ST2-expressing Th2-committed T cell compartment in vivo. *J. Immunol.* 167, 724-732.

Nawijn, M. C., Ferreira, R., Dingjan, G. M., Kahre, O., Drabek, D., Karis, A., Grosveld, F., and Hendriks, R. W. (2001b). Enforced expression of GATA-3 during T cell development inhibits maturation of CD8 single-positive cells and induces thymic lymphoma in transgenic mice. *J. Immunol.* 167, 715-723.

North, T. E., de Bruijn, M. F., Stacy, T., Talebian, L., Lind, E., Robin, C., Binder, M., Dzierzak, E., and Speck, N. A. (2002). Runx1 expression marks long-term repopulating hematopoietic stem cells in the midgestation mouse embryo. *Immunity.* 16, 661-672.

Nutt, S. L., Heavey, B., Rolink, A. G., and Busslinger, M. (1999). Commitment to the B-lymphoid lineage depends on the transcription factor Pax5. *Nature.* 401, 556-562.

Ono, Y., Fukuhara, N., and Yoshie, O. (1997). Transcriptional activity of TAL1 in T cell acute lymphoblastic leukemia (T-ALL) requires RBTN1 or -2 and induces TALLA1, a highly specific tumor marker of T-ALL. *J. Biol. Chem.* 272, 4576-4581.

Ono, Y., Fukuhara, N., and Yoshie, O. (1998). TAL1 and LIM-only proteins synergistically induce retinaldehyde dehydrogenase 2 expression in T-cell acute lymphoblastic leukemia by acting as cofactors for GATA3. *Mol. Cell Biol.* 18, 6939-6950.

Oosterwegel, M., Timmerman, J., Leiden, J., and Clevers, H. (1992). Expression of GATA-3 during lymphocyte differentiation and mouse embryogenesis. *Dev. Immunol.* 3, 1-11.

Osawa, M., Hanada, K., Hamada, H., and Nakauchi, H. (1996a). Long-term lymphohematopoietic reconstitution by a single CD34-low/negative hematopoietic stem cell. *Science.* 273, 242-245.

Osawa, M., Nakamura, K., Nishi, N., Takahasi, N., Tokuomoto, Y., Inoue, H., and Nakauchi, H. (1996b). In vivo self-renewal of c-Kit+ Sca-1+ Lin(low/-) hemopoietic stem cells. *J. Immunol.* 156, 3207-3214.

Ouyang, W., Lohning, M., Gao, Z., Assenmacher, M., Ranganath, S., Radbruch, A., and Murphy, K. M. (2000). Stat6-independent GATA-3 autoactivation directs IL-4-independent Th2 development and commitment. *Immunity.* 12, 27-37.

Ouyang, W., Ranganath, S. H., Weindel, K., Bhattacharya, D., Murphy, T. L., Sha, W. C., and Murphy, K. M. (1998). Inhibition of Th1 development mediated by GATA-3 through an IL-4-independent mechanism. *Immunity.* 9, 745-755.

Owen, J. J., and Ritter, M. A. (1969). Tissue interaction in the development of thymus lymphocytes. *J. Exp. Med.* 129, 431-442.

Pai, S. Y., Truitt, M. L., and Ho, I. C. (2004). GATA-3 deficiency abrogates the development and maintenance of T helper type 2 cells. *Proc. Natl. Acad. Sci. U S A.* 101, 1993-1998.

Pai, S. Y., Truitt, M. L., Ting, C. N., Leiden, J. M., Glimcher, L. H., and Ho, I. C. (2003). Critical roles for transcription factor GATA-3 in thymocyte development. *Immunity.* 19, 863-875.

Palomero, T., Lim, W. K., Odom, D. T., Sulis, M. L., Real, P. J., Margolin, A., Barnes, K. C., O'Neil, J., Neuberg, D., Weng, A. P., et al. (2006). NOTCH1 directly regulates c-MYC and activates a feed-forward-loop transcriptional network promoting leukemic cell growth. *Proc. Natl. Acad. Sci. U S A.*

Pan, X., Minegishi, N., Harigae, H., Yamagiwa, H., Minegishi, M., Akine, Y., and Yamamoto, M. (2000). Identification of human GATA-2 gene distal IS exon and its expression in hematopoietic stem cell fractions. *J. Biochem.* (Tokyo) 127, 105-112.

Pan, X., Ohneda, O., Ohneda, K., Lindeboom, F., Iwata, F., Shimizu, R., Nagano, M., Suwabe, N., Philipsen, S., Lim, K. C., et al. (2005). Graded levels of GATA-1 expression modulate survival, proliferation, and differentiation of erythroid progenitors. *J. Biol. Chem.* 280, 22385-22394.

Pandolfi, P. P., Roth, M. E., Karis, A., Leonard, M. W., Dzierzak, E., Grosveld, F. G., Engel, J. D., and Lindenbaum, M. H. (1995). Targeted disruption of the GATA3 gene causes severe abnormalities in the nervous system and in fetal liver haematopoiesis. *Nat. Genet.* 11, 40-44.

Park, H., Li, Z., Yang, X. O., Chang, S. H., Nurieva, R., Wang, Y. H., Wang, Y., Hood, L., Zhu, Z., Tian, Q., and Dong, C. (2005). A distinct lineage of CD4 T cells regulates tissue inflammation by producing interleukin 17. *Nat. Immunol.* 6, 1133-1141.

Passegue, E., Wagers, A. J., Giuriato, S., Anderson, W. C., and Weissman, I. L. (2005). Global analysis of proliferation and cell cycle gene expression in the regulation of hematopoietic stem and progenitor cell fates. *J. Exp. Med.* 202, 1599-1611.

Pedone, P. V., Omichinski, J. G., Nony, P., Trainor, C., Gronenborn, A. M., Clore, G. M., and Felsenfeld, G. (1997). The N-terminal fingers of chicken GATA-2 and GATA-3 are independent sequence-specific DNA binding domains. *Embo. J.* 16, 2874-2882.

Persons, D. A., Allay, J. A., Allay, E. R., Ashmun, R. A., Orlic, D., Jane, S. M., Cunningham, J. M., and Nienhuis, A. W. (1999). Enforced expression of the GATA-2 transcription factor blocks normal hematopoiesis. *Blood.* 93, 488-499.

Peterkin, T., Gibson, A., Loose, M., and Patient, R. (2005). The roles of GATA-4, -5 and -6 in vertebrate heart development. Semin. *Cell Dev. Biol.* 16, 83-94.

Petrie, H. T., and Kincade, P. W. (2005). Many roads, one destination for T cell progenitors. *J. Exp. Med.* 202, 11-13.

Philipsen, S., Pruzina, S., and Grosveld, F. (1993). The minimal requirements for activity in transgenic mice of hypersensitive site 3 of the beta globin locus control region. *Embo J.* 12, 1077-1085.

Porcher, C., Swat, W., Rockwell, K., Fujiwara, Y., Alt, F. W., and Orkin, S. H. (1996). The T cell leukemia oncoprotein SCL/tal-1 is essential for development of all hematopoietic lineages. *Cell.* 86, 47-57.

Porritt, H. E., Rumfelt, L. L., Tabrizifard, S., Schmitt, T. M., Zuniga-Pflucker, J. C., and Petrie, H. T. (2004). Heterogeneity among DN1 prothymocytes reveals multiple progenitors with different capacities to generate T cell and non-T cell lineages. *Immunity.* 20, 735-745.

Radtke, F., Wilson, A., Mancini, S. J., and MacDonald, H. R. (2004). Notch regulation of lymphocyte development and function. *Nat. Immunol.* 5, 247-253.

Richter, A., Lohning, M., and Radbruch, A. (1999). Instruction for cytokine expression in T helper lymphocytes in relation to proliferation and cell cycle progression. *J. Exp. Med.* 190, 1439-1450.

Robb, L., Elwood, N. J., Elefanty, A. G., Kontgen, F., Li, R., Barnett, L. D., and Begley, C. G. (1996). The scl gene product is required for the generation of all hematopoietic lineages in the adult mouse. *Embo J.* 15, 4123-4129.

Robert-Moreno, A., Espinosa, L., de la Pompa, J. L., and Bigas, A. (2005). RBPjkappa-dependent Notch function regulates Gata2 and is essential for the formation of intra-embryonic hematopoietic cells. *Development.* 132, 1117-1126.

Rodrigues, N. P., Janzen, V., Forkert, R., Dombkowski, D. M., Boyd, A. S., Orkin, S. H., Enver, T., Vyas, P., and Scadden, D. T. (2005). Haploinsufficiency of GATA-2 perturbs adult hematopoietic stem-cell homeostasis. *Blood.* 106, 477-484.

Rodriguez, P., Bonte, E., Krijgsveld, J., Kolodziej, K. E., Guyot, B., Heck, A. J., Vyas, P., de Boer, E., Grosveld, F., and Strouboulis, J. (2005). GATA-1 forms distinct activating and repressive complexes in erythroid cells. *Embo J.* 24, 2354-2366.

Rolink, A. G., Nutt, S. L., Melchers, F., and Busslinger, M. (1999). Long-term in vivo reconstitution of T-cell development by Pax5-deficient B-cell progenitors. *Nature.* 401, 603-606.

Rothenberg, E. V. (2000). Stepwise specification of lymphocyte developmental lineages. *Curr. Opin. Genet. Dev.* 10, 370-379.

Rothenberg, E. V., and Taghon, T. (2005). Molecular genetics of T cell development. *Annu. Rev. Immunol.* 23, 601-649.

Russell ES, B. E. (1966). *Biology of the laboratory Animal.* (New York, McGraw-Hill).

Sakaguchi, S., Ono, M., Setoguchi, R., Yagi, H., Hori, S., Fehervari, Z., Shimizu, J., Takahashi, T., and Nomura, T. (2006). Foxp3+ CD25+ CD4+ natural regulatory T cells in dominant self-tolerance and autoimmune disease. *Immunol. Rev.* 212, 8-27.

Samson, S. I., Richard, O., Tavian, M., Ranson, T., Vosshenrich, C. A., Colucci, F., Buer, J., Grosveld, F., Godin, I., and Di Santo, J. P. (2003). GATA-3 promotes maturation, IFN-gamma production, and liver-specific homing of NK cells. *Immunity.* 19, 701-711.

Schwarz, B. A., and Bhandoola, A. (2004). Circulating hematopoietic progenitors with T lineage potential. *Nat. Immunol.* 5, 953-960.

Schwarz, B. A., and Bhandoola, A. (2006). Trafficking from the bone marrow to the thymus: a prerequisite for thymopoiesis. *Immunol. Rev.* 209, 47-57.

Shimizu, R., Kuroha, T., Ohneda, O., Pan, X., Ohneda, K., Takahashi, S., Philipsen, S., and Yamamoto, M. (2004). Leukemogenesis caused by incapacitated GATA-1 function. *Mol. Cell Biol.* 24, 10814-10825.

Shimizu, R., Takahashi, S., Ohneda, K., Engel, J. D., and Yamamoto, M. (2001). In vivo requirements for GATA-1 functional domains during primitive and definitive erythropoiesis. *Embo J.* 20, 5250-5260.

Shinkai, Y., Rathbun, G., Lam, K. P., Oltz, E. M., Stewart, V., Mendelsohn, M., Charron, J., Datta, M., Young, F., Stall, A. M., and et al. (1992). RAG-2-deficient mice lack mature lymphocytes owing to inability to initiate V(D)J rearrangement. *Cell.* 68, 855-867.

Smith, L. G., Weissman, I. L., and Heimfeld, S. (1991). Clonal analysis of hematopoietic stem-cell differentiation in vivo. *Proc. Natl. Acad. Sci. U S A.* 88, 2788-2792.

Spangrude, G. J., Smith, L., Uchida, N., Ikuta, K., Heimfeld, S., Friedman, J., and Weissman, I. L. (1991). Mouse hematopoietic stem cells. *Blood.* 78, 1395-1402.

Spilianakis, C. G., and Flavell, R. A. (2004). Long-range intrachromosomal interactions in the T helper type 2 cytokine locus. *Nat. Immunol.* 5, 1017-1027.

Spilianakis, C. G., Lalioti, M. D., Town, T., Lee, G. R., and Flavell, R. A. (2005). Interchromosomal associations between alternatively expressed loci. *Nature.* 435, 637-645.

Stewart, M., Cameron, E., Campbell, M., McFarlane, R., Toth, S., Lang, K., Onions, D., and Neil, J. C. (1993). Conditional expression and oncogenicity of c-myc linked to a CD2 gene dominant control region. *Int. J. Cancer.* 53, 1023-1030.

Szabo, S. J., Kim, S. T., Costa, G. L., Zhang, X., Fathman, C. G., and Glimcher, L. H. (2000). A novel transcription factor, T-bet, directs Th1 lineage commitment. Cell 100, 655-669.

Szabo, S. J., Sullivan, B. M., Peng, S. L., and Glimcher, L. H. (2003). Molecular mechanisms regulating Th1 immune responses. *Annu. Rev. Immunol.* 21, 713-758.

Taghon, T., De Smedt, M., Stolz, F., Cnockaert, M., Plum, J., and Leclercq, G. (2001). Enforced expression of GATA-3 severely reduces human thymic cellularity. *J. Immunol.* 167, 4468-4475.

Ting, C. N., Olson, M. C., Barton, K. P., and Leiden, J. M. (1996). Transcription factor GATA-3 is required for development of the T-cell lineage. *Nature*. 384, 474-478.

Tong, Q., Tsai, J., Tan, G., Dalgin, G., and Hotamisligil, G. S. (2005). Interaction between GATA and the C/EBP family of transcription factors is critical in GATA-mediated suppression of adipocyte differentiation. *Mol. Cell Biol.* 25, 706-715.

Trainor, C. D., Ghirlando, R., and Simpson, M. A. (2000). GATA zinc finger interactions modulate DNA binding and transactivation. *J. Biol. Chem.* 275, 28157-28166.

Trainor, C. D., Omichinski, J. G., Vandergon, T. L., Gronenborn, A. M., Clore, G. M., and Felsenfeld, G. (1996). A palindromic regulatory site within vertebrate GATA-1 promoters requires both zinc fingers of the GATA-1 DNA-binding domain for high-affinity interaction. *Mol. Cell Biol.* 16, 2238-2247.

Tsai, F. Y., Keller, G., Kuo, F. C., Weiss, M., Chen, J., Rosenblatt, M., Alt, F. W., and Orkin, S. H. (1994). An early haematopoietic defect in mice lacking the transcription factor GATA-2. *Nature*. 371, 221-226.

Tsai, F. Y., and Orkin, S. H. (1997). Transcription factor GATA-2 is required for proliferation/survival of early hematopoietic cells and mast cell formation, but not for erythroid and myeloid terminal differentiation. *Blood*. 89, 3636-3643.

Tsai, S. F., Martin, D. I., Zon, L. I., D'Andrea, A. D., Wong, G. G., and Orkin, S. H. (1989). Cloning of cDNA for the major DNA-binding protein of the erythroid lineage through expression in mammalian cells. *Nature*. 339, 446-451.

Tsang, A. P., Visvader, J. E., Turner, C. A., Fujiwara, Y., Yu, C., Weiss, M. J., Crossley, M., and Orkin, S. H. (1997). FOG, a multitype zinc finger protein, acts as a cofactor for transcription factor GATA-1 in erythroid and megakaryocytic differentiation. *Cell*. 90, 109-119.

Tsuzuki, S., Towatari, M., Saito, H., and Enver, T. (2000). Potentiation of GATA-2 activity through interactions with the promyelocytic leukemia protein (PML) and the t(15;17)-generated PML-retinoic acid receptor alpha oncoprotein. *Mol. Cell Biol.* 20, 6276-6286.

Usary, J., Llaca, V., Karaca, G., Presswala, S., Karaca, M., He, X., Langerod, A., Karesen, R., Oh, D. S., Dressler, L. G., et al. (2004). Mutation of GATA3 in human breast tumors. *Oncogene*. 23, 7669-7678.

Usui, T., Nishikomori, R., Kitani, A., and Strober, W. (2003). GATA-3 suppresses Th1 development by downregulation of Stat4 and not through effects on IL-12Rbeta2 chain or T-bet. *Immunity*. 18, 415-428.

Usui, T., Preiss, J. C., Kanno, Y., Yao, Z. J., Bream, J. H., O'Shea, J. J., and Strober, W. (2006). T-bet regulates Th1 responses through essential effects on GATA-3 function rather than on IFNG gene acetylation and transcription. *J. Exp. Med.* 203, 755-766.

van der Wees, J., van Looij, M. A., de Ruiter, M. M., Elias, H., van der Burg, H., Liem, S. S., Kurek, D., Engel, J. D., Karis, A., van Zanten, B. G., et al. (2004). Hearing loss following Gata3 haploinsufficiency is caused by cochlear disorder. *Neurobiol. Dis.* 16, 169-178.

Van Esch, H., Groenen, P., Nesbit, M. A., Schuffenhauer, S., Lichtner, P., Vanderlinden, G., Harding, B., Beetz, R., Bilous, R. W., Holdaway, I., et al. (2000). GATA3 haplo-insufficiency causes human HDR syndrome. *Nature*. 406, 419-422.

Veldhoen, M., Hocking, R. J., Atkins, C. J., Locksley, R. M., and Stockinger, B. (2006a). TGFbeta in the context of an inflammatory cytokine milieu supports de novo differentiation of IL-17-producing T cells. *Immunity.* 24, 179-189.

Veldhoen, M., Hocking, R. J., Flavell, R. A., and Stockinger, B. (2006b). Signals mediated by transforming growth factor-beta initiate autoimmune encephalomyelitis, but chronic inflammation is needed to sustain disease. *Nat. Immunol.*

von Boehmer, H. (2005). Unique features of the pre-T-cell receptor alpha-chain: not just a surrogate. *Nat. Rev. Immunol.* 5, 571-577.

Vosshenrich, C. A., Garcia-Ojeda, M. E., Samson-Villeger, S. I., Pasqualetto, V., Enault, L., Goff, O. R., Corcuff, E., Guy-Grand, D., Rocha, B., Cumano, A., et al. (2006). A thymic pathway of mouse natural killer cell development characterized by expression of GATA-3 and CD127. *Nat. Immunol.* 7, 1217-1224.

Wakana, K., Akiyama, Y., Aso, T., and Yuasa, Y. (2006). Involvement of GATA-4/-5 transcription factors in ovarian carcinogenesis. *Cancer Lett.* 241, 281-288.

Wechsler, J., Greene, M., McDevitt, M. A., Anastasi, J., Karp, J. E., Le Beau, M. M., and Crispino, J. D. (2002). Acquired mutations in GATA1 in the megakaryoblastic leukemia of Down syndrome. *Nat. Genet.* 32, 148-152.

Weng, A. P., Ferrando, A. A., Lee, W., Morris, J. P. t., Silverman, L. B., Sanchez-Irizarry, C., Blacklow, S. C., Look, A. T., and Aster, J. C. (2004). Activating mutations of NOTCH1 in human T cell acute lymphoblastic leukemia. *Science.* 306, 269-271.

Weng, A. P., Millholland, J. M., Yashiro-Ohtani, Y., Arcangeli, M. L., Lau, A., Wai, C., Del Bianco, C., Rodriguez, C. G., Sai, H., Tobias, J., et al. (2006). c-Myc is an important direct target of Notch1 in T-cell acute lymphoblastic leukemia/lymphoma. *Genes Dev.* 20, 2096-2109.

Weng, A. P., Nam, Y., Wolfe, M. S., Pear, W. S., Griffin, J. D., Blacklow, S. C., and Aster, J. C. (2003). Growth suppression of pre-T acute lymphoblastic leukemia cells by inhibition of notch signaling. *Mol. Cell Biol.* 23, 655-664.

Whyatt, D. J., deBoer, E., and Grosveld, F. (1993). The two zinc finger-like domains of GATA-1 have different DNA binding specificities. *Embo J.* 12, 4993-5005.

Wieser, R., Volz, A., Vinatzer, U., Gardiner, K., Jager, U., Mitterbauer, M., Ziegler, A., and Fonatsch, C. (2000). Transcription factor GATA-2 gene is located near 3q21 breakpoints in myeloid leukemia. *Biochem. Biophys. Res. Commun.* 273, 239-245.

Yamagata, T., Mitani, K., Oda, H., Suzuki, T., Honda, H., Asai, T., Maki, K., Nakamoto, T., and Hirai, H. (2000). Acetylation of GATA-3 affects T-cell survival and homing to secondary lymphoid organs. *Embo J.* 19, 4676-4687.

Yamamoto, M., Ko, L. J., Leonard, M. W., Beug, H., Orkin, S. H., and Engel, J. D. (1990). Activity and tissue-specific expression of the transcription factor NF-E1 multigene family. *Genes Dev.* 4, 1650-1662.

Yamashita, M., Ukai-Tadenuma, M., Miyamoto, T., Sugaya, K., Hosokawa, H., Hasegawa, A., Kimura, M., Taniguchi, M., DeGregori, J., and Nakayama, T. (2004). Essential role of GATA3 for the maintenance of type 2 helper T (Th2) cytokine production and chromatin remodeling at the Th2 cytokine gene loci. *J. Biol. Chem.* 279, 26983-26990.

Yang, H. Y., and Evans, T. (1992). Distinct roles for the two cGATA-1 finger domains. *Mol. Cell Biol.* 12, 4562-4570.

Yang, Z., Gu, L., Romeo, P. H., Bories, D., Motohashi, H., Yamamoto, M., and Engel, J. D. (1994). Human GATA-3 trans-activation, DNA-binding, and nuclear localization activities are organized into distinct structural domains. *Mol. Cell Biol.* 14, 2201-2212.

Yoder, M. C., and Hiatt, K. (1997). Engraftment of embryonic hematopoietic cells in conditioned newborn recipients. *Blood.* 89, 2176-2183.

Yoder, M. C., Hiatt, K., Dutt, P., Mukherjee, P., Bodine, D. M., and Orlic, D. (1997). Characterization of definitive lymphohematopoietic stem cells in the day 9 murine yolk sac. *Immunity.* 7, 335-344.

Yokota, T., Huang, J., Tavian, M., Nagai, Y., Hirose, J., Zuniga-Pflucker, J. C., Peault, B., and Kincade, P. W. (2006). Tracing the first waves of lymphopoiesis in mice. *Development.* 133, 2041-2051.

Young, N. S. (1999). Acquired aplastic anemia. *Jama.* 282, 271-278.

Young, N. S., and Maciejewski, J. (1997). The pathophysiology of acquired aplastic anemia. *N. Engl. J. Med.* 336, 1365-1372.

Zeng, W., Chen, G., Kajigaya, S., Nunez, O., Charrow, A., Billings, E. M., and Young, N. S. (2004). Gene expression profiling in CD34 cells to identify differences between aplastic anemia patients and healthy volunteers. *Blood.* 103, 325-332.

Zhang, D. H., Cohn, L., Ray, P., Bottomly, K., and Ray, A. (1997). Transcription factor GATA-3 is differentially expressed in murine Th1 and Th2 cells and controls Th2-specific expression of the interleukin-5 gene. *J. Biol. Chem.* 272, 21597-21603.

Zheng, W., and Flavell, R. A. (1997). The transcription factor GATA-3 is necessary and sufficient for Th2 cytokine gene expression in CD4 T cells. *Cell.* 89, 587-596.

Zhou, M., Ouyang, W., Gong, Q., Katz, S. G., White, J. M., Orkin, S. H., and Murphy, K. M. (2001). Friend of GATA-1 represses GATA-3-dependent activity in CD4+ T cells. *J. Exp. Med.* 194, 1461-1471.

Zhu, J., Min, B., Hu-Li, J., Watson, C. J., Grinberg, A., Wang, Q., Killeen, N., Urban, J. F., Jr., Guo, L., and Paul, W. E. (2004). Conditional deletion of Gata3 shows its essential function in T(H)1-T(H)2 responses. *Nat. Immunol.* 5, 1157-1165.

Ziegler, S. F. (2006). FOXP3: of mice and men. *Annu. Rev. Immunol.* 24, 209-226.

Zon, L. I., Mather, C., Burgess, S., Bolce, M. E., Harland, R. M., and Orkin, S. H. (1991). Expression of GATA-binding proteins during embryonic development in Xenopus laevis. *Proc. Natl. Acad. Sci. U S A.* 88, 10642-10646.

Zon, L. I., Yamaguchi, Y., Yee, K., Albee, E. A., Kimura, A., Bennett, J. C., Orkin, S. H., and Ackerman, S. J. (1993). Expression of mRNA for the GATA-binding proteins in human eosinophils and basophils: potential role in gene transcription. *Blood.* 81, 3234-3241.

Zuniga-Pflucker, J. C., and Schmitt, T. M. (2005). Unraveling the origin of lymphocyte progenitors. *Eur. J. Immunol.* 35, 2016-2018.

In: Stem Cell Research Developments
Editor: Calvin A. Fong, pp. 107-134

ISBN: 978-1-60021-601-5
© 2007 Nova Science Publishers, Inc.

Chapter III

Protein Tyrosine Phosphatase Shp-2 in Cytokine Signalings and Stem Cell Regulations

Gang-Ming Zou[*]

Department of Pathology, Johns Hopkins University School of Medicine.
1550 Orleans Street. CRB-2. Baltimore. MD. 21231. USA.

ABSTRACT

Shp-2 is a cytoplasmic protein tyrosine phosphatase that contains two SH2 domains and a tyrosine phosphatase domain. This phosphatase exhibits either a positive or negative regulatory role in a number of cytokine receptor signaling pathways, including several that are critical in stem cell regulation. For instance, it is involved in LIF receptor signaling and has a positive regulatory role in embryonic stem (ES) cell differentiation and proliferation. Maintenance of balance between activation of the JAK-STAT and Shp-2-Ras-MAPK pathways is critical to sustain the pluripotency of ES cells. Shp-2 is necessary for hematopoiesis in a mouse model expressing a mutant residual protein (Shp-$2^{\Delta/\Delta}$). We recently used siRNA to reduce Shp-2 expression and examined the consequences on ES cell-derived hematopoietic development and observed Shp-2 expression is essential for ES cell derived-hemangioblast, primitive, and definitive hematopoietic progenitor development. We further demonstrated that reduction of Shp-2 expression using siRNA blocked the bFGF-induced increase in hemangioblast development. Recently, it has been demonstrated that trophoblast stem cells require FGF4 for self-renewal and to prevent differentiation. Shp-2 prevents apoptosis in trophoblast stem cells, by activation of Erk and subsequent phosphorylation and destabilization of the pro-apoptotic protein Bim. In neural stem/progenitor cell, a recent study reveal that Shp-2-binding sites on FRS2α play an important role in NSPC proliferation but are dispensable for NSPC self-renewing capacity after FGF2

---

[*] Corresponding Author: Gang-Ming Zou, MD, PhD; Department of Pathology; Johns Hopkins University School of Medicine; 1550 Orleans Street. CRB2, M341. Baltimore MD 21231. USA; Tel: 410-955 3511; Fax: 410-614 0671; Email: gzou1@jhmi.edu

stimulation. In this review, the role of Shp-2 signaling in cytokine receptor and various stem cells, including both embryonic stem cells and adult stem cells is extensively reviewed and appropriately discussed.

Key words: Shp-2, Stem cells, Adult stem cells, Embryonic stem cell, Cytokine, Protein tyrosine phosphatase, *PTPN11*, Signal transduction, LIGHT, CD258.

ABBREVIATIONS

BMMSC	Bone marrow-derived Mesenchymal stem cells
EGF	Epidermal growth factor
EPC	Endothelial progenitor cells
EPO	Erythropoietin
ES cells	Embryonic stem cells
FGF	Fibroblast growth factor
GM-CSF	Granulocyte macrophage colony-stimulating factor
HGF	Hepatocyte growth factor
HPC	Hematopoietic progenitor cells
HSC	Hematopoietic stem cells
IL-2	Interleukin 2
IL-3	Interleukin 3
IL-6	Interleukin 6
JAK	Janus kinase
LIF	Leukemia inhibitory factor
MAPK	Mitogen-activated protein kinases
MSC	Mesenchymal stem cells
PDGF	Platelet-derived growth factor
PECAM	Platelet endothelial cell adhesion molecule-1
PI3K	Phosphatidylinositol 3-kinase
PLCγ	Phospholipase C gamma
PTP	Protein tyrosine phosphatase
SCF	Stem cell factor
SOCS3	Suppressor of cytokine signaling 3
STAT	Signal transducers and activators of transcription
VEGF	Vascular endothelial growth factor

INTRODUCTION

Shp-2 is a cytoplasmic protein tyrosine phosphatase encoded by the *PTPN11* gene (Feng, 1999; Qu, 2000). This nonreceptor tyrosine phosphatase (PTPase) relays signals from activated growth factor receptor to p21^{ras}(RAS), Src family kinase, and other signaling molecules. Shp-2 was previously termed Syp, Shp2, PTP1D, SH-PTP2, PTP2C (Saxton et al,

1997). Csw in Drophilia is a likely homolog of Shp-2 (Perkins et al, 1992). Shp-2 plays an essential role in a number of growth factor and integrin signaling pathways, and its mutation causes developmental defects and/or malignancies (Zhang et al, 2004). For instance, Shp-2 has been described to participate in several hematopoietic growth factor-stimulated signal transduction pathways including those of stem cell factor (SCF), interleukin-3 (IL-3), macrophage-colony stimulating factor (M-CSF), erythropoietin, and leukemia inhibitory factor (LIF) (Tauchi et al, 1994; 1995; Wheadon et al, 2002; Burdon et al, 1999; Qu et al, 1997) and has been implicated in controlling the cellular functions of cell cycle progression, proliferation, survival, and migration (Yu et al, 1998; Yuan et al, 2003; Zhang et al, 2002). Shp-2 protein has two SH2 domains (N-terminal SH2 and C-terminal SH2 domain) and a PTP domain (see figure 1). Shp-2 can be activated through phosphorylation. EGF stimulation induces tyrosine phosphorylation of Shp-2 (Thien et al, 1997). Activation of the Ras-ERK1/2 signaling pathway via gp130 in stem cells is dependent on phosphorylation of Shp-2 (Forrai et al, 2006). Tyrosine phosphorylation of a single tyrosine residue (Y757) in murine gp130 is essential for recruitment of Shp-2, leading to its tyrosine phosporylation in a JAK1-dependent manner (Schaper et al, 1998).

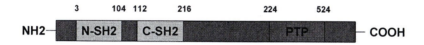

Figure 1. The cartoon represents the structural domain of Shp-2 protein: N-SH2: N-terminal SH2 domain; C-SH2: C-terminal SH2 domain; PTP: PTP domain.

INTERPLAY BETWEEN SHP-2 AND SHP-1

Shp-1 and Shp-2 are two SH2 domain-containing tyrosine phosphatases with major implications in cellular signaling. Both Shp-1 and Shp-2 have been shown to interact with a diverse array of cytosolic and membrane-bound signaling proteins. Generally, Shp-1 and Shp-2 perform opposing roles in signaling processes; Shp-1 acts as a negative regulator of transduction in hematopoietic cells, whereas Shp-2 acts as a positive regulator. Intriguingly, Shp-1 has been proposed to play a positive regulating role in nonhematopoietic cells, although the mechanisms for this are not understood. Craggs and Kellie (2001) observed that green fluorescent protein-tagged Shp-1 is unexpectedly localized within the nucleus of transfected HEK293 cells. In contrast, the highly related Shp-2 protein is more abundant within the cytoplasm of transfected cells. In accordance with this, endogenous Shp-1 is localized within the nucleus of several other nonhematopoietic cell types, whereas Shp-2 is distributed throughout the cytoplasm. In contrast, Shp-1 is confined to the cytoplasm of hematopoietic cells, with very little nuclear Shp-1 evident. These findings reveal that Shp-1 and Shp-2 are distinctly localized within nonhematopoietic cells. In a recent study, Wang et al (2006) investigated the interaction of these two enzymes in a single cell system by knocking down their expressions with siRNAs and analyzing the effects on epidermal growth factor signaling. They demonstrated that knockdown of either Shp-1 or Shp-2 caused significant reduction in the activation of ERK1/2 but not Akt. Furthermore, Shp-1, Shp-2, and Gab1 formed a signaling complex, and Shp-1 and Shp-2 interact with each other in this complex. The interaction of Shp-1 with Gab1 is mediated by Shp-2 since it was abrogated by knockdown of Shp-2. Shp-2, but not Shp-1, binds directly to tyrosine phosphorylated Gab1. This indicates that both Shp-1 and Shp-2 might have a positive role in epidermal growth factor-induced ERK1/2 activation and that they act cooperatively rather than antagonistically.

STEM CELLS

Stem cells exhibits 3 important features: 1) the capacity of self-renewal, which allows maintenance of the undifferentiated stem cell pool over the lifetime of the host; 2) self-regulation of stem cell numbers through balancing self-renewal against differentiation of dividing daughter cells; and 3) the ability to undergo differentiation and maturation sufficient for the reconstitution and long-term survival of all functional elements in a given cell collection (Schulenburg et al, 2006). Self-renewal is a process by which a daughter cell maintains the same properties of its parent. It indicates cell proliferation without any differentiation or maturation and without loss of proliferative capacity. One of best example of self-renewing cells are long-term hematopoietic stem cells (LT-HSC), which maintain themselves as a population for the lifetime of the organism. Stem cells can be classified to three major groups: ES cells, embryonic germ cells, and adult stem cells. ES cells are cells derived from the inner cell mass of developing blastocysts. They are self-renewing, pluripotent, and theoretically immortal. They have the potential to differentiate to three germlayer: ectoderm, mesoderm, and endoderm. Embryonic germ cells have characteristics similar to embryonic stem cells. They are collected from the fetus later in the developmental process from a region known as the gonadal ridge. Though these cells can give rise to the three germ layers that make all the specific organs of the body, the cell types that can develop from embryonic germ cells are slightly more limited than those that develop from embryonic stem cells. Adult stem cells are found in different tissues of the developed, adult organism that remain in an undifferentiated, or unspecialized, state. These stem cells can give rise to specialized cell types of the tissue from which they came. These can also be referred to as multipotent stem cells, as the numbers of cell types which they can differentiate are limited. They replace cells that need to be replaced on a regular basis in a living organism, such as blood and other connective tissues. Adult stem cell therapies will complement but not replace embryonic stem cell therapies. One advantage of adult stem cells is that they offer the opportunity to utilize small samples of adult tissues of a patient's own cells for expansion and subsequent implantation. This avoids the ethical issues of embryonic stem cells. In the past, stem cells with self-renewal capacity but with more limited potencies for differentiation are usually called progenitors. However, those cells recently have been defined closely to Unipotent stem cells that self-renewal as well as give rise to a single mature cell type by International Society for Stem Cell Research (ISSCR). The up-to-date definition for progenitor cell is an early descendant of a stem cell that can only differentiate, whereas it cannot renew itself anymore. This new definition indicates progenitor cell does no any longer belong to stem cells since they have no self-renew potential.

CYTOKINES IN STEM CELL REGULATION

As described, stem cells exhibit some specific characteristics that distinguish them from non-stem cells, like self-renewal and differentiation. However, stem cells also have several characteristics share with non-stem cells, such as survival, mitogenesis, migration etc. Cytokines play a critical role in these activities. Cytokines regulate the differentiation of hematopoietic stem cells (Spangrude, 1991). HSCs release VEGF in an autocrine manner to regulate their survival (Gerber et al, 2002). Mouse ES cells autocrine a number of cytokines that enhance the survival of other stem cells, such as bone marrow HSC (Guo et al, 2006). Certainly, cytokines produced by the stem cell microenviromental also regulate stem cell self-renewal and mobilization. For instance, bone marrow stromal cells secrets SCF and IL-6 to sustain and expand hematopoietic stem cell/progenitor cells. In addition to HSC, cytokines also play important roles in other stem cell regulation, like in neuronal stem cells, LIF promote self-renewal of neuronal stem cells in adult brain (Bauer et al, 2006), and IL-17A enhances the expansion of mesenchymal stem cells (Huang et al, 2006).

CYTOKINES IN REGULATION OF STEM CELL NICHE

A specific physiological microenvironment which functions to house and regulate stem cells is termed the niche (Schofield, 1978; Scadden, 2006). Adult stem cell niches vary in their cellular composition, structure, and location in different tissues. HSC niche contains the periosteum, blood vessel, osteoblasts, lining trabecular bone, and endothelial cells. How do stem cells communicate with their niche? A special cell-cell junction has been proposed between germ stem cells and its niche cells (Xie and Sprading, 2000). Tie-2/Ang-1 signaling pathway plays a critical role in the maintenance of HSC in a quiescent state in the bone marrow niche (Hofmeister et al, 2007). Recent studies reveal niche cells may also control stem cell behavior through shedding of some soluble factors, such as TGF-β, BMP, FGF, IGF, and VEGF (Li and Xie, 2005; Gargeett, 2006). Niche cells maintain adult stem cells in a dormant state (G_0) through signaling pathways inhibitory for growth and differentiation, often involving TGF-β and BMP family members (Li and Xie, 2005). One of the key functions of niche cells is to sense the need for tissue replacement and communicate proliferative and differentiation signals to resident stem cells (Moore and Lemischka, 2006). FGF2, IGF, and VEGF have the regulatory role in certain niches (Gargeett, 2006). Normal stem cells in the adult somatic tissue and cancer stem cells share the common feature of self-renewal and slow cycling (Li and Neaves, 2006). Cancer stem cells may indeed arise from normal stem cells by mutation of genes that make the stem cells cancerous, but this may not be the case in all tumors (Clarke et al, 2006). In regard to niche hypothesis about cancer stem cells, Li and Neaves (2006) recently propose the hypothesis that cancer stem cells may also arise from a microenviroment with dominant growth promoting signaling rather than growth-inhibiting signal.

SHP-2 IN CYTOKINE SIGNALING: OVERVIEW

As described in figure 2, a cytokine binds to its receptor leading to receptor autophosphorylation. Shc bind to the phospho-tyrosine residue in the receptor. They recruit Grb-2, which further activates GEF. Activated GEF triggers the activation of the Ras/Raf/Erk cascade. Shp-2 activates Src through direct dephosphorylation. Src then activates Ras. In other regard, Sprouty is an inhibitor of Ras, and Shp-2 inactivates it through dephosphorylation, subsequently, enhancing Ras activation. In the early literature, Shp-2 was thought to exert a uniquely positive regulatory role of signaling in hematopoietic cell lineage. Mammalian Shp-2 and its homologues in C. elegans and Drosophila have been shown to act as positive regulators of the Ras/ERK pathway in a number of cytokine receptor signaling pathways (Neel, 2003). Recent evidence shows that Shp-2 exert both positive and negative regulatory roles on cytokine receptor signal transduction (Salmond and Alexander, 2006). Shp-2 has an essential role in stem cell regulation based on its involvement in a number of cytokine signaling pathway. We will summarize the role of Shp-2 in different cytokine pathways in the following:

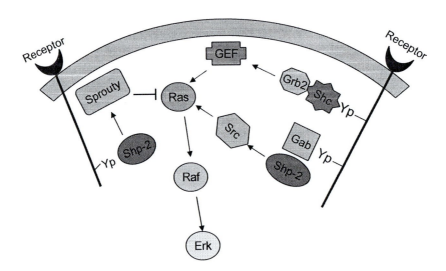

Figure 2. Shp-2 involvement in cytokine receptor signaling. Cytokine binds to its receptor leading to receptor autophosphorylation. Shc binds to the phospho-tyrosine residue in the receptor. They then recruit Grb-2, which further activates GEF. GEF then triggers the activation of the Ras/Raf/Erk cascase. Shp-2 activates Src through direct dephosphorylation which then activates Ras. In other regard, Sprouty is an inhibitor of Ras, and Shp-2 inactivate it through dephosphorytlation, subsequently, enhancing Ras activation.

IL-1

IL-1 alone does not affect hematopoietic stem cell function (Gardner et al, 2003). But in the neural system, it promotes mitotic arrest and differentiation of oligodendrocyte progenitors (Vela et al, 2002). IL-1 receptor include IL-1R1 (type 1) and IL-1RII (type II). IL-1 triggers intracellular signaling cascade by binding to IL-1RI, while IL-1RII functions as a ligand sink (Bankers-Fulbright JL et al, 1996). Shp-2 is involved in IL-1 mediated NF-kB activation, because IL-1 stimulated NF-kB DNA binding activity and Inhibitor of kB (IkB) phosphorylation was dramatically decreased in Shp-2$^{-/-}$ cells and this NF-kB activation is by a MAP kinase-independent fashion (You et al, 2001).

IL-2

IL-2 induces CD34$^+$ hematopoietic cells to differentiate into NK cells in vitro. This was show by Culturing of G-CSF mobilized peripheral blood CD34$^+$ cells in the presence of SCF and IL-2. After three weeks culture, a diversity of CD56$^+$ subsets which possessed granzyme A could be observed, but the cytotoxic apparatus required for classical NK-like cytotoxicity was lacked. These CD56$^+$ cells had the unusual property of inhibiting proliferation of K562 and P815 cell lines in a cell-contact dependent fashion (Sconocchia et al. 2005). IL-2 also promotes monocyte differentiation from G-CSF-mobilized CD34$^+$ cells (Sconocchia et al, 2004). Shp-2 is involved in IL-2 induced activation of MAPK and the STAT proteins in the human CTCL cell line MyLa2059. MyLa2059 cells were stably transfected with wild-type Shp-2 or inactive Shp-2. The cells transfected with inactive Shp-2 revealed reduced MAPK activation upon IL-2 stimulation, suggesting that Shp-2 upregulates IL-2 induced MAPK activation in T cells. Using CTLL-20 as a model system, Yu et al (2000) provide evidence that tyrosine dephosphorylation of STAT5 subsequent to IL-2-induced phosphorylation occurs in the absence of STAT5 nuclear translocation and new protein synthesis. They further demonstrate that Shp-2, but not Shp-1, directly dephosphorylates STAT5 in an in vitro tyrosine phosphatase assay with purified proteins.

IL-3

IL-3 is a multiple-lineage colony stimulating factor which positively regulates proliferation, differentiation and survival of HSCs (Garland and Crompton, 1983; Guan et al, 2006). It induces tyrosine phosphorylation of the SH2/SH3-containing adapter protein CrkL and its transient association with tyrosine-phosphorylated Shp-2 in a murine IL-3-dependent cell line, 32D (Chin et al, 1997). In BaF/3 cells, expression of C459S mutant Shp-2 protected the β-chain of the murine IL-3R and Gab2 from tyrosine dephosphorylation. The tyrosine phosphorylation of a 135 kDa transmembrane protein was also protected upon expression of C459S Shp-2. Expression of WT, C459S and D425A mutant forms of Shp-2 had limited effect on IL-3-driven proliferation, STAT5 phosphorylation, or activation of protein kinase B. However, expression of WT Shp-2 on those cells increased ERK activation. In addition, expression of C459S mutant Shp-2 decreased cell survival in suboptimal IL-3 and upon IL-3 withdrawal suggesting that Shp-2 plays an important role in mediating the anti-apoptotic effect of IL-3. Shp-2 plays an essential role in IL-3 signal transduction in both catalytic-dependent and -independent manners and that overexpression of WT Shp-2 attenuate IL-3-mediated hematopoietic cell function through accelerated dephosphorylation of STAT5. These results raised the possibility that Shp-2-associated leukemias are not solely attributed to the increased catalytic activity of gain-of-function (GOF) mutant Shp-2. GOF mutant Shp-2 must have gained additional capacities. To test this hypothesis, Yu et al (2006b) investigated effects of a GOF mutation of Shp-2 (Shp-2 E76K) on hematopoietic cell function and IL-3 signal transduction by comparing with those of overexpressed WT Shp-2. They observed that Shp-2 E76K mutation caused myeloproliferative disease in mice, while overexpression of WT Shp-2 decreased hematopoietic potential of the transduced cells in recipient animals. The E76K mutation in the N-terminal SH2 domain increased interactions of mutant Shp-2 with Grb2, Gab2, and p85 leading to hyperactivation of IL-3-induced Erk and PI3K pathways. Catalytically inactive Shp-2 E76K with an additional C459S mutation retained the capability to increase the interaction with Gab2 and to enhance the activation of the PI3K pathway.

IL-6

Recombinant murine IL-6 support multilineage colony formation by spleen cells from 5-fluorouracil (5-FU)-treated mice. In mice, IL-6 had a direct effect on the growth and development of murine granulocyte-macrophage progenitors. By contrast, human rIL-6 did not support colony formation by human bone marrow mononuclear cells, and IL-6 may not show an independent activity for human hematopoiesis of myeloid lineage (Suda et al, 1988). To investigate the in vivo effect of human recombinant IL-6 on hematopoietic stem cells, Suzuki et al (1989) perfused IL-6 to normal mice for 7 days and revealed an 8 fold enhancement in the number of spleen CFU-S 7 days after starting perfusion. IL-6 also regulates neural stem cell differentiation (Taga and Fukuda, 2005). IL-6 binds to the receptor gp130 and activates gp130-Shp-2-RAS-MAPK signaling which triggers liver protection in T cell-mediated liver injury (Klein et al, 2005). It activates the Jak/STAT pathway as well as the mitogen-activated protein kinase cascade. Tyrosine 759 of the IL-6 signal-transducing receptor subunit gp130 has been identified as being involved in negative regulation of IL-6-induced gene induction and activation of the Jak/STAT pathway. Since this site is known to be a recruitment motif for the Shp-2, it has been suggested that Shp-2 is the mediator of tyrosine 759-dependent signal attenuation. SOCS3 also acts through the tyrosine motif 759 of gp130. The receptor- and membrane-targeted Shp-2 counteracts IL-6 signaling independent of SOCS3 binding to gp130. In other regard, SOCS3 inhibits signaling in cells expressing a truncated Shp-2 protein, which is not recruited to gp130. So, there are two largely distinct modes of negative regulation of gp130 activity, despite the fact that both SOCS3 and Shp-2 are recruited to the same site within gp130 (Lehmann et al, 2003). IL-6 induces B-cell proliferation by binding to receptor complexes composed of a specific alpha-receptor (gp80; CD126) and the signal transducing receptor subunit gp130 (CD130). Immediately after receptor complex activation, STAT1, STAT3, and the Shp-2 are recruited to gp130 and subsequently tyrosine phosphorylated. The activated dimerized STATs translocate to the nucleus and bind to enhancer elements of IL-6-inducible genes. Shp-2 acts as an adapter and links the Jak/STAT pathway to the Ras/Raf/MAPK cascade but it is also involved in signal attenuation. Whereas STAT3 activation appears to be crucial for all biological activities of IL-6, the requirement of Shp-2-activation depends on the individual biological response. The presence of a single STAT-recruitment site within gp130 is sufficient for IL-6- induced proliferation of Ba/F3 cells (Schmitz et al, 2000).

EGF

EGF is a growth factor with a molecular weight of 6 kDa. Both human and murine EGF contain 53 amino acids. It is a strong activator of ERK5. Cells transfected with mutant ERK5 do not enter S phase of the cell cycle in response to EGF stimulation. EGF activates MEKK3 and this active MEKK3 then further activates ERK5. EGFR is expressed in bone marrow-derived mesenchymal stem cells (BMMSC) (Satomura et al, 1998). The signaling of EGFR drove proliferation and migration of human BMMSCs while not adversely affecting cell survival; and EGF might be used to expand BMMSC in vivo (Tamama et al, 2006). Furthermore, EGF also stimulates human MSC differentiation into bone forming cells (Kratchmarova et al, 2005). It stimulates proliferation of mouse ES cells via PLC/PKC, Ca2+ influx, and the p44/42 MAPK signal pathway through EGFR tyrosine kinase phosphorylation (Heo et al, 2006). Shp-2 is a positive mediator of the mitogenic signal transduction induced by EGF (Zhao et al, 1995; Bennett et al, 1996). Both Gab1 and Shp-2 associate with tyrosine-phosphorylated EGFR upon EGF stimulation in the tumorigenic SHE line, and Shp-2 is involved in EGFR signaling via the formation of the EGFR-Gab1-Shp-2 complex (Kameda et al, 2001). EGF stimulation increases the association of Shp-2 with p85 PI3K in rat pulmonary hepatocytes (Kong et al, 2000). Ras activation is induced in epidermal cells along with phosphorylation of the multisubstrate docking protein Gab1 and it binds to Shp-2. EGF-activated Ras promote epidermal proliferation and opposes differentiation, suggesting that Gab1 and Shp-2 promote the undifferentiated epidermal cell state by faciliting Ras/MAPK signaling (Cai et al, 2002). Major vault protein (MVP) is the predominant component of vaults that are cytoplasmic ribonucleoprotein complexes of unknown function. Kolli et al (2004) identified that MVP protein is a novel substrate for Shp-2 in EGF signaling. MVP may function as a novel scaffold protein for both Shp-2 and ERK. The regulation of MVP tyrosyl phosphorylation by Shp-2 may play an important role in cell survival signaling.

EPO

In hematopoiesis, erythroid progenitor cells are derived from myeloid stem cells. These progenitor cells develop in two phases: erythroid burst-forming units (BFU-E) followed by erythroid erythroid colony-forming units (CFU-E). BFU-E differentiates into CFU-E upon stimulation by EPO, and further differentiates into erythroblasts when stimulated by other

factors. EPO regulates both proliferation and differentiation of erythroid progenitor precursor
cells via its cell surface receptors. Signaling through the EPO receptor (EPOR) is promoted
by tyrosine phosphorylation of the cytosolic domain and the recruitment of secondary
signaling molecules such as the PI3K and Shp-2 to the activated receptor (Klingmuller,
1997), and subsequently activates GATA-1 (figure 3). The EPO receptor (EPOR) transduces
its signals by activating physically associated tyrosine kinases, mainly Jak2 and Lyn, and
thereby inducing tyrosine phosphorylation of various substrates including the EPOR itself. In
EPO-stimulated cells, CrkL, an adapter protein, becomes tyrosine-phosphorylated, physically
associates with Shc, Shp-2, and Cbl, and plays a role in activation of the Ras/Erk signaling
pathway. EPO induces binding of CrkL to the tyrosine-phosphorylated EPOR and SHIP1 in
32D/EpoR-Wt cells overexpressing CrkL. In vitro binding studies showed that the CrkL SH2
domain directly mediates the EPOR binding, which was specifically inhibited by a synthetic
phosphopeptide corresponding to the amino acid sequences at Tyr(460) in the cytoplasmic
domain of EPOR. The CrkL SH2 domain was also required for tyrosine phosphorylation of
CrkL in EPO-stimulated cells (Arai et al, 2001). In the cell line, CTLL-EPOR, which
contains functional cell-surface receptors for EPO, EPO stimulation activated the tyrosine
phosphorylation of the adaptor protein, Shp-2, and the association of Shp-2/Grb2/cytokine
receptor complexes. In addition, EPO, IL-2, and IL-15 activated Raf1 and ERK2, which
demonstrates that the Raf1/MEK/MAPK pathway is activated (Barber et al, 1997).

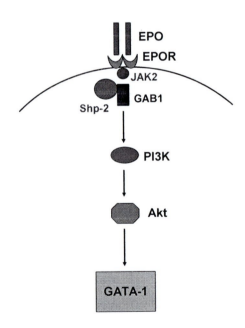

Figure 3. Shp-2 in EPO receptor signaling. The EPO receptor (EPOR) transduces its signals by activating
physically associated tyrosine kinases, mainly Jak2, and thereby inducing tyrosine phosphorylation of
various substrates including the EPOR itself. In EPO-stimulated cells, GAB1 become phosphorylated and
associates with Shp-2 and PI3K and activates PI3K. PI3K then activate the GATA1 transcription factor.

FGF

Fibroblast growth factors (FGFs) comprise a large family of signaling molecules with various functions in development as well as in adult physiology and pathology. These factors also have significant regulatory role in both embryonic stem cells and adult stem cells (Dvorak et al, 2006; Yeoh et al, 2006; Zaragosi et al, 2006). FGF1 and 2 were shown to preserve long-term repopulating hematopoietic stem cells (Yeoh et al, 2006). Primordial germ cells are reprogrammed in vitro to form pluripotent stem cells in response to exogenous FGF2 (Durcova-Hills et al, 2006). FGF4 promote neural stem cell proliferation and neural differentiation in the postnatal brain (Kosaka et al, 2006). It also cooperates with HGF to induce differentiation of human umbilical cord blood-derived mesenchymal stem cells into hepatocytes (Kang et al, 2005). Our recent work reveals a positive regulatory role for FGF in the formation of hemangioblasts in vitro (Zou et al, 2006a). Shp-2 is required for FGF mediated MAPK activation (Saxton et al, 1997). FGFs stimulate their receptors (FGFRs), which do not directly recruit Grb-2/SOS or Shp-2. Grb-2/SOS and Shp-2 bind to membrane-associated adaptor proteins termed SNTs following FGF-induced SNT tyrosine phosphorylation. Grb-2/SOS recruitment to SNT promotes Ras activation, whereas Shp-2 may be activated by SNT engagement (Xu et al, 1998). In Xenopus, Shp-2 is essential for FGF-induced MAPK activation and mesoderm induction (O'Reilly et al, 2000). In mouse fibroblast, Ca^{2+} oscillations in response to FGF2 require the phosphatase activity of Shp-2 (Uhlen et al, 2006). Our recent work demonstrates that knockdown of Shp-2 with siRNA blocks the FGF-induced increase in hemangioblast formation in an *in vitro* ES cell differentiation system. This indicates that Shp-2 is essential for FGF signaling in hemangioblast growth regulation (Zou et al, 2006a).

FLT3L

Flt3L is a ligand for the tyrosine receptor Flt3/Flk-2. Flt3 receptor was detected on the surface of human bone marrow cells that were enriched for $CD34^+$ expression. The addition of Flt3L to irradiated long-term marrow culture seeded with $CD34^+$ cells augmented both total and progenitor cell production. In vitro expression studies with isolated $CD34^+$ bone marrow cells demonstrated that Flt3L alone supported maintenance of both CFU-GM and CFU-HPP progenitors over 3 to 4 weeks. Flt3L stimulates both primitive multipotent and lineage-committed hematopoietic progenitor cells (McKenna et al, 1995). It also has a potent regulatory role in B cell progenitor cells as Flt3L plus IL-7 supported the expansion of murine thymic B cell progenitors (McKenna et al, 1998). In a human Flt3 signaling study, it has been demonstrated that Shp-2, but not Shp-1, was tyrosine-phosphorylated by Flt3L stimulation. Shp-2 did not associate with Flt3, but binds directly to Grb2. Shp-2 and SHIP form complexes with adaptor proteins Grb2 and Shc, then further modulate MAP kinase activation (Zhang et al. 1999). A murine IL-3-dependent hematopoietic cell line BaF3 stably expressing full-length human Flt-3 receptor showed that Human Flt3 underwent autophosphorylation and associate with Grb2 in response to Flt3L stimulation. Shp-2 is tyrosine-phosphorytlated by FLt3L stimulation. Shp-2 does not associate with Flt-3; it binds to Grb2 directly. Therefore, Shp-2 is an important component in the human Flt3 signaling.

GM-CSF

GM-CSF promotes the survival, proliferation, and differentiation of myeloid progenitor cells. This cytokine also plays a major role in dendritic cell ontogeny (Zou and Tam, 2002; Zou et al, 2004). The peptidase CD26 negatively regulates HSC/HPC and that inhibition of CD26 improves the chemotactic ability and trafficking of HSC/HPC. Treatment of cord blood HSC/HPC ($CD34^+CD38^-$) with GM-CSF upregulates CD26 expression (Christopherson II et al, 2006). In collaboration with other cytokines, GM-CSF exhibits the ability to expand HSCs (Liu et al, 2006). In a HSC transplantation assay, host GM-CSF signaling strongly modulates the ability of donor hematopoietic cells to radioprotect lethally irradiated mice (Katsumoto et al, 2005). Shp-2 and Shc were phosphorylated by IL-3/GM-CSF stimulation in BA/F3 cells; however, these phosphorylation events can be inhibited by the expression of delta JAK2. The biologic actions of GM-CSF are mediated by its binding to the alpha and beta subunits of the GM-CSF receptor (GM-CSFRα and βc, respectively). The treatment of Mouse WT19 cell lines with hGM-CSF stimulated the phosphorylation of ERK and induced the tyrosine-phosphorylation of Shp-2 and STAT5 (Matsuguchi et al. 1998). A recent report demonstrates that mutation in *PTPN11* induce hematopoietic progenitor hypersensitivity to GM-CSF due to hyperactivation of the Ras signaling axis (Chan et al. 2005). Proteins that bear immunoreceptor tyrosine based inhibitory motifs (ITIM) are suggested to participate in the repression of cell activation via phosphatases such as Shp-1, Shp-2 and/or SHIP-1. CLECSF6, also called DCIR, is a transmembrane protein expressed on leukocytes and predominantly on neutrophils that contains one ITIM pattern. GM-CSF reduces the binding of Shp-2 to the ITIM of CLECSF6 while enhancing the phosphorylation level of Shp-2. Upon binding of GM-CSF to its receptor, Shp-2 is recruited and phosphorylated. Phosphorylation of Shp-2 by GM-CSF receptor promotes the binding of Shp-2 to the GM-CSF receptor to the disadvantage of CLECSF6. Therefore, upon treatment with GM-CSF, Shp-2 could move from a CLECSF6 associated signalosome with a repressor function to a GM-CSF receptor associated signalosome with an activator function (Richard et al, 2006)

HGF

HGF is one of the major growth factors in the bone marrow microenvironments. It plays a strong role in the migration of BMMSC. Recently, Oyagi et al (2006) transplanted BMMSCs to test their effect in liver-injured rats. Their work reveals that transplantation of BMMSCs cultured with HGF effectively treats liver injury in rats. Short-term exposure of mesenchymal stem cells to HGF can induce the activation of its cognate Met receptor and the downstream effectors ERK1/2, p38MAPK, and PI3K/Akt, while long-term exposure to HGF resulted in cytoskeletal rearrangement, cell migration, and marked inhibition of proliferation through the arrest at the G1-S checkpoint. Both PI3K and MAPK were involved in this HGF-induced migration. HGF/c-Met signal regulates the apoptosis and migration of BMMSC (Liu et al. 2005). HGF's effect on mesenchymal stem cells proliferation was reversed by the p38 inhibitor SB203580, while the effects on cell migration were abrogated by the PI3K inhibitor Wortmannin, suggesting that HGF acts through different pathways to determine its complex effects on mesenchymal stem cells (Forte et al, 2006). Circulating endothelial progenitor cells (EPCs) play a pivotal role in angiogenesis. HGF induces EPC mobilization from the bone marrow in vivo (Ishizawa et al, 2004). It promotes neuronal differentiation of neural stem cells derived from mouse embryonic brain or ES cells (Kato et al. 2004). Cardiac stem cells and early committed cells (CSCs-ECCs) express c-Met, and HGF mobilizes CSCs-ECCs. It also induces hepatic stem cell differentiation in liver development (Suzuki et al, 2003). The Shp-2-Rho small G protein signaling pathway is involved in HGF-induced cell scattering (Kodama et al, 2000). Shp-2 catalytic activity is required for the activation of Erk and epithelial morphogenesis by the Met receptor and it is a positive modulator of Erk activity and epithelial morphogenesis downstream from the Met receptor (Maroun et al, 2000). It is also required for the HGF-induced activation of sphingosine kinase-1 (SPK1), a highly conserved lipid kinase that plays an important role in cell migration. Loss-of-function mutation of Shp-2 did not affect the expression of SPK1, whereas this mutation resulted in blockage of HGF-induced migration in embryonic fibroblasts (Duan et al, 2006). In a Trk-Met-Gab1-specific branching morphogenesis assay, association of Gab1 with Shp-2 was essential to induce a biological response in MDCK cells. Overexpression of a Gab1 mutant deficient in Shp-2 interaction could also block HGF-induced activation of the MAPK pathway, suggesting that Shp-2 is critical for c-Met/Gab1-specific signaling (Schaeper et al. 2000).

TNF-α

TNF-α is a key cytokine and major mediator of inflammation, immunity and apoptosis (Locksley et al, 2001). It is also involved in stem cell regulation. For instance, it modulate neuronal cell fate in embryonic progenitor cultures (Liu et al, 2005). In competitive repopulation assays, hematopoietic progenitors from recipients with AML or MDS possess resistantance to TNF-α-induced apoptosis (Li et al, 2005). Mouse ES cells release TNF-α and irradiation of ES cells enhances this release (Guo et al, 2006). Human neural precursor cells express both TNFRI (p55) and TNFRII (p75) and TNF-α induces chemokine production and apoptosis in these cells (Sheng et al, 2005). TNF-α-mediated JNK, c-Jun, and NF-κB activation required Src and Shp-2 activity (Lerner-Marmarosh et al, 2003). TNF induce IL-6 expression through activation of NF-kB and Shp-2 is essential for this course (You et al, 2001). TNF-α induces the expression of SOCS3 and inhibits IL-6-induced STAT3 activation in macrophages. This course depends on the activation of p38 MAPK. Recruitment of Shp-2 to the receptor subunit gp130 attenuates IL-6-mediated STAT-activation. Bode et al (2003) observed that stimulation of macrophages and fibroblast cell lines with TNF-α causes the recruitment of Shp-2 to the gp130 signal-transducing subunit and leads to tyrosine phosphorylation of Shp-2 and gp130. In this context the cytoplasmic Shp-2/SOCS3 recruitment site of gp130 tyrosine 759 is important for the inhibitory effects of TNF-α, since mutation of this residue completely restores IL-6-stimulated activation of STAT3. Therefore, functional Shp-2 and its recruitment to gp130 are key events in inhibition of IL-6-dependent STAT activation by TNF-α.

LIGHT (CD258)

LIGHT, also named CD258, is a type II transmembrane protein belonging to the TNF family that was originally identified as a weak inducer of apoptosis. The receptors for LIGHT are HVEM and LT-β receptor (Zou et al, 2004). LIGHT possesses a regulatory role in stem cells since it promotes ES cell differentiation in vitro (Zou et al, 2006b). But we do not know whether this cytokine also regulates other stem cells, like HSC or neuronal stem cells since currently there is no information about LIGHT receptor expression in these stem cells. Our recent work also confirms LIGHT's role in inducing maturation of dendritic cells (DCs), such as upregulating CD80 and CD86 expression on DCs. We observed that DCs derived from ES cell differentiation (esDCs) express CCR7 and CCR10 (the receptor of CCL27) upon LIGHT stimulation. LIGHT also upregulates CCL27 but not CCL19 and CCL21 expression in esDC (Zou et al, 2007). The esDC migration potential is increased after LIGHT activation compared to control cells. We have identified that LIGHT activates NF-kB in esDC and inhibition of NF-kB activation by a specific NF-κB inhibitor can partly attenuate the effect of LIGHT in regulation of CCL27 expression. Moreover, Shp-2 is required for LIGHT-dependent activation of NF-kB since Shp-2 knockdown by siRNA affects NF-kB activation, which consequently influences LIGHT-mediated CCL27 expression. We are the first group to demonstrate that Shp-2 is involved in LIGHT signaling (Zou et al, 2007).

PDGF

Adult neural stem cells and early hematopoietic/endothelial (hemangio) precursors express PDGF receptors (Kesari and Stiles, 2006; Rolny et al, 2006). PDGF-AA, -AB and – BB initiate calcium signaling and produce a robust increase in neurite outgrowth of human neural precursor cells (Richards et al, 2006). Activation of the PDGFR-β on the hemangioprecursors accelerated differentiation of endothelial cells, whereas differentiation of the hematopoietic lineages was suppressed (Rolny et al, 2006). PDGF enhances expansion of umbilical cord blood CD34$^+$ cells (Su et al, 2005), and induced proliferation and migration of mesenchymal stem cells derived from human adipose tissues (Kang et al, 2005b). PDGF receptor is a physiological substrate of Shp-2 and Shp-2 has a positive role in PDGF-stimulated activation of MAP kinase (Zhao and Zhao, 1999). Upon binding of PDGF, the PDGF β receptor (PDGFRβ) undergoes autophosphorylation on distinct tyrosine residues and binds several SH2-domain-containing signal relay enzymes, including PI3K, PLCγ, RasGAP, and Shp-2 (Klinghoffer et al, 1996). Following binding of PDGF, the PDGF α receptor (PDGFRα) becomes tyrosine phosphorylated and associates with a number of signal transduction molecules, including PLCγ-1, PI3K, Shp-2, Grb2, and Src (Bazenet et al, 1996).

Shp-2 binds to Tyr763 and Tyr1009 in the PDGF β-receptor and activate Ras/MAP kinase pathway and chemotaxis (Ronnstrand et al, 1999). Actually, Shp-2 not only participates in transmission of signals from growth factor receptors but also plays a specific role in the control of the PDGFR-β expression. This is an important mechanism for the positive control of cell proliferation by Shp-2 (Lu et al, 1998). Ligand stimulation of PDGF receptors leads to the activation of p38. Activation of p38 is required for PDGF-induced cell motility responses such as cell migration and actin reorganization, but it is not required for PDGF-stimulated DNA synthesis. PDGF induced a rapid Gab1 phosphorylation, which depended on the recruitment of Grb2. PDGF also enhanced the binding of Gab1 to Shp-2, but not to p85 (Kallin et al, 2004).

SCF

SCF-Kit pathway plays an important role as a survival factor for many progenitor cell type including primordial germ cells (Dolci et al, 1991), hematopoietic stem cells (Caceres-Cortes et al, 1999), and neuronal stem cells (Erlandsson et al, 2004). SCF is also a survival factor for differentiating mouse ES cells (Bashamboo et al, 2006). Upon SCF binding kit, dimerlizes and activates Src family kinase and PI3K via Y567 and Y719 respectively, which converge on the activation of Rac/JNK pathway. Stimulation with SCF leads to a significant increase in interaction between Kit and p85 as well as in receptor associated PI3K activity in CHRF myeloid leukemia cells, and both Shp-1 and Shp-2 exhibit a basal association with c-Kit (Scholl et al, 2004). The adapter protein APS preferentially associate with phosphorylated Tyr-568 and Tyr-936 in c-Kit. Tyr-568 acts as the binding site of the Src family of tyrosine kinases, the Csk-homologous kinase CHK, and Shp-2 (Wollberg et al, 2003). Gab2 requires Shp-2 for SCF-evoked Rac/JNK, Ras activation, and mast cell proliferation (Yu et al, 2006a). Upon binding to SCF, c-Kit dimerizaes, autophosphorylates, and recruits signaling proteins. The juxtamembrane sequence of c-Kit contains recruitment sites for the Fyn and Lyn, as well as Shp-1 and Shp-2. To characterize the role of Fyn in c-Kit signaling, Samayawardhena et al (2006) generated bone marrow-derived mast cells (BMMCs) from wild-type and Fyn knock-out mice. Fyn-deficient mast cells showed a significant reduction in phosphorylation of Shp-2 phosphatase and p38 MAPK. Defects in Shp-2 and p38 phosphorylation were restored in Fyn-deficient mast cells transduced with a Fyn-expressing retrovirus (Fyn-rescue). They offer evidence that recruitment of both Shp-2 and Fyn to juxtamembrane sites in c-Kit results in Shp-2 phosphorylation, downstream signaling to p38 MAPK, and enhanced chemotaxis of mast cells.

VEGF

VEGF family of ligands and receptors has been the focus of attention in vascular biology for more than a decade. This family consists of five mammalian and one parapoxvirus-encoded member. The VEGFs bind to three different VEGF-receptor tyrosine kinases. Binding of the VEGF to their receptors induce receptor dimerization and activation, which transduce signals that direct cellular function (Cross et al, 2003). VEGF A is an endothelium-specific growth factor that binds to two distinct receptor tyrosine kinases: Flt-1 and KGR/Flk-1. Recently, there is increasing evidence that these factors regulate stem cell functions. Our work demonstrated it is a critical factor in hemanigioblast growth in vitro (Zou et al, 2006a). VEGF-A induce differentiation of human bone marrow progenitor cells (Fons et al, 2004) and enhances primitive erythropoiesis (Martin et al, 2004). Interestingly, it inhibits primitive neural stem cell survival but promotes definitive neural stem cell survival (Wada et al, 2006). It stimulates autophosphorylation of both Flk-1 and Flt-1, whereas their signal transduction properties are not fully understood currently. In porcine aortic endothelial (PAE) cells, VEGF-induced stimulation of Flk-1 results in the association and phosphorylation of Shc and the induction of the formation of the Shc-Grb2 complex. VEGF activates MAPK through Flk-1, but not Flt-1. Both Shp-1 and Shp-2 physically associate with Flk-1 secondary to VEGF stimulation (Kroll et al, 1997). Igarashi et al (1998) examined the interaction of certain proteins with a SH2-domain with Flt-1 and Flk-1 using a yeast two-hybrid system and they demonstrated that Shp-2 binds to Flt-1 at Y1212. Collagen I downregulates VEGF A-mediated Flk-1 activation, and this activity requires Shp-2, which is recruited to the activated Flk-1. Shp-2 binds directly to tyrosine 1173 in the Flk-1 and regulates Flk-1 internalization (Mitola et al, 2006).

SHP-2 AND ES CELLS

ES cells are pluripotent stem cells derived from day 3.5 embryos without use of immortalizing or transforming agents. They usually maintain a stable euploid karyotype. ES cell differentiation provides a defined cell population for pharmacological testing and cellular transplantation. ES cell study presents an excellent opportunity for experimental analysis of gene regulation and function during self-renewal, cell commitment and differentiation. LIF is required to maintain pluripotency and permit self-renewal of murine ES cells. LIF binds to a receptor complex of LIF-R and gp130 and signals via the JAK-STAT pathway, with signaling attenuated by suppressor of cytokine signaling (SOCS) proteins. Recent in vivo studies have highlighted the role of SOCS-3 in the negative regulation of signaling via gp130. SOCS-3-null ES cell lines exhibited less self-renewal and greater differentiation into primitive endoderm. The absence of SOCS-3 enhanced JAK-STAT and ERK-1/2 signal transduction via gp130, with higher levels of phosphorylated STAT-1, STAT-3, Shp-2, and ERK-1/2 in steady state and in response to LIF stimulation. Attenuation of ERK signaling by the addition of MAPK/ERK kinase (MEK) inhibitors to SOCS-3-null ES cell cultures rescued the differentiation phenotype, but did not restore proliferation to wild-type levels (Forrai et al, 2006). Homozygous mutant mice with a targeted deletion of 65 amino acid in the N-terminal SH2 domain of Shp-2 dies in utero at mid-gestation, with multiple defects in mesodermal patterning. To surpass the embryonic lethality in dissecting the Shp-2 function in cell growth and differentiation, Qu and Feng (1998) established homozygous Shp-2 mutant ES cell lines. They described the development of cardiac muscle cells was dramatically delayed and impaired in embryoid bodies (EBs) of Shp-2 mutant origin. Shp-2 mutant ES cells failed to differentiate into epithelial and fibroblast cells in vitro, whereas higher efficiency of secondary EB formation was observed from the mutant than the wild-type ES cells. Further, mutant ES cells were more sensitive than wild-type cells to the differentiation suppressing effect of LIF. In addition, Shp-2 mutant ES cells possess a reduced growth rate compared to wild-type cells. These results suggest that the Shp-2 tyrosine phosphatase is a positive regulator for both cell differentiation and proliferation, in contrast to the Src-family kinases which promote cell growth but block differentiation. (Qu and Feng, 1998). The propagation of pluripotent mouse ES cells depends on signals transduced through the cytokine receptor subunit gp130. Signaling molecules activated downstream of gp130 in ES cells include STAT3, Shp-2, and the ERK1/2. A chimaeric receptor in which tyrosine 118 in the gp130 cytoplasmic domain was mutated did not engage Shp-2 and failed to activate ERKs. The intracellular domain of gp130 plays an important role in self-renewal of ES cells. Mutational analysis of the cytoplasmic domain of gp130 revealed that the tyrosine residue of gp130 is responsible for STAT3 activation and self-renewal of ES cells, while that required for Shp-2 and MAP kinase activation was dispensable. (Matsuda et al, 1999).

SHP-2 AND HEMATOPOIETIC STEM/PROGENITOR CELLS

Shp-2 is necessary for proficient hematopoietic stem cell differentiation at multiple levels of the hematopoietic hierarchy. These findings support the notion that the residual mutant protein (Shp-2$^{\Delta 46-110}$) is biologically inert and re-emphasizes the importance of Shp-2 function in controlling normal hematopoiesis. $PTPN11^{\Delta/\Delta}$ ES cells possess a severe block in differentiation to primitive erythroid, definitive erythroid, and myeloid lineages both *in vitro* and *in vivo* (Qu et al, 1997; 1998; 2001). Chan et al (2003) further defined that re-introduction of wild-type (WT) $PTPN11$ into $PTPN11^{\Delta/\Delta}$ ES partially normalized these hematopoietic defects. Additionally, they observed reduced differentiation of $PTPN11^{\Delta/\Delta}$ ES cells to mesoderm and to the multi-potential precursor for both hematopoietic and endothelial cells, the hemangioblast. We recently used an RNA interference approach to knockdown Shp-2 expression in murine EB-derived cells. Consistent with studies using the $PTPN11^{\Delta/\Delta}$ ES cell model, we observed that reduction of Shp-2 expression by siRNA causes diminished hemangioblast and primitive and definitive hematopoietic progenitor formation (Zou et al, 2006a). Furthermore, consistent with reduced bFGF-induced signaling in $PTPN11^{\Delta/\Delta}$ murine embryonic fibroblasts (Saxton et al, 1997), we observed that reduction of Shp-2 expression using siRNA ablates bFGF induction of hemangioblast formation (Zou et al, 2006a). These studies validate the findings of the $PTPN11^{\Delta/\Delta}$ ES cell and mouse model and further suggest that Shp-2 is not only needed for the initial formation of mesoderm, but is also required for proficient hematopoietic differentiation from hematopoietic progenitor cells. Importantly, we did not observe an increase in the level of apoptosis following transfection with the siRNA, suggesting that the hematopoietic progenitors were viable, but still failed to differentiate and grow into a detectable colony. Altogether, these works validate the previous findings generated using the $PTPN11^{\Delta/\Delta}$ mouse model and highlight the importance of Shp-2 in hematopoietic stem cell differentiation. Shp-2 heterozygous hematopoietic stem cells have deficient repopulating ability due to diminished self-renewal. Reduced Shp-2 function in the form of Shp-2 haploinsufficiency, causes reduced HSC self-renewal. Shp-2 acts to downregulate self-renewal promoting pathways within murine ES cells, but functions to upregulate those pathways within murine HSC, implying that Shp-2 plays distinct roles in embryonic and somatic stem cell population (Chan et al, 2006)

SHP-2 AND TROPHOBLAST STEM CELLS

In mice, *PTPN11* Null embryos die peri-implantation, much earlier than mice that express Shp-2 truncation (Yang et al, 2006). *PTPN11* null blastocysts initially develop normally, but they subsequently exhibit inner cell mass death, diminished numbers of trophoblast giant cells, and failure to yield trophoblast stem cell lines. Molecular markers reveal that the trophoblast lineage, which requires FGF4, is specified but fails to expand normally. Moreover, deletion of *PTPN11* in trophoblast stem cells causes rapid apoptosis. Shp-2 is required for FGF4-evoked activation of the Src/Ras/Erk pathway that culminates in phosphorylation and destabilization of the proapoptotic protein Bim. Bim depletion substantially blocks apoptosis and significantly restores *PTPN11* null trophoblast stem cell proliferation, thereby establishing a key mechanism by which FGF4 controls stem cell survival (Yang et al, 2006).

SHP-2 AND NEURAL STEM/PROGENITOR CELLS

The molecular mechanisms underlying the regulation of neural stem cells and intermediate progenitor cells as well as their contribution to overall corticogenesis remain unknown. The docking protein FRS2α is a major mediator of signaling by means of FGFs and neurotrophins. FRS2α mediates many of its pleiotropic cellular responses by recruiting the adaptor protein Grb2 and the protein tyrosine phosphatase Shp-2 upon ligand stimulation. Targeted disruption of Shp-2-binding sites in FRS2α leads to severe impairment in cerebral cortex development in mutant mice. The defect in corticogenesis appears to be due to the abnormalities in intermediate progenitor cells. Genetic evidence is provided that FRS2α plays critical roles in the maintenance of intermediate progenitor cells and in neurogenesis in the cerebral cortex. Moreover, FGF2-responsive neurospheres, which are cell aggregates derived from neural stem/progenitor cells from *FRS2α*-mutant mice were smaller than those of WT mice. However, mutant neural stem/progenitor cells were able to self-renew, demonstrating that Shp-2-binding sites on FRS2α play an important role in NSPC proliferation but are dispensable for NSPC self-renewing capacity after FGF2 stimulation (Yamamoto, 2005).

CONCLUSIONS

Stem cells are regulated by a number of cytokines in their self-renewal, proliferation, differentiation, and survival. These cytokines might be produced by the stem cell microenvironment or via autocrine pathways. As reviewed here, Shp-2 has been involved in signaling of many cytokine receptors (see table 1) that are related to stem cell self-renewal, differentiation, proliferation, and apoptosis. Therefore, this phosphatase exhibits important roles in stem cell regulation. The abnormal expression or mutation of this phosphatase in stem cells might affect cytokine receptor signaling and subsequently affect their development at different stage.

Table 1. List of cytokines where Shp-2 is involved in receptor signaling

Cytokine name	Abbreviation
Interleukin-1	IL-1
Interleukin-2	IL-2
Interleukin-3	IL-3
Interleukin-4	IL-4
Interleukin-5	IL-5
Interleukin-6	IL-6
Epidermal growth factor	EGF
Erythropoietin	EPO
Fibroblast growth factor	FGF
Granulocyte macrophage colony-stimulating factor	GM-CSF
Hepatocyte growth factor	HGF
Insulin-like growth factor	IGF
Interferon α	IFN-α
Leukemia inhibitory factor	LIF
LIGHT	LIGHT
Platelet-derived growth factor	PDGF
Stem cell factor	SCF
Tumor necrosis factor	TNF
Vascular endothelial growth factor	VEGF

ACKNOWLEDGEMENTS

I would greatly appreciate Anne Yang for her encouragement and support during I prepare this manuscript.

REFERENCES

Arai A, Kanda E, Nosaka Y, Miyasaka N, Miura O. CrkL is recruited through its SH2 domain to the erythropoietin receptor and plays a role in Lyn-mediated receptor signaling. *J. Biol. Chem.* 2001. 276:33282-33290.

Bankers-Fulbright JL, Kalli KR, McKean DJ. Interleukin-1 signal transduction. *Life Sci.* 1996. 59:61-83.

Barber DL, Corless CN, Xia K, Roberts TM, D'Andrea AD. Erythropoietin activates Raf1 by an Shc-independent pathway in CTLL-EPO-R cells. *Blood.* 1997. 89:55-64.

Bashamboo A, Taylor AH, Samuel K, Panthier JJ, Whetton AD, Forrester LM. The survival of differentiating embryonic stem cells is dependent on the SCF-KIT pathway. *J. Cell Sci.* 2006. 119(Pt 15):3039-3046.

Bauer S, Patterson PH. Leukemia inhibitory factor promotes neural stem cell self-renewal in the adult brain. *J. Neurosci.* 2006. 26:12089-12099.

Bazenet CE, Gelderloos JA, Kazlauskas A. Phosphorylation of tyrosine 720 in the platelet-derived growth factor alpha receptor is required for binding of Grb2 and Shp-2 but not for activation of Ras or cell proliferation. *Mol. Cell Biol.* 1996. 16:6926-6936.

Bennett AM, Hausdorff SF, O'Reilly AM, Freeman RM, Neel BG. Multiple requirements for SHPTP2 in epidermal growth factor-mediated cell cycle progression. *Mol. Cell Biol.* 1996. 16:1189-202.

Bode JG, Schweigart J, Kehrmann J, Ehlting C, Schaper F, Heinrich PC, Haussinger D. TNF-alpha induces tyrosine phosphorylation and recruitment of the Src homology protein-tyrosine phosphatase 2 to the gp130 signal-transducing subunit of the IL-6 receptor complex. *J. Immunol.* 2003. 171:257-66.

Burdon T, Stracey C, Chambers I, Nichols J, Smith A. Suppression of Shp-2 and ERK signalling promotes self-renewal of mouse embryonic stem cells. *Dev. Biol.* 1999. 210:30-43.

Caceres-Cortes JR, Santiago-Osorio E, Monroy-Garcia A, Mora-Garcia L, Weiss-Steider B. Stem cell factor (SCF) supports granulocyte progenitor survival in mouse bone marrow cultures. *Rev. Invest. Clin.* 1999. 51:107-116.

Cai T, Nishida K, Hirano T, Khavari PA. Gab1 and Shp-2 promote Ras/MAPK regulation of epidermal growth and differentiation. *Cell Biol.* 2002. 159:103-112.

Chan RJ, Leedy MB, Munugalavadla V, Voorhorst CS, Li Y, Yu M, Kapur R. Human somatic *PTPN11* mutations induce hematopoietic-cell hypersensitivity to granulocyte-macrophage colony-stimulating factor. *Blood.* 2005. 105:3737-3742.

Chan RJ, Johnson SA, Li Y, Yoder MC, Feng GS. A definitive role of Shp-2 tyrosine phosphatase in mediating embryonic stem cell differentiation and hematopoiesis. *Blood.* 2003. 102:2074-2080.

Chan RJ, Li Y, Hass MN, Walter A, Voorhorst CS, Shelley WC, Yang Z, Orschell CM, Yoder MC. Shp-2 heterozygous hematopoietic stem cells have deficient repopulating ability due to diminished self-renewal. *Exp. Hematol.* 2006. 34:1229-1238.

Chin H, Saito T, Arai A, Yamamoto K, Kamiyama R, Miyasaka N, Miura O. Erythropoietin and IL-3 induce tyrosine phosphorylation of CrkL and its association with Shc, Shp-2, and Cbl in hematopoietic cells. *Biochem. Biophys. Res. Commun.* 1997. 239:412-417.

Christopherson KW 2nd, Uralil SE, Porecha NK, Zabriskie RC, Kidd SM, Ramin SM. G-CSF- and GM-CSF-induced upregulation of CD26 peptidase downregulates the functional chemotactic response of CD34+CD38- human cord blood hematopoietic cells. *Exp. Hematol.* 2006. 34:1060-1068.

Clarke MF, Dick JE, Dirks PB, Eaves CJ, Jamieson CH, Jones DL, Visvader J, Weissman IL, Wahl GM. Cancer Stem Cells--Perspectives on Current Status and Future Directions: AACR Workshop on Cancer Stem Cells. *Cancer Res.* 2006 66:9339-9344.

Craggs G, Kellie S. A functional nuclear localization sequence in the C-terminal domain of Shp-1. *J. Biol. Chem.* 2001. 276:23719-23725.

Cross MJ, Dixelius J, Matsumoto T, Claesson-Welsh L. VEGF-receptor signal transduction. *Trends Biochem. Sci.* 2003. 28:488-494.

Dolci S, Williams DE, Ernst MK, Resnick JL, Brannan CI, Lock LF, Lyman SD, Boswell HS, Donovan PJ. Requirement for mast cell growth factor for primordial germ cell survival in culture. *Nature.* 1991. 352(6338):809-811.

Duan HF, Qu CK, Zhang QW, Yu WM, Wang H, Wu CT, Wang LS. Shp-2 tyrosine phosphatase is required for hepatocyte growth factor-induced activation of sphingosine kinase and migration in embryonic fibroblasts. *Cell Signal.* 2006. 18:2049-2055.

Durcova-Hills G, Adams IR, Barton SC, Surani MA, McLaren A. The role of exogenous fibroblast growth factor-2 on the reprogramming of primordial germ cells into pluripotent stem cells. *Stem Cells.* 2006. 24:1441-1449.

Dvorak P, Dvorakova D, Hampl A. Fibroblast growth factor signaling in embryonic and cancer stem cells. *FEBS Lett.* 2006. 580:2869-2874.

Erlandsson A, Larsson J, Forsberg-Nilsson K. Stem cell factor is a chemoattractant and a survival factor for CNS stem cells. *Exp. Cell Res.* 2004. 301:201-210.

Feng GS. Shp-2 tyrosine phosphatase: signaling one cell or many. *Exp. Cell Res.* 1999. 253:47-54.

Fons P, Herault JP, Delesque N, Tuyaret J, Bono F, Herbert JM. VEGF-R2 and neuropilin-1 are involved in VEGF-A-induced differentiation of human bone marrow progenitor cells. *J. Cell Physiol.* 2004. 200:351-359.

Forrai A, Boyle K, Hart AH, Hartley L, Rakar S, Willson TA, Simpson KM, Roberts AW, Alexander WS, Voss AK, Robb L. Absence of suppressor of cytokine signalling 3 reduces self-renewal and promotes differentiation in murine embryonic stem cells. *Stem Cells.* 2006. 24:604-614.

Forte G, Minieri M, Cossa P, Antenucci D, Sala M, Gnocchi V, Fiaccavento R, Carotenuto F, De Vito P, Baldini PM, Prat M, Di Nardo P. Hepatocyte growth factor effects on mesenchymal stem cells: proliferation, migration, and differentiation. *Stem Cells.* 2006. 24:23-33.

Gardner RV, McKinnon E, Poretta C, Leiva L. Hemopoietic function after use of IL-1 with chemotherapy or irradiation. *J. Immunol.* 2003. 171:1202-1206.

Garland JM, Crompton S. A preliminary report: preparations containing Interleukin-3 (IL-3) promote proliferation of multipotential stem cells (CFUs) in the mouse. *Exp. Hematol.* 1983. 11:757-761.

Gargett CE. Uterine stem cells: What is the evidence? *Hum. Reprod. Update.* 2006 Sep 15; [Epub ahead of print]

Gerber HP, Malik AK, Solar GP, Sherman D, Liang XH, Meng G, Hong K, Marsters JC, Ferrara N. VEGF regulates haematopoietic stem cell survival by an internal autocrine loop mechanism. *Nature.* 2002. 417:954-958.

Guan T, Wang SL, Wang YP. Signal transduction of IL-3 in regulating hematopoietic stem cell proliferation and differentiation. Sheng Li Ke Xue Jin Zhan. 2006. 37:117-120.

Guo Y, Graham-Evans B, Broxmeyer HE. Murine embryonic stem cells secrete cytokines/growth modulators that enhance cell survival/anti-apoptosis and stimulate colony formation of murine hematopoietic progenitor cells. *Stem Cells.* 2006. 24:850-856.

Heo JS, Lee YJ, Han HJ. EGF stimulates proliferation of mouse embryonic stem cells: involvement of Ca2+ influx and p44/42 MAPKs. *Am. J. Physiol. Cell Physiol.* 2006. 290:C123-33.

Hofmeister CC, Zhang J, Knight KL, Le P, Stiff PJ. Ex vivo expansion of umbilical cord blood stem cells for transplantation: growing knowledge from the hematopoietic niche. *Bone Marrow Transplant.* 2007. 39:11-23.

Huang W, La Russa V, Alzoubi A, Schwarzenberger P. Interleukin-17A: a T-cell-derived growth factor for murine and human mesenchymal stem cells. *Stem Cells.* 2006. 24:1512-1518.

Igarashi K, Isohara T, Kato T, Shigeta K, Yamano T, Uno I. Tyrosine 1213 of Flt-1 is a major binding site of Nck and Shp-2. *Biochem. Biophys. Res. Commun.* 1998. 246:95-99.

Ishizawa K, Kubo H, Yamada M, Kobayashi S, Suzuki T, Mizuno S, Nakamura T, Sasaki H. Hepatocyte growth factor induces angiogenesis in injured lungs through mobilizing endothelial progenitor cells. *Biochem. Biophys. Res. Commun.* 2004. 324:276-80.

Kallin A, Demoulin JB, Nishida K, Hirano T, Ronnstrand L, Heldin CH. Gab1 contributes to cytoskeletal reorganization and chemotaxis in response to platelet-derived growth factor. *J. Biol. Chem.* 2004. 279:17897-17904.

Kameda H, Risinger JI, Han BB, Baek SJ, Barrett JC, Glasgow WC, Eling TE. Identification of epidermal growth factor receptor- Grb2-associated binder-1-Shp-2 complex formation and its functional loss during neoplastic cell progression. *Cell Growth Differ.* 2001. 12:307-318

Kang XQ, Zang WJ, Bao LJ, Li DL, Song TS, Xu XL, Yu XJ. Fibroblast growth factor-4 and hepatocyte growth factor induce differentiation of human umbilical cord blood-derived mesenchymal stem cells into hepatocytes. *World J. Gastroenterol.* 2005a. 11:7461-7465.

Kang YJ, Jeon ES, Song HY, Woo JS, Jung JS, Kim YK, Kim JH. Role of c-Jun N-terminal kinase in the PDGF-induced proliferation and migration of human adipose tissue-derived mesenchymal stem cells. *J. Cell Biochem.* 2005b. 95:1135-1145.

Kato M, Yoshimura S, Kokuzawa J, Kitajima H, Kaku Y, Iwama T, Shinoda J, Kunisada T, Sakai N. Hepatocyte growth factor promotes neuronal differentiation of neural stem cells derived from embryonic stem cells. *Neuroreport.* 2004. 15:5-8.

Katsumoto TR, Duda J, Kim A, Wardak Z, Dranoff G, Clapp DW, Shannon K. Granulocyte/macrophage colony-stimulating factor and accessory cells modulate radioprotection by purified hematopoietic cells. *J. Exp. Med.* 2005. 201:853-858.

Kesari S, Stiles CD. The bad seed: PDGF receptors link adult neural progenitors to glioma stem cells. *Neuron.* 2006. 51:151-153.

Klein C, Wustefeld T, Assmus U, Roskams T, Rose-John S, Muller M, Manns MP, Ernst M, Trautwein C. The IL-6-gp130-STAT3 pathway in hepatocytes triggers liver protection in T cell-mediated liver injury. *J. Clin. Invest.* 2005. 115:860-869.

Klinghoffer RA, Duckworth B, Valius M, Cantley L, Kazlauskas A. Platelet-derived growth factor-dependent activation of phosphatidylinositol 3-kinase is regulated by receptor binding of SH2-domain-containing proteins which influence Ras activity. *Mol. Cell Biol.* 1996. 16:5905-5914.

Klingmuller U. The role of tyrosine phosphorylation in proliferation and maturation of erythroid progenitor cells--signals emanating from the erythropoietin receptor. *Eur. J. Biochem.* 1997. 249:637-647.

Kodama A, Matozaki T, Fukuhara A, Kikyo M, Ichihashi M, Takai Y. Involvement of an Shp-2-Rho small G protein pathway in hepatocyte growth factor/scatter factor-induced cell scattering. *Mol. Biol. Cell.* 2000. 11:2565-2575.

Kolli S, Zito CI, Mossink MH, Wiemer EA, Bennett AM. The major vault protein is a novel substrate for the tyrosine phosphatase Shp-2 and scaffold protein in epidermal growth factor signaling. *J. Biol. Chem.* 2004. 279:29374-29385.

Kong M, Mounier C, Wu J, Posner BI. Epidermal growth factor-induced phosphatidylinositol 3-kinase activation and DNA synthesis. Identification of Grb2-associated binder 2 as the major mediator in rat hepatocytes. *J. Biol. Chem.* 2000 . 275:36035-36042.

Kosaka N, Kodama M, Sasaki H, Yamamoto Y, Takeshita F, Takahama Y, Sakamoto H, Kato T, Terada M, Ochiya T. FGF-4 regulates neural progenitor cell proliferation and neuronal differentiation. *FASEB J.* 2006. 20:1484-1485.

Kratchmarova I, Blagoev B, Haack-Sorensen M, Kassem M, Mann M. Mechanism of divergent growth factor effects in mesenchymal stem cell differentiation. *Science.* 2005. 308(5727):1472-1477.

Kroll J, Waltenberger J. The vascular endothelial growth factor receptor KDR activates multiple signal transduction pathways in porcine aortic endothelial cells. *J. Biol. Chem.* 1997. 272:32521-32527.

Lehmann U, Schmitz J, Weissenbach M, Sobota RM, Hortner M, Friederichs K, Behrmann I, Tsiaris W, Sasaki A, Schneider-Mergener J, Yoshimura A, Neel BG, Heinrich PC, Schaper F. Shp-2 and SOCS3 contribute to Tyr-759-dependent attenuation of interleukin-6 signaling through gp130. *J. Biol. Chem.* 2003. 278:661-671.

Lerner-Marmarosh N, Yoshizumi M, Che W, Surapisitchat J, Kawakatsu H, Akaike M, Ding B, Huang Q, Yan C, Berk BC, Abe J. Inhibition of tumor necrosis factor-[alpha]-induced Shp-2 phosphatase activity by shear stress: a mechanism to reduce endothelial inflammation. *Arterioscler. Thromb. Vasc. Biol.* 2003. 23:1775-1781

Li L, Neaves WB. Normal stem cells and cancer stem cells: the niche matters. *Cancer Res.* 2006. 66:4553-4557.

Li L, Xie T. Stem cell niche: structure and function. *Annu. Rev. Cell Dev. Biol.* 2005. 21:605-631. Review.

Li X, Le Beau MM, Ciccone S, Yang FC, Freie B, Chen S, Yuan J, Hong P, Orazi A, Haneline LS, Clapp DW. Ex vivo culture of Fancc-/- stem/progenitor cells predisposes cells to undergo apoptosis, and surviving stem/progenitor cells display cytogenetic abnormalities and an increased risk of malignancy. *Blood.* 2005. 105:3465-3471.

Liu Y, Liu T, Fan X, Ma X, Cui Z. Ex vivo expansion of hematopoietic stem cells derived from umbilical cord blood in rotating wall vessel. *J. Biotechnol.* 2006. 124:592-601.

Liu YP, Lin HI, Tzeng SF. Tumor necrosis factor-alpha and interleukin-18 modulate neuronal cell fate in embryonic neural progenitor culture. *Brain Res.* 2005. 1054:152-158.

Locksley RM, Killeen N, Lenardo MJ. The TNF and TNF receptor superfamilies: integrating mammalian biology. *Cell.* 2001. 104:487-501.

Lu X, Qu CK, Shi ZQ, Feng GS. Downregulation of platelet-derived growth factor receptor-beta in Shp-2 mutant fibroblast cell lines. *Oncogene*. 1998. 17:441-448.

Maroun CR, Naujokas MA, Holgado-Madruga M, Wong AJ, Park M. The tyrosine phosphatase Shp-2 is required for sustained activation of extracellular signal-regulated kinase and epithelial morphogenesis downstream from the met receptor tyrosine kinase. *Mol. Cell Biol.* 2000. 20:8513-8525.

Martin R, Lahlil R, Damert A, Miquerol L, Nagy A, Keller G, Hoang T. SCL interacts with VEGF to suppress apoptosis at the onset of hematopoiesis. *Development.* 2004. 131:693-702.

Matsuda T, Nakamura T, Nakao K, Arai T, Katsuki M, Heike T, Yokota T. STAT3 activation is sufficient to maintain an undifferentiated state of mouse embryonic stem cells. *EMBO J.* 1999. 18:4261-4269.

Matsuguchi T, Lilly MB, Kraft AS. Cytoplasmic domains of the human granulocyte-macrophage colony-stimulating factor (GM-CSF) receptor beta chain (hbetac) responsible for human GM-CSF-induced myeloid cell differentiation. *J. Biol. Chem.* 1998. 273:19411-19418.

McKenna HJ, de Vries P, Brasel K, Lyman SD, Williams DE. Effect of flt3 ligand on the ex vivo expansion of human CD34+ hematopoietic progenitor cells. *Blood.* 1995. 86:3413-3420.

McKenna HJ, Morrissey PJ. Flt3 ligand plus IL-7 supports the expansion of murine thymic B cell progenitors that can mature intrathymically. *J. Immunol.* 1998. 160:4801-4809.

Mitola S, Brenchio B, Piccinini M, Tertoolen L, Zammataro L, Breier G, Rinaudo MT, den Hertog J, Arese M, Bussolino F. Type I collagen limits VEGFR-2 signaling by a Shp-2 protein-tyrosine phosphatase-dependent mechanism 1. *Circ. Res.* 2006. 98:45-54.

Moore KA, Lemischka IR. Stem cells and their niches. *Science.* 2006. 311(5769):1880-1885. Review.

Neel BG, Gu H, Pao L. The 'Shp'ing news: SH2 domain-containing tyrosine phosphatases in cell signaling. *Trends Biochem. Sci.* 2003. 28:284-293.

O'Reilly AM, Pluskey S, Shoelson SE, Neel BG. Activated mutants of Shp-2 preferentially induce elongation of Xenopus animal caps. *Mol. Cell Biol.* 2000. 20:299-311.

Oyagi S, Hirose M, Kojima M, Okuyama M, Kawase M, Nakamura T, Ohgushi H, Yagi K. Therapeutic effect of transplanting HGF-treated bone marrow mesenchymal cells into CCl4-injured rats. *J. Hepatol.* 2006. 44:742-748.

Perkins LA, Larsen I, Perrimon N. corkscrew encodes a putative protein tyrosine phosphatase that functions to transduce the terminal signal from the receptor tyrosine kinase torso. *Cell.* 1992. 70:225-236.

Qu CK, Feng GS. Shp-2 has a positive regulatory role in ES cell differentiation and proliferation. *Oncogene*. 1998. 17:433-439.

Qu CK, Yu WM, Azzarelli B, Cooper S, Broxmeyer HE, Feng GS. Biased suppression of hematopoiesis and multiple developmental defects in chimeric mice containing Shp-2 mutant cells. *Mol. Cell Biol.* 1998. 18:6075-6082.

Qu CK, Nguyen S, Chen J, Feng GS. Requirement of Shp-2 tyrosine phosphatase in lymphoid and hematopoietic cell development. *Blood.* 2001. 97:911-914.

Qu CK, Shi ZQ, Shen R, Tsai FY, Orkin SH, Feng GS. A deletion mutation in the SH2-N domain of Shp-2 severely suppresses hematopoietic cell development. *Mol. Cell Biol.* 1997. 17:5499-5507.

Qu CK. The Shp-2 tyrosine phosphatase: signaling mechanisms and biological functions. *Cell Res.* 2000. 10:279-288.

Richard M, Thibault N, Veilleux P, Gareau-Page G, Beaulieu AD. Granulocyte macrophage-colony stimulating factor reduces the affinity of Shp-2 for the ITIM of CLECSF6 in neutrophils: a new mechanism of action for Shp-2. *Mol. Immunol.* 2006. 43:1716-21.

Richards GR, Smith AJ, Cuddon P, Ma QP, Leveridge M, Kerby J, Roderick HL, Bootman MD, Simpson PB. The JAK3 inhibitor WHI-P154 prevents PDGF-evoked process outgrowth in human neural precursor cells. *J. Neurochem.* 2006. 97:201-210.

Rolny C, Nilsson I, Magnusson P, Armulik A, Jakobsson L, Wentzel P, Lindblom P, Norlin J, Betsholtz C, Heuchel R, Welsh M, Claesson-Welsh L. Platelet-derived growth factor receptor-{beta} promotes early endothelial cell differentiation. *Blood.* 2006 May 11; [Epub ahead of print]

Ronnstrand L, Arvidsson AK, Kallin A, Rorsman C, Hellman U, Engstrom U, Wernstedt C, Heldin CH. Shp-2 binds to Tyr763 and Tyr1009 in the PDGF beta-receptor and mediates PDGF-induced activation of the Ras/MAP kinase pathway and chemotaxis. *Oncogene.* 1999. 18:3696-3702.

Salmond RJ, Alexander DR. Shp-2 forecast for the immune system: fog gradually clearing. *Trends Immunol.* 2006. 27:154-160.

Samayawardhena LA, Hu J, Stein PL, Craig AW. Fyn kinase acts upstream of Shp2 and p38 mitogen-activated protein kinase to promote chemotaxis of mast cells towards stem cell factor. *Cell Signal.* 2006. 18:1447-1454.

Satomura K, Derubeis AR, Fedarko NS, Ibaraki-O'Connor K, Kuznetsov SA, Rowe DW, Young MF, Gehron Robey P. Receptor tyrosine kinase expression in human bone marrow stromal cells. *J. Cell Physiol.* 1998. 177:426-438.

Saxton TM, Henkemeyer M, Gasca S, Shen R, Rossi DJ, Shalaby F, Feng GS, Pawson T. Abnormal mesoderm patterning in mouse embryos mutant for the SH2 tyrosine phosphatase Shp-2. *EMBO J.* 1997. 16:2352-2364.

Scadden DT. The stem-cell niche as an entity of action. *Nature.* 2006. 441:1075-1079.

Schaper F, Gendo C, Eck M, Schmitz J, Grimm C, Anhuf D, Kerr IM, Heinrich PC. Activation of the protein tyrosine phosphatase Shp-2 via the interleukin-6 signal transducing receptor protein gp130 requires tyrosine kinase Jak1 and limits acute-phase protein expression. *Biochem. J.* 1998. 335 (Pt 3):557-565.

Schaeper U, Gehring NH, Fuchs KP, Sachs M, Kempkes B, Birchmeier W. Coupling of Gab1 to c-Met, Grb2, and Shp2 mediates biological responses. *J. Cell Biol.* 2000. 149:1419-1432.

Schmitz J, Dahmen H, Grimm C, Gendo C, Muller-Newen G, Heinrich PC, Schaper F. The cytoplasmic tyrosine motifs in full-length glycoprotein 130 have different roles in IL-6 signal transduction. *J. Immunol.* 2000. 164:848-854.

Schofield R. The relationship between the spleen colony-forming cell and the haemopoietic stem cell. *Blood Cells.* 1978. 4:7-25.

Scholl S, Kirsch C, Bohmer FD, Klinger R. Signal transduction of c-Kit receptor tyrosine kinase in CHRF myeloid leukemia cells. *J. Cancer Res. Clin. Oncol.* 2004. 130:711-718.

Schulenburg A, Ulrich-Pur H, Thurnher D, Erovic B, Florian S, Sperr WR, Kalhs P, Marian B, Wrba F, Zielinski CC, Valent P. Neoplastic stem cells: A novel therapeutic target in clinical oncology. *Cancer.* 2006. 107:2512-2520.

Sconocchia G, Fujiwara H, Rezvani K, Keyvanfar K, El Ouriaghli F, Grube M, Melenhorst J, Hensel N, Barrett AJ. G-CSF-mobilized CD34+ cells cultured in interleukin-2 and stem cell factor generate a phenotypically novel monocyte. *J. Leukoc. Biol.* 2004. 76:1214-1219.

Sconocchia G, Provenzano M, Rezvani K, Li J, Melenhorst J, Hensel N, Barrett AJ. CD34+ cells cultured in stem cell factor and interleukin-2 generate CD56+ cells with antiproliferative effects on tumor cell lines. *J. Transl. Med.* 2005. 3:15.

Sheng WS, Hu S, Ni HT, Rowen TN, Lokensgard JR, Peterson PK. TNF-alpha induced chemokine production and apoptosis in human neural precursor cells. *J. Leukoc. Biol.* 2005. 78:1233-1241.

Spangrude GJ. Hematopoietic stem-cell differentiation. *Curr. Opin. Immunol.* 1991. 3:171-178.

Su RJ, Li K, Zhang XB, Pan Yuen PM, Li CK, James AE, Liu J, Fok TF. Platelet-derived growth factor enhances expansion of umbilical cord blood CD34+ cells in contact with hematopoietic stroma. *Stem Cells Dev.* 2005. 14:223-230.

Suda T, Yamaguchi Y, Suda J, Miura Y, Okano A, Akiyama Y. Effect of interleukin 6 (IL-6) on the differentiation and proliferation of murine and human hemopoietic progenitors. *Exp. Hematol.* 1988. 16:891-895.

Suzuki C, Okano A, Takatsuki F, Miyasaka Y, Hirano T, Kishimoto T, Ejima D, Akiyama Y. Continuous perfusion with interleukin 6 (IL-6) enhances production of hematopoietic stem cells (CFU-S). *Biochem. Biophys. Res. Commun.* 1989. 159:933-938.

Suzuki A, Iwama A, Miyashita H, Nakauchi H, Taniguchi H. Role for growth factors and extracellular matrix in controlling differentiation of prospectively isolated hepatic stem cells. *Development.* 2003. 130:2513-2524.

Taga T, Fukuda S. Role of IL-6 in the neural stem cell differentiation. *Clin. Rev. Allergy Immunol.* 2005. 28:249-256.

Tamama K, Fan VH, Griffith LG, Blair HC, Wells A. Epidermal growth factor as a candidate for ex vivo expansion of bone marrow-derived mesenchymal stem cells. *Stem Cells.* 2006. 24:686-695.

Tauchi T, Feng GS, Marshall MS, et al. The ubiquitously expressed Syp phosphatase interacts with c-kit and Grb2 in hematopoietic cells. *J. Biol. Chem.* 1994. 269:25206-25211.

Tauchi T, Feng GS, Shen R, et al. Involvement of SH2-containing phosphotyrosine phosphatase Syp in erythropoietin receptor signal transduction pathways. *J. Biol. Chem.* 1995. 270:5631-5635.

Thien CB, Langdon WY. Tyrosine kinase activity of the EGF receptor is enhanced by the expression of oncogenic 70Z-Cbl. *Oncogene.* 1997. 15:2909-2919.

Uhlen P, Burch PM, Zito CI, Estrada M, Ehrlich BE, Bennett AM. Gain-of-function/Noonan syndrome Shp-2/Ptpn11 mutants enhance calcium oscillations and impair NFAT signaling. *Proc. Natl. Acad. Sci. U S A.* 2006. 103:2160-2165.

Vela JM, Molina-Holgado E, Arevalo-Martin A, Almazan G, Guaza C. Interleukin-1 regulates proliferation and differentiation of oligodendrocyte progenitor cells. *Mol. Cell Neurosci.* 2002. 20:489-502.

Wada T, Haigh JJ, Ema M, Hitoshi S, Chaddah R, Rossant J, Nagy A, van der Kooy D. Vascular endothelial growth factor directly inhibits primitive neural stem cell survival but promotes definitive neural stem cell survival. *J. Neurosci.* 2006. 26:6803-6812.

Wang N, Li Z, Ding R, Frank GD, Senbonmatsu T, Landon EJ, Inagami T, Zhao ZJ. Antagonism or synergism: Role of tyrosine phosphatases Shp-1 and Shp-2 in growth factor signaling. *J. Biol. Chem.* 2006. 281:21878-21883.

Wheadon H, Paling NR, Welham MJ. Molecular interactions of SHP1 and Shp-2 in IL-3-signalling. *Cell Signal.* 2002. 14:219-229.

Wollberg P, Lennartsson J, Gottfridsson E, Yoshimura A, Ronnstrand L. The adapter protein APS associates with the multifunctional docking sites Tyr-568 and Tyr-936 in c-Kit. *Biochem J.* 2003. 370(Pt 3):1033-1038

Xie T, Spradling AC. A niche maintaining germ line stem cells in the Drosophila ovary. *Science.* 2000. 290(5490):328-330.

Xu H, Lee KW, Goldfarb M. Novel recognition motif on fibroblast growth factor receptor mediates direct association and activation of SNT adapter proteins. *J. Biol. Chem.* 1998. 273:17987-17990.

Yamamoto S, Yoshino I, Shimazaki T, Murohashi M, Hevner RF, Lax I, Okano H, Shibuya M, Schlessinger J, Gotoh N. Essential role of Shp2-binding sites on FRS2alpha for corticogenesis and for FGF2-dependent proliferation of neural progenitor cells. *Proc. Natl. Acad. Sci. U S A.* 2005. 102:15983-15988.

Yang W, Klaman LD, Chen B, Araki T, Harada H, Thomas SM, George EL, Neel BG. An Shp2/SFK/Ras/Erk signaling pathway controls trophoblast stem cell survival. *Dev. Cell.* 2006. 10:317-327.

Yeoh JS, van Os R, Weersing E, Ausema A, Dontje B, Vellenga E, de Haan G. Fibroblast growth factor-1 and -2 preserve long-term repopulating ability of hematopoietic stem cells in serum-free cultures. *Stem Cells.* 2006. 24:1564-1572.

You M, Flick LM, Yu D, Feng GS. Modulation of the nuclear factor kappa B pathway by Shp-2 tyrosine phosphatase in mediating the induction of interleukin (IL)-6 by IL-1 or tumor necrosis factor. *J. Exp. Med.* 2001. 193:101-110.

Yu CL, Jin YJ, Burakoff SJ. Cytosolic tyrosine dephosphorylation of STAT5. Potential role of Shp-2 in STAT5 regulation. *J. Biol. Chem.* 2000. 275:599-604.

Yu M, Luo J, Yang W, Wang Y, Mizuki M, Kanakura Y, Besmer P, Neel BG, Gu H. The scaffolding adapter Gab2, via Shp-2, regulates kit-evoked mast cell proliferation by activating the Rac/JNK pathway. *J. Biol. Chem.* 2006a. 281:28615-28626.

Yu WM, Daino H, Chen J, Bunting KD, Qu CK. Effects of a leukemia-associated gain-of-function mutation of Shp-2 phosphatase on interleukin-3 signaling. *J. Biol. Chem.* 2006b. 281:5426-5434.

Yu DH, Qu CK, Henegariu O, Lu X, Feng GS. Protein-tyrosine phosphatase Shp-2 regulates cell spreading, migration, and focal adhesion. *J. Biol. Chem.* 1998. 273:21125-21131.

Yuan L, Yu WM, Qu CK. DNA damage-induced G2/M checkpoint in SV40 large T antigen-immortalized embryonic fibroblast cells requires Shp-2 tyrosine phosphatase. *J. Biol. Chem.* 2003. 278:42812-42820.

Zaragosi LE, Ailhaud G, Dani C.Autocrine FGF2 signaling is critical for self-renewal of Human Multipotent Adipose-Derived Stem Cells. *Stem Cells.* 2006. 24:2412-2419.

Zhang S, Mantel C, Broxmeyer HE. Flt3 signaling involves tyrosyl-phosphorylation of Shp-2 and SHIP and their association with Grb2 and Shc in Baf3/Flt3 cells. *J. Leukoc. Biol.* 1999. 65:372-380.

Zhang SQ, Tsiaras WG, Araki T, Wen G, Minichiello L, Klein R, Neel BG. Receptor-specific regulation of phosphatidylinositol 3'-kinase activation by the protein tyrosine phosphatase Shp2. *Mol. Cell Biol.* 2002. 22:4062-4072.

Zhang SQ, Yang W, Kontaridis MI, Bivona TG, Wen G, Araki T, Luo J, Thompson JA, Schraven BL, Philips MR, Neel BG. Shp2 regulates SRC family kinase activity and Ras/Erk activation by controlling Csk recruitment. *Mol. Cell.* 2004. 13:341-355.

Zhao R, Zhao ZJ. Tyrosine phosphatase Shp-2 dephosphorylates the platelet-derived growth factor receptor but enhances its downstream signalling. *Biochem. J.* 1999. 338 (Pt 1):35-39.

Zhao Z, Tan Z, Wright JH, Diltz CD, Shen SH, Krebs EG, Fischer EH. Altered expression of protein-tyrosine phosphatase 2C in 293 cells affects protein tyrosine phosphorylation and mitogen-activated protein kinase activation. *J. Biol. Chem.* 1995. 270:11765-11769.

Zou GM, Chan RJ, Shelley WC, Yoder MC. Reduction of Shp-2 expression by small interfering RNA reduces murine embryonic stem cell-derived in vitro hematopoietic differentiation. *Stem Cells.* 2006a. 24:587-594.

Zou GM, Chen JJ, Ni J. LIGHT induces differentiation of mouse embryonic stem cells associated with activation of ERK5. *Oncogene.* 2006b. 25:463-469.

Zou GM, Hu WY, Wu W. TNF family molecule LIGHT regulates chemokine CCL27 expression on mouse embryonic stem cell-derived dendritic cells through NF-kappaB activation. *Cell Signal.* 2007. 19:87-92.

Zou GM, Martinson J, Hu WY, Tam Y, Klingemann HG. The effect of LIGHT in inducing maturation of monocyte-derived dendritic cells from MDS patients. *Cancer Immunol. Immunother.* 2004. 53:681-689.

Zou GM, Tam YK. Cytokines in the generation and maturation of dendritic cells: recent advances. *Eur. Cytokine Netw.* 2002. 13:186-199.

In: Stem Cell Research Developments
Editor: Calvin A. Fong, pp. 135-160

ISBN: 978-1-60021-601-5
© 2007 Nova Science Publishers, Inc.

Chapter IV

Stem Cells for Neural Tissue Engineering

Sherri S. Schultz[*]

Albert Einstein College of Medicine; 1300 Morris Park Avenue
Bronx, New York 10461

ABSTRACT

Neurodegenerative diseases and the nervous system's inability to repair following injury, create a growing need for the replacement of neural tissue. The non-immunogenic environment of the nervous system lends itself to accepting cell grafts more readily than the majority of the organs in the body. Stem cells may integrate into the host tissue and act beneficially in ways additional to adding to neuron numbers. Replacing a damaged cell with a phenotypically exact cell may not be necessary or most practical. An immature cell or neural stem cell (NSC) may be beneficial by exerting a trophic support for the mobilization of endogenous progenitors in the niche. In fact, a specified heterogeneous mix of cells may provide one or more roles for regeneration. Therefore, NSCs from a variety of sources may hold great potential for integration into a damaged human nervous system environment, promoting cognitive and behavioral recovery. NSCs have been derived from a variety of sources; fetal, embryonic, and adult stem cells and are cultured in different ways. Beyond deciphering the mechanisms, the availability and safety of implementing stem cell therapies, amongst such diverse stem cell types are among the many considerations that need to be accounted for. There is a need to solve these issues to be able to start implementing life saving therapies.

---

[*] Sherri S. Schultz: sschultz@aecom.yu.edu; 914-954-2101

I. INTRODUCTION

Tissue engineering is the science of designing and constructing live functional organs and parts for regeneration or replacement of diseased or damaged tissue. The basic elements are scaffoldings, cells, and the chemicals that mediate their biological interactions. The scaffolds serve as a framework and also coordinate the growth of three-dimensional tissue. The scaffolds range from a nearly bioinert biocomposite permanent to polyglycolic or polylactic acids polymers that biodegrade for reabsoption. However, the non-resorbed material will never be completely inert and will inevitably result in some degree of scar tissue.[91] In some situations, the biological environment may not demand a physical network for their delivery and direct injection is more conducive for regeneration.

The scaffolding and cell source should be optimized for the regeneration of a specific biological environment, such as central nervous system (CNS). For example, neuronal growth could be enhanced when a gelatin polymer scaffold coated with basic fibroblast growth factor (bFGF) is used as a culture scaffold, due to increased cross-linking of the gelatin gel functional group (-NH) in the presence of bFGF.[19]

There are a wide range of cell sources to choose from but the population of cells must be homogeneous, numerous, and be able to maintain the appropriate phenotype for eliciting the necessary biological function. Primary cells are mature cells that are harvested from organs and could be implanted specifically in the organ that it originated from (e.g. spinal cord neurons for transplantation into an injured spinal cord). These cells are post-mitotic, slowly proliferating, and sparse following isolation from the tissue. Fetal cell from embryonic mesencephalic tissue have been implanted in Parkinson's patients, although similar to primary cells, there is a limit in tissue availability and a difficulty in standardizing such an application. [60] Thus, stem cells have recently been recognized as alternatives to primary cells or whole organ transplants.

Stem cells are self-renewing cells that can be cultured in relatively large quantities. The ability of stem cells to generate cell lineage diversity is their hallmark. Neuroectodermal induced stem cells are referred to as neural stem cells (NSCs). Essentially, these cells are capable of identical renewal of themselves and also capable of differentiating into neurons, astrocytes, and oligodendrocytes; the basic categories that comprise the main specialized cells in the brain. NSCs typically derive from several sources, including adult and embryonic.

Cell implantation entails replacing damaged cells with cells that potentially offer different growth factors to endogenous cells or provide a source of trophic factors for the differentiation of endogenous primitive neural progenitor cells of the CNS. NSCs may offer the most advantages for restoring a damaged CNS environment. These cells range from NSCs isolated from the CNS, to NSCs engineered to express an excess of growth factor, and to multipotent stem cells with differentiation capacities beyond that of the ectodermal lineage. Maximal success for regenerating the brain or the spinal cord would depend largely on the selection of the most appropriate stem cell to form those tissues.

II. STEM CELLS

A. Embryonic Stem Cells

Embryonic stem cells are derived from the inner cell mass (ICM) of a blastocyst. The research started in the 1970s in embryocarcinoma (EC) cells of teratocarcinomas from mice. Those cells were found to differentiate into all three germ layers, ectoderm, mesoderm, and endoderm, as well as form tumors when implanted *in vivo*. When introduced into the ICM, the EC cells were able to contribute to development of the mouse embryo. In 1981, Evans et al. cultured embryonic stem cells directly from the ICM since the EC cells acquired mutations (presumably associated with coming from a teratocarcinoma), that disabled the pluripotent capacity of the cells.[135] Human embryonic stem cells (hESCs) were developed more than a decade following the advent of the mouse embryonic stem cell. Shortly following, government funding has been designated to select cell lines created before August 2001, which would ultimately dictate which hESC lines receive the most research (some favored lines: H1, H7, H9, provided by WiCell Research Institute, Wisconsin).

Current human embryonic stem cell (hESC) research has focused on overall characterization and application in animal models. In determining how to implement hESC therapy, the focus has been primarily on how to identify, maintain, differentiate, and implant stem cells. Some effort has been channeled into deciphering signal transduction pathways and the expression of key genes and proteins that maintain an undifferentiated pluripotent state or trigger differentiation. Since cell therapy is not a standardly used strategy in disease and injury treatments and hESCs are not found in nature, it is unknown how many or what factors in animal models, known and unknown, hold a role in determining the feasibility of using hESCs in a therapeutic setting. Therefore, a stringent evaluation of hESC for human application may prove worthwhile.

Current characterization has started with gene expression using microarrays and evolved into epigenetic studies. A few specific genes have been associated with maintaining pluripotency in hESCs. Transcription of the Oct4 gene results in multiple downstream events that maintain hESCs in a pluripotent state. The Oct4 protein binds to multiple sites in cooperation with the transcription factors, Sox2 and Nanog, in order to maintain the genome in a pluripotent state. Each transcription factor occupies the promoters of more than 1000 genes. [9]

Epigenetic information and chromatin structure are remodeled during early development. hESCs are blocked at a stage of development when the structural remodeling of chromatin is still in progress. The most studied epigenetic marks are DNA methylation and histone modifications. Specific nuclear proteins, such as polycomb group proteins (PcGs) associated with transcriptional silencing and have been implicated in the maintenance of the pluripotent state.[10] PcGs are targeted to specific chromatin domains with features called "bivalent domains" (H3K27 and H3K4 are methylated in mouse ES cells) that repress the genes, allowing development and differentiation.[6]

hESCs have a great capacity for differentiation but the cell culture conditions for maintaining undifferentiation are somewhat elucive. Different hESCs are obtained from different embryos and each have also been exposed to a range of different culture conditions in different laboratories. However small some of the nuances may be, there are precise conditions for maintaining their undifferentiated state. At our current level of technology, they require a layer of feeder cells; irradiated mouse embryonic fibroblasts (MEFs) that are routinely used although this practice should soon be eliminated due to xenogenic contamination. (The exposure of the hESCs to live animal cells presents a risk of contamination with retroviruses and other pathogens that could be transmitted the patients). The irradiated MEFs only survive 10-14 days and hESCs may either be plated directly onto freshly irradiated MEFs or grown on Matrigel, depending on the situations. Karyotyping should be routine because multiple culture passages renders any culture at risk for chromosomal damage or mutations.

It is essential for hESCs to be completely differentiated prior to implantation because they will inevitably result in the formation of a teratoma when implant en masse *in vivo*. hESC implantation may result in tumor formation in immunodeficient animals and benign teratoma could form at the site of injection and at other locations. [135] Long-term experiments need to address this situation if hESCs are going to be feasible, especially since the formation of any type of tumor in the brain or spinal cord can detrimentally impinge on surrounding healthy tissue and impair the function of neighboring CNS cells.

Genetic and epigenetic abnormalities were detected in some hESC cultures. Genetic translocations were discovered in some of the NIH-endorsed cell lines and a non-human animal protein in hESC lines grown on animal feeder layers was also discovered. [28,29,72]. NSCs derived from hESCs could potentially have abnormal gene expression as has been found with low levels of the metabolic gene, CPT1A (a gene linked with hypoglycemia in humans). Shen et al. (2006) discovered differences in the DNA cytosine methylation patterns between NSCs differentiated from hESCs at different passages and in undifferentiated cells. Abnormal DNA methylation is a characteristic that is shared with cancer cells. This could possibly result from a number of factors ranging from a poor differentiation procedure or unstable hESCs, prior to differentiation.[110] In light of these concerns, the expansion of adult stem cells or the mobilization of endogenous brain stem cells may be an attractive option for treating CNS injury and neurodegenerative diseases.

B. Adult Stem Cells

Adult stem cells have been identified as cells that are capable of self-renewal and differentiating into a phenotype. Adult stem cells have been cultured from organs throughout the body, in bone marrow stroma [46,79,136], skeletal muscle [67,105,142], cardiac muscle [130], liver [69], intestine [24,103], and adipose tissue [69,144]. Different research groups have focused on the characterization of adult stem cells, which includes the molecular genetics, the identification through cell surface markers, the ability to uptake Hoescht dye, and the extent of their differentiation potential. The high degree of potentiality some adult stem cells possess allow them to differentiate across lineages other than the organs which they originated from. For example, adult stem cells originating from mesodermal organs have been differentiated into NSCs through the administration of specified chemicals or growth factors. Despite the traditionally accepted theory that neurogenesis arrests past the developmental stage, there are adult stem cells or zones of neogenesis throughout the body that are referred to as niches. [98,106,137]

Niches are supportive environments to stem cells. Studies on intestinal epithelium, the epidermis, and the bone marrow have generated some common themes for stem cell niches. The anatomical organization manages the spatiotemporal function of stem cells. Positive and negative cellular signaling is processed in niches and there are intercellular signaling pathways within the niche. They sequester stem cells from apoptotic and differentiation stimuli. Niches presumably help prevent excessive stem cell production that could lead to tumor initiation and growth.

Disturbance of the niche may result in disturbance of the stem cells. Brain cancer patients undergoing irradiation have a decrease in neurogenesis because the irradiation disturbs the structural microenvironment of the "stem cell niche" between the stem cells and blood vessels in the hippocampus.[50,81] The basic premise of the stem cell niche is that the permissive microenvironment appears precedent to the regionally different properties of the stem cells. [82]

1. Reported Areas of Neurogenic Niches in the Brain

Endogenous NSCs are self-renewing, proliferating, mitototic (although cell cycles may be quite long), and multipotent for the different neuroectodermal lineages, astroglial, oligodendrocyte, neuronal, or glial. [31,38,76,132]. Some of the NSCs have restriction to only one or two of the neuroectodermal lineages. This partial fate restriction may even allow for more efficient production of the desired cell types. [31] The activation of endogenous NSCs results in their proliferation, migration, differentiation, and integration. The endogenous stem cells may need to increase in number above their average homeostasis. They must migrate to the appropriate site were the cells are needed. They must also differentiate appropriately to replace the activity where it was lost.

Inductive signals may motivate endogenous stem cells to proliferate and migrate. Soluble proteins, extracellular matrix proteins, synthetic agents, or other as of yet unidentified substances may activate signal pathways that promote mitosis in quiescent cells or drive cellular motor proteins into locomotion. There could also be signals that are linked specifically to apoptosis for example, Magavi et al. (2000) showed neurogenesis occurred only in response to apoptosis.[15,68] A decrease in ambient oxygen (2-5%) has been shown to trigger stem cell proliferation and differentiation in the CNS.[118,143]

Recently, adult stem cells have been identified within the brain in the subventricular zone (SVZ) in the wall of the lateral ventricle and the subgranular zone of the hippocampal dentate gyrus (DG).[8,53]. In addition, the substantia nigra or cerebellar white matter of the adult brain may also possess some types of neural progenitor cells. [20,80,100]

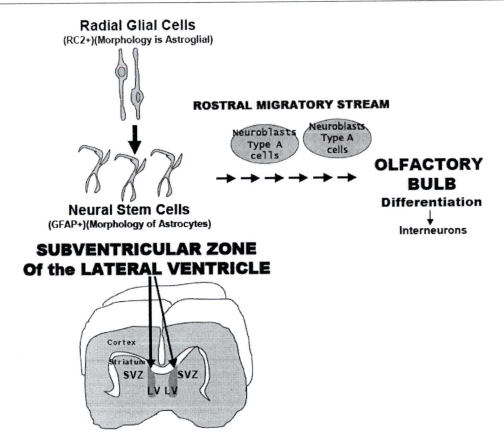

Figure 1. Adult stem cells in the SVZ. The radial glial cells start in the path of neurogenesis and migration of the NSCs continue from the SVZ of the lateral ventricle (LV) (The SVZ locations is depicted in this drawing of a sagittal section of the brain). The type A neuroblast cells travel to the olfactory bulb were they eventually reach terminal neuronal differentiation.

The SVZ is a vestige of a larger periventricular germinative area that narrowed during development. The ventricular zone generates neurons early in development and glial cells, oligodendrocytes, and astrocytes arise from the SVZ in a second proliferating layer in late embryonic development. Neural progenitor stem cells migrate from the lateral wall of the lateral ventricle to the SVZ of the lateral ventricle wall through the rostral migratory stream (RMS) to the olfactory bulb (OB). The stem cells acquire different morphological characteristics along this migratory pathway (Figure 1). The majority of the SVZ cells are type A neuroblasts migratory cells that also proliferate. The majority of the cells that are generated in the SVZ will also die before they fully mature into neurons. Interestingly, dopaminergic deafferentation will decrease neuronal proliferation in the SVZ in Parkinson's Disease, resulting in less interneurons in the olfactory bulb. [134] The slowly proliferating GFAP positive cells of the SVZ are termed type B cells and ensheath the type A cells. [2,78]. The type B cells differentiate into the rapidly dividing immature progenitors, type C cells. Type C cells form clusters and migrate through the RMS to the OB and are the least common but most actively proliferating cells.[88,109]

SVZ cells react in response to injury but do not result in massive replacement and the newly generated neurons are not stable and many die. The death of the new neurons may be a part of the apoptotic response during embryonic neurogenesis. Alternatively, the death of neurons may be due to the cessation of neuronal signal that supported the immature neuron amongst a population of mature neurons. [88]

In addition to the SVZ, the other commonly known area of adult neurogenesis is the dentate gyrus of the hippocampus. NSCs from the DG of the hippocampus migrate from the subgranular zone (SGZ) to the granular cell layer (GCL) to differentiate into granule neurons with axons that extend into the CA3 region of the hippocampus. The SGZ has weakly proliferative GFAP-positive cells, referred to as type B cells, that differentiate into a transitional small dark type D cell that differentiate into neurons of the GCL.

Endogenous adult NSCs remain quiescent under normal physiological conditions and there are a few in the non-neurogenic areas of the brain. Injury may play an important role in neurogenesis throughout the entire brain. The local environment may become inducive towards proliferation, migration, and neuronal or glial differentiation.[128]

Multiple groups have also reported evidence of stem cells in the spinal cord. The presence of NSCs has been detected in the periventricular area, parenchyma, ependyma, parenchyma, the lumbar/sacral region. [132,139] Fawcett and Asher reported that the endogenous NSCs in the spinal cord do not penetrate the volume of the injury from the ventricular zone in the medial portion of the cord.[32] However, the spinal cord does not regenerate following injury, probably because there are too few endogenous NSCs and/or they can not migrate to the injury site for spinal cord repair. [4,32,42,104,108]

2. Monitoring and Culturing NSCs

The current research in neuroectodermal differentiation of stem cells and NSCs are pertinent for nervous tissue regeneration, due to the numerous damage conditions and diseases in the CNS. There are several methods that have been typically used for the *in vivo* identification of NSCs. Constitutive neurogenesis in the hippocampus and olfactory bulb was demonstrated by using [^{3}H] thymidine, which incorporates and localizes to the nuclei.[1] Bromodeoxyuridine (BrdU) is a thymidine analogue that incorporates into the DNA of cells in S phase of mitotic cycle (not division). *In vivo* monitoring of the dividing cells in the rat or animal brain is typical done with bromodeoxyuridine (BrdU). BrdU is a thymidine analogue that incorporates and localizes to the nuclei [1]. It is delivered through intraperitoneal injections of roughly 120 mg/kg of BrdU [36,73]. However, BrdU reactivity could include proliferating newborn neurons or glial cells, inflammatory cells, and cells with DNA damage.[73] It is possible that dying neurons could enter S-phase and still incorporate BrdU [40,140]. However, long-term experiments should eliminate that confusion. [94] Other NSC labels are doublecortin which identifies migrating neuroblasts, and proliferating cell nuclear antigen (PCNA) [88]. In addition, endogenous cells may also be measured with immunohistochemistry of brain slices. *In vivo* neurogenesis is most typically confirmed by both the BrdU labeling and double staining cells that label with multiple antibodies to proteins identified with early development or stem cells (Table 1).

There are different mechanisms for tracking exogenously transplanted cells. Implanted cells can also be identified either by transfection of a GFP-expressing retrovirus, which require a complete cell division rather than only S-phase for integration. [94,124] Transducting or transfecting stem cells prior to implantation may pose the risk of transforming the adult stem cells to tumor cells; and/or inhibiting the ability of the stem cells to differentiate into one or more phenotypes.[74,124] Alternatively, an endogenous expressing marker in cells expressing a nuclear marker, such as ß -galactosidase, will allow for detection of individual cells derived from ROSA mice. ROSA mice are transgenic for bacterial ß-galactosidase, having the $LacZ^+$ gene in every cell in their body. [37,74]

The criteria commomly used to identify NSCs in culture are: 1) the expression of standard neural antigens; 2) a morphological resemblance to the neuroectodermal phenotypes; 3) self-renewal; 4) calcium fluxes; 5) the ability to propagate an action potential; and 6) the expression of neurotransmitters or enzymes (ex: dopamine-associated enzyme, tyrosine hydroxylase) specific to that biological function. Many papers have tested hypotheses of directing primitive or minimally differentiated neural cells towards further differentiation based upon these criteria. [17,22,51,56,65,83,98,106,116,120,125,127, 132,137] NSCs have been cultured from the caudal portion of the SVZ [85], the striatum [85], optic nerve, septum, corpus callosum, spinal cord, retina, and hypothalamus [31,40,70,85,111,132]. However, some NSCs *in vivo* may have difficulty maintaining their inherent properties when separated from their neurogenic niche microenvironment due to insufficiencies of the *in vitro* environment.[31]

NSCs may be *in vitro* propagated, in the form of 3-dimensional floating spheres referred to as neurospheres, and in a flat adherent form. Neurospheres have previously been used to assess the proliferative activity of the NSCs, based on diameter, the resultant number of neurospheres, and the multipotency of forming all the multiple neural phenotypes. However, those particular features may not accurately reflect the potential of the NSCs proliferation, self-renewal, and multipotency. [112,129]

Culture systems of neurons, astrocytes, and oligodendrocytes have long relied upon growth factors as a primary nutrient. Different mitogens interact in determining the fate of cell division or terminal differentiation in specific types of stem cells. Neurotrophic factors can affect neurogenesis through cell survival, transmitter metabolism, synthesis of cytoskeletal proteins, and cell surface glycoproteins. Synergistic interactions of growth factors may be essential for maintaining homeostasis in the CNS while other combinations of growth factors may be necessary to regeneration and development. Specified culture conditions for different types of neural progenitors are generated as an effort to simulate the in vivo environment of the cell. *In vitro* experiments have shown that basic fibroblast growth factor (bFGF), epidermal growth factor (EGF), transforming growth factor (TGF), insulin growth factor-1 (IGF-1), and monoamines increase proliferation, while glutamate, GABA, and opioid peptides decrease proliferation. Platelet-derived growth factor (PDGF), ciliary neurotrophic factor (CNTF), and vasoactive intestinal peptide (VIP) also affect proliferation and differentiation. [14,41,109]

Table 1. Antibodies used to detect the proteins associated with NSCs using immunohistochemistry

Antibody: Immunohistochemistry	Differentiation Stage Specificity	Antigen	Reference
Tenascin	Immature	Extracellular matrix proteins (ECM) for neuronal and oligodendrocyte precursors	[26]
PSA-NCAM (polysialic acid -neural cadherin adhesion molecule)	Immature	ECM for oligodendrocyte and neuronal (Type A neuroblasts) precursors	[26,125]
Rat401 (nestin)	Immature	Neuronal, microglia	[141]
Hu	Immature	Early neuronal marker	[68]
RC2	Immature	Radial glia	[26]
3CB2	Immature	Cytoskeletal component of radial glia	[26]
B-tubulin III (Tuj1)	Immature	Type A migrating neuroblasts	[27]
GFAP	Immature Inflamm/ Reactive	Immature and Reactive astrocytes Postnatal NSC (mostly SVZ)	[5]
CD44	Immature	Progenitor astrocyte	[64]
Dcx (doublecortin)	Immature	Migrating neuroblasts	[88,115]
Meis2	Immature	Medium-sized spiny neurons of the striatum	[88]
Prox-1 and calbindin	Immature	Progenitor in dentate gyrus	
NG2 proteoglycan chondroitin /AN2	Immature Embryonic/ postnatal	Immature oligodendrocytes Postnatal progenitors	[26] [5,57]
PSA-NCAM + PDGFαR	More immature	Forerunner of NG2 precursor	[77]
PDGF-α receptor	Immature/mature	Oligodendrocytes; PDGF is chemotactic and promotes migration	[26]
O2A	Immature	Oligodendrocyte	[26]
A2B5	Immature / cancer	Coexpress with NCAM to NSC	[125]
CD133	Immature [125]/ cancer	Tumor NSCs	[113] [43,114]
^{125}I-NGF	Immature/ Inflammation	Proliferation and mobilization of SVZ: response to inflammation / demyelination	[88]
GABA (neurotransmitter) and tyrosine hydroxylase (dopamine associated enzyme	Immature	Precursor in the olfactory bulb.	[52]

A few different agents have been used to differentiate stem cells into NSCs and neurons. Retinoic acid (RA) has been used to differentiate the hESCs into neurons, at high levels. However, the teratogenicity of RA deter it from becoming a possible usage with stem cells in therapeutic applications. [97,117,135] Culturing NSCs with bFGF and EGF has become a common practice for the maintenance of NSCs derived from different parts of the nervous system as well as neuroectodermally induced stem cells from non-ectodermal lineage organs. FGF promotes mesodermal and neuroectodermal cell proliferation, differentiation, and mediates maintenance and tissue repair in adults. FGF molecular signaling occurs through either a low-affinity binding heparan sulfate proteoglycan or a high-affinity binding with tyrosine transmembrane receptors. Alternative splicing of the FGF receptors regulate the ligand-binding specificity with some FGF receptors binding a variety of FGFs. Main sources of FGF-2 and FGF receptors are in sensory neurons, Schwann cells, and macrophages. [41]

The practice of culturing with bFGF and EGF includes differentiating stem cells from non-neuroectodermal lineages into a neural lineage.[98,137] The specificity of EGF and FGF in the specific induction and growth of NSCs is surprising since EGF and FGF receptors operate in most of the cells of the human body and result in the activation of a signal transduction pathway that activates the Ras-MAPK cascade. The use of specific culture conditions also raises the possibility that the culture conditions may selectively promote the survival and proliferation of individual progenitor cells in the cultures and not detect the existence of one or more additional populations of primitive stem cells. In addition,when hESCs are cultured with bFGF in prolonged conditions at high density to create neurospheres, it may also result in the formation of a clonal population, possibly leading to cancer. [96] Interestingly, glioblastoma cells are also maintained in culture with EGF and bFGF. Furthermore, stem cell implantation requires thorough investigation on an *in vitro* level prior to implantation. By evaluating what genes are being activated or what proteins are being expressed within a healthy and/or multiplying population, key molecules can be identified in what is necessary to maintain those cells or decipher what motivates neurogenesis.

III. CNS DISEASES WITH POTENTIAL FOR STEM CELL THERAPY

Stem cells may present a form of regenerative therapy for neurodegenerative diseases. Neurodegenerative diseases have complicated pathologies and a few more common neurodegenerative diseases are briefly charted above (Table 2). The success could depend upon the extent of damage and the course of disease progression. Different types of neurons are dying with variation in the numbers of damaged and dying cells, variation in the location of cell loss, and the loss of those synaptic connections.

In particular, animal models for Alzheimer's Disease (AD) have revealed particular complexities in using stem cell therapy for treatment. For example, AD has been examined in overexpressing amyloid- precursor protein (APP) transgenic mice that received NSCs, ectodermally induced adult stem cells (induction through overexpression of Nanog). Excessive APP or recombinant APP treatment causes glial differentiation of stem cells. *In vitro* studies with NSCs also showed that APP resulted in glial differentiation rather than neuronal. [55,119] The resultant glial differentiation may function to eliminate the APP protein, but ultimately, new neurons are necessary to replace degenerating neurons. The amyloid beta peptide (Abeta), implicated in AD, impairs neurogenesis and migration of NSCs in the neurogenic zone of the brain of APP mice in the subventricular zone.[44] NSC differentiation is suppressed and apoptosis is induced when Abeta is introduced to cultured NSCs from human embryonic cerebral cortex. The complexities involved in stem cell therapy for AD, may require a combinatorial therapy of stem cells with, for example, a neurosteroid allopregnanolone to promote the proliferation of endogenous NSCs in the AD mouse brain.[11]

Table 2. Neurodegenerative diseases.

Disorder	Chromosomal Location	Clinical Symptoms	Mode of Inheritance	Disease Mechanisms
Alzheimer's Disease	1. AD4: 1q31-42, 2. AD3: 14q24.3, 3. AD2: 19q13.2, 4. AD1: 21q21.3-22.05	Dementia, memory loss	1. Autosomal Dominant (AD) 2. AD 3. Codominant 4. AD	Mutations in the proteins : 1. presenilin-2 or 2.presenilin-1 gene (membrane protein in intracellular protein transport) 3. Apolipoprotein E4 (supports cellular functions that require lipoprotein mobilization) 4. Amyloid precursor protein (APP) for APP metabolism
Huntington's Disease	4p16.3	Chorea, depression, dementia	AD	CAG triplet repeats in a gene that encodes huntingtin protein. The polyglutamate tract in the protein result in toxic accumulations
Parkinson's Disease	4q21-23, 6q25-27, 2p13, 4p14, 1p35-p36, 1p36, 12p11-q13, 2q22-23, 5q23	Tremors, rigidity, Depression,	1. AD, 2. Autosomal Recessive (AR), 3. Mitochondrial	Interference with the ubiquitin-proteasome system. Mutations in PARK1 (alpha-synuclein), PARK2 (parkin), and PARK7 (DJ-1). Also, UCH-L1, Nurr1 (NR4A2), Synphilin-1 (SNCAIP), and Mitochondria (NADH complex I)

The mutated genes associated with Alzheimer's Disease results in accumulations of proteins that form plaques, neurofibrillary tangles, and lesions that culminate in the diffuse atrophy of the cerebral cortex with secondary enlargement of the ventricular system. Huntington's Disease is a polyglutamine aggregation that affects the proteolytic processes and other cell processes that may trigger mitochondrial or metabolic toxicity to induce apoptosis. There is a large decrease in neurotransmitters: gamma aminobutyric acid (GABA) and glutamic acid decarboxylase. The striatum is predominantly affected although there is also gliosis and neuronal loss of medium-spiny neurons in the caudate and the putamen. Parkinson's Disease is caused by the loss of nerve cells in the substantia nigra pars compacta, the locus coeruleus in the midbrain, the globus pallidus, and the putamen. Dopaminergic neurons (which input in the striatum of the basal ganglia) and cholinergic striatal interneurons that modulate GABA-inhibition to the thalamus are destroyed. [3,7,71,86]

Parkinson's Disease (PD) requires the replacement of midbrain dopaminergic neurons. hESCs differentiated into NSCs reach terminal differentiation into dopaminergic neurons through treatment with sonic hedgehog (SHH) and FGF-8. Perrier et al. (2004) showed the differentiation of hESCs towards a midbrain dopamine neuron had the sequential expression of the transcription factors, Pax2, Pax5, engrailed (En1), dopamine release, the presence of tetrodotoxin-sensitive action potentials, and the visualization of tyrosine-hydroxylase-positive synaptic terminals. [87,99] Roy et al. (2006) used the 6-hydroxydopamine-lesioned rat brain model for PD and also exposed SHH and FGF-8 treated NSCs to telomerase-immortalized fetal midbrain astrocytes for an increase in TH+ neurons. The glial cells were used as paracrine agents for the TH+ neurons in heterogeneous cultures. Although the enrichment of TH+ neurons had a high level of engraftment when assessed 10 weeks following transplantation ($136,726 +/- 23,515/mm^3$ cells engrafted) as well as improved motor skills, the dopaminergic antigenicity of those neurons decreased after a few months, and the data suggested there was a graft associated tumorigenesis, likely due the presence of incompletely differentiated hESCs. Human trials with intrastriatal transplantation of embryonic mesencephalic tissues in PD patients did show that the graft could reinnervate the striatum, restore dopamine release for up to 10 years, yet the results from these trials, had a lot of variation, with some people having no improvement. [35,52,59,60,60,89,92].

Stem cell therapy for Huntington's Disease (HD) is also complicated. Excitotoxic lesions from quinolinic acid destroyed the medium sized spiny neurons in the striatum of adult mice, and NSC neurospheres were injected into the brain. Earlier injection of the NSCs (2 days) versus later (7 and 14 days) had greater cell transplant survival [47]. NSCs secreting GDNF (high expression in the striatum) with some degree of integration in quinolinic-lesioned nude mouse striata and reduced amphetamine-induced rotational behavior in mice with unilateral lesions. [90] In the long run, it is essential for the striatal tissue to restore the function in the striato-cortical neural loops to show a behavioral restoration that can be maintained on a long term level in the clinic.

IV. CNS Injury with Potential for Cell Therapy

Brain Injury

Neurodegenerative diseases are inherited through known and unknown genetic variants. Neurodegeneration could also result from direct or indirect trauma to the spinal cord and brain. Brain damage is usually an irreversible injury of varying magnitude, with indirect injury being more common, such as with cardiac arrest, aneurysms, bleeding, near-drowning, or carbon monoxide poisoning. The neurons of the brain are particularly sensitive to hypoxic conditions and result in cell death.

One example of brain injury is global ischemia, a vascular injury that effects the environment of the CNS. It is the permanent occlusion of the vertebral arteries and transient occlusion of the common carotid arteries to the entire brain. The entire forebrain is deprived of oxygen and glucose resulting in patterns of global ischemia-induced cell death. [145] The most prominent damage occurs to the pyramidal neurons of the CA1 region of the hippocampus. There is still some injury to the hilar neurons of the dentate gyrus, the pyramidal neurons of the neocortical layers, and the Purkinje neurons of the cerebellum. The inhibitory interneurons of the CA1 and the neurons in the nearby CA2 (transition zone), CA3, and dorsal ganglia all survive.

The ischemic injury also results in compensatory neurogenesis in some areas that participate in adult neurogenesis. [143] There are multiple animal experiments that demonstrate neurogenesis following global ischemia. [61,102,109] Following transient global ischemia in gerbils, the DG had proliferative cells based on BrdU labeling. Double-labeling of BrdU with NeuN became apparent by day 26 following ischemia. The SGZ cells also migrated to the dentate hilus and differentiated into astrocytes. Long-term survival of differentiated neurons was only demonstrated in non-injured hippocampus. [88] Sharp et al. (2002) subjected adult gerbils to 10 minutes of global ischemia. At 15 days post-ischemia, BrdU labeled cells did not stain for neuronal or astrocytic markers in the SGZ. At 26 and 40 days post-ischemia, 27% and 67% of the BrdU positive cells were also NeuN positive, respectively. The BrdU positive cells were distributed throughout the granule cell layer and the dentate hilus. PCNA staining with NeuN confirmed the BrdU findings.

The patterns of neurogenesis and apoptosis also appear to have a great deal of overlap on a temporal level. Kuhn et al. (1997) showed differential and site-specific effects on progenitor cells *in vivo*.[54] It is unknown exactly what motivates neurogenesis and cell death in these situations. These signals could be either driven by internal cues or receive some type of external motivation.

Stem cell therapy may be more practical following the 48 hour post-injury period if excitotoxicity is going to destroy the cells in that region. The brain is exceptionally sensitive to the deprivation of oxygen or glucose. This results in apoptotic and necrotic cell death of neurons in specific areas of the brain. In a four-vessel occlusion model in rats, there is histological evidence of neuronal death by 48 hours. Jomura et al. (2006) implanted Oct-4+-umbilical cord matrix cells in the thalamic nucleus, hippocampus, corpus callosum, and cortex, 3 days prior to cardiac arrest in rats. A 25-32% decrease in neuronal loss was mostly found outside of the CA1 hippocampal region, the region of the most damage. More research needs to be conducted to figure out if implanting stem cells are a realistic option. [48]

Spinal Cord Injury

Another example of CNS injury is spinal cord injury. Initially, there is a mechanical disruption that is accompanied by an initial loss of neurons at that region and only occasionally is the inner gray matter containing cell bodies affected, initially.[75] This initial injury results in cellular disturbances, loss of hemostasis, and ionic and neurotransmitter imbalances. The loss of hemostasis prevents the delivery of nutrients and oxygen to cells, resulting in apoptosis and necrosis of starved cells.[63] Catecholamines, glutamate, and serotonin accumulate in the extracellular space. Free radicals are introduced to the injured CNS through radical oxygen synthesized by neutrophils, mitochondrial disruption, oxidized hemoglobin, and the arachidonic acid cascade. The radicals disrupt the cell membranes and lead to cell death.[23,33] Excitotoxic neuronal death ensues due to the accumulation of neurotransmitters intracellularly, resulting in rapid membrane damage and death to nerve and glial cells.[58,75,101]

The secondary injury or distant damage is the cumulative effect of the primary mechanical injury that leads to significant tissue destruction. The secondary injury usually runs its course over several days. The ultimate result is the formation of a glial scar rimming a cavitation that becomes a fluid-filled cyst that causes regenerative failure.[34]

Multiple endogenous cells contribute to the secondary injury and prevent spinal cord regeneration. Reactive astrocytes create a major physical obstacle for the regeneration of axons that were damaged. [13,95] The astrocytes divide and fill in the vacant spaces that the axons of pre-injury neurons occupied and presumably, where regenerating axons would be. The vascular damage produces a massive macrophage recruitment that continues over many weeks.[121]'[12,107] In general, the type of immunoreactivity seen in spinal cord injury is similar to that seen in excitotoxic brain lesions.[123]

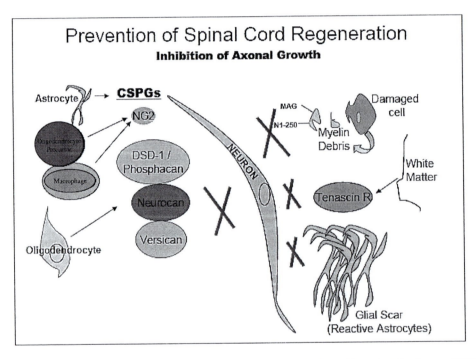

Figure 2. Molecules that prevent spinal cord regeneration. The chondroitin sulfate phosphoglycans (CSPGs) are inhibitors of axonal regrowth in spinal cord injury. They are released by oligodendrocyte precursors, macrophages, and oligodendrocytes. There are other molecules (myelin debris and tenascin R) and cells (reactive astrocytes) that also have anti-growth properties.

Multiple endogenous cells contribute to the secondary injury and prevent spinal cord regrneration. (Figure 2). Chondroitin sulphate proteoglycans (CSPG) are extracellular matrix molecules that are neurite growth inhibitors produced by astrocytes, oligodendrocyte precursor cells, and meningeal cells. Oligodendrocytes, cells that myelinate neurons in healthy conditions, produce DSD-1/phosphacan, neurocan, and versican, which inhibit axonal growth and are upregulated 7 days after injury. [121] The myelin debris from dying or damaged neurons contain inhibitory molecules N1-250 and MAG, expressed immediately after injury.[18] The debris may remain for several months due to the slow microglia /macrophage phagocytic activity. Tenascin R is another inhibitory protein and is located in the extracellular matrix of the CNS, particularly in white matter. It inhibits axonal growth by interacting with the axon surface molecule F3/11. [49]

Stem cell implantation has heralded some significant improvement in spinal cord injury as seen in rat models of spinal cord injury. Embryonic stem cells have been implanted in injured rat spinal cords with statistically significant functional improvement.[16,62,74,133] Similarly, adult stem cells from the CNS [66,122,138,139]: olfactory ensheathing glial cells [93], Schwann cells [39,131], NSCs cultured from the spinal cord [126], or even from bone marrow [21,45,84], were transplanted into the contused spinal cord and reduced functional deficits.

V. CONCLUSION

Treatment for CNS damage may be optimized by concentrating efforts on one or more regenerative molecular mechanism that are best influenced by one or a combination of treatments. Steps towards repairing different parts of the CNS have been approached from various angles. Some groups have tried chemical treatments and growth factors. Limiting damage may be done by blocking inhibitors of axonal growth or through the prevention of excitotoxicity, apoptosis, and/ or free radical formation and propagation. A variety of agonist have been tested in animal models and a few have also undergone preliminary clinical testing. The glutamate receptor class of AMPA receptors in excitotoxicity may be blocked antagonistically. Anti-apoptotic drugs may also prevent some cell death.[75,121]. Anti-inflammatories, such as the antibiotic, minocycline, has been used to suppress cytokines, Il-1β and IL-6, tumor necrosis factor alpha, as well as oxygen biproducts, nitric oxide, and reactive oxygen species – all of which are released by microglia from inflammation resultant of AD, PD, AIDS dementia – resulting from brain ischemic events that suppress the resultant neurogenesis.[30] These treatments as well as others may be combined with stem cell therapy to provide the most efficient route for regenerating a healthy CNS. Figuring out what exactly is needed to regain the pre-injury or pre-disease homeostasis in the CNS is necessary for its restoration.

Stem cell therapy may offer more specificity than adding unknown amounts of putative necessary growth factors for regeneration. A stem cell can integrate, adapt, and possibility support and/or be supported by a biological environment. Adult and/or embryonic stem cells could aid the survival of endogenous cells to preserve the brain or spinal cord. Implanted stem cells may or may not actually replace the damaged and dieing cells but express extracellular matrix proteins to provide a framework for the attachment and growth of endogenous neural cells or stem cells. Appropriate ratios of growth factors/cytokines can be implied as supportive or conducive for cell life or the proliferation of cells. The addition of these supportive factors may be specific to particular time points during brain ischemia or glial scar formation in the spinal cord or the disease course of PD and HD, requiring inductive factors at different time points in different geographical locations, for recovery. In essence, we need to find ways to promote the degenerating environment into a regenerating environment.

Given the complexity of CNS damage, the greatest improvement from stem cells may result from their potential plasticity to provide all the necessary and highly specific support and nutrients. The stem cells may also deliver their own anti-inflammatory properties to deter microglia or suppress the byproducts of microglia, the chemokines and reactive oxygen species, that elicit inflammation, that would obstruct neurogenesis. [104] Although the CNS offers an inhospitable environment for regeneration it also has immunopriveledging that would probably allow for the acceptance of a non-autologous cell therapy treatment than other systems in the human body.

Stem cell biology and tissue engineering have evolved as a potential treatment for diseases. The most recent synthetic biomaterials strive to mimic natural extracellular matrix for the purpose of directing stem cell differentiation and restructuring the organ. The prospect of stem cells as a regenerative medicine has expanded from the scientific community into the lay community. The therapeutic possibilities for disease management range from cardiac failure to neural degenerative diseases.

Cell therapies should be considered for implementation in optimized biological settings, with or without a scaffolding. There are essential factors to be considered: 1. Replication of the architecture and the complex cellular interdependence of the normal tissue, 2. Angiogenesis is necessary to supply nutrience to the cells during integration, 3. The host tissue must interface with the grafted cells, 4. There must be specific in vivo functioning ability, and 5. The realistic application (low-cost, sterility prior to implantation, and maintained during storage/transport). 6. Any specialized biological functions must be within the range of their regular behavior [91]

REFERENCES

[1]   Altman J and Das GD. Autoradiographic and histological evidence of postnatal hippocampal neurogenesis in rats. *Journal of Comparative Neurology.* 124, 319-335. 1965.

[2]   Alvarez-Buylla A, Seri B, and Doetsch F. Identification of neural stem cells in the adult vertebrate brain. *Brain Research Bulletin.* 57(6), 751-758. 2002.

[3]   Arminoff MJ. 1998. Parkinson's Disease and Other Extrapyrimidal Disorders *In* Fauci AS, Braunwald E, Isselbacher KJ, Wilson JD, Martin JB, Kasper DJ, Hauser SL, and Longo DL (ed.), *Harrison's Principles of Internal Medicine.* McGraw Hill Health Profession Division, New York.

[4]   Behar O, Mizuno K, Neumann S, and Woolf CJ. Putting the spinal cord together again. *Neuron.* 26, 291-293. 2000.

[5]   Belachew S, Chittajallu R, Aguirre AA, Yuan X, Kirby M, Anderson S, and Gallo V. Postnatal NG2 proteoglycan-expressing progenitor cells are intrinsically multipotent and generate functional neurons. *The Journal of Cell Biology.* 161(1), 169-186. 2003.

[6]   Bernstein BE, Mikkelsen TS, Xie X, Kamal M, Huebert DJ, Cuff J, Fry B, Meissner A, Wernig M, Plath K, Jaenisch R, Wagschal A, Feil R, Schreiber SL, and Lander ES. A bivalent chromatin structure marks key developmental genes in embryonic stem cells. *Cell.* 125(2), 315-326. 2006.

[7]   Bird TD. 1998. Alzheimer's Disease and other Primary Dementias *In* Fauci AS, Braunwald E, Isselbacher KJ, Wilson JD, Martin JB, Kasper DJ, Hauser SL, and Longo

DL (ed.), *Harrison's Principles of Internal Medicine.* McGraw Hill Health Profession Division, New York.

[8] Bottai D, Fiocco R, Gelain F, Defilippis L, Galli R, Gritti A, and Vescovi A. Neural stem cells in the adult nervous system. *Journal of Hematotherapy and Stem Cell Research.* 12, 655-670. 2003.

[9] Boyer LA, Lee TI, Cole MF, Johnstone SE, Levine SS, Zucker JP, Guenther MG, Kumar RM, Murray HL, Jenner RG, Gifford DK, Jaenisch R, and Young RA. Core transcriptional regulatory circuitry in human embryonic stem cells. *Cell.* 122(6), 947-956. 2005.

[10] Boyer LA, Plath K, Zeitlinger J, Brambrink T, Medeiros LA, Lee TI, Levine SS, Wernig M, Tajonar A, Ray MK, Bell GW, Ote AP, Vidal M, Gifford DK, Young RA, and Jaenisch R. Polycomb complexes repress developmental regulators in murine embryonic stem cells. *Nature.* 441(7091), 349-353. 2006.

[11] Brinton RD and Wang JM. Therapeutic potential of neurogenesis for prevention and recovery from Alzheimer's disease: allopregnanolone as a proof of concept neurogeneic agent. *Current Alzheimer Research.* 3(3), 185-190. 2006.

[12] Brodal P. 1998. The central nervous system. Oxford University Press, Inc., Oxford.

[13] Bush TG, Puvanachandra N, Horner CH, Svendsen CN, Mucke L, Johnson MH, and Sofroniew MV. Leukocyte infiltration, neuronal degeneration, and neurite outgrowth after ablation of scar-forming, reactive astrocytes in adult transgenic mice. *Neuron.* 23, 297-308. 1999.

[14] Cameron HA, Hazel TG, and McKay RD. Regulation of neurogenesis by growth factors and neurotransmitters. *Journal of Neurobiology.* 36, 287-306. 1998.

[15] Cao Q, Benton RL, and Whittemore SR. Stem cell repair of central nervous system injury. *Journal of Neuroscience Research.* 68, 501-510. 2002.

[16] Cao Q, Zhang YP, Howard RM, Walters WM, Tsoulfas P, and Whittemore SR. Pluripotent stem cells engrafted into the normal or lesioned adult rat spinal cord are restricted to a glial lineage. *Experimental Neurology.* 167, 48-58. 2001.

[17] Carpenter MK, Hu Z, Jackson J, Sherman S, Seiger A, and Wahlberg LU. In vitro expansion of a multipotent population of human neural progenitor cells. *Experimental Neurology.* 158, 265-278. 1999.

[18] Chen Q. Molecular basis of behavioral recovery following spinal cord decompression: an immunocytochemical study. *Chinese Medical Journal.* 113(8), 737-742. 2000.

[19] Chen YW, Chiou SH, Wong TT, Ku HH, Lin HT, Chung SH, Yen SH, and Kao CL. Using gelatin scaffold with coated basic fibroblast growth factor as a transfer system for transplantation of human neural stem cells. *Transplantation Proceedings.* 38, 1616-1617. 2006.

[20] Chichung Lie D, Dziewczapolski G, Willhoite AR, Kaspar BK, Shults CW, and Gage FH. The adult substantia nigra contains progenitor cells with neurogenic potential. *Journal of Neuroscience.* 22(15), 6639-6649. 2002.

[21] Chopp M, Zhang XH, Li Y, Wang L, Chen J, Lu D, Lu M, and Rosenblum M. Spinal cord injury in rat: treatment with bone marrow stromal cell transplantation. *Neuroreport.* 11(13), 3001-3005. 2000.

[22] Ciccolini F. Identification of two distinct types of multipotent neural precursors that appear sequentially during CNS development. *Molecular and Cellular Neuroscience.* 17, 895-907. 2001.

[23] Clark WM, Hazel S, and Coull BM. Lazaroids. *Drugs.* 50(6), 971-983. 1995.

[24] Crosnier C, Stamataki D, and Lewis J. Organizing cell renewal in the intestine: stem cells, signals, and combinatorial control. *Nature Review in Genetics* 7(5), 349-359. 2006.

[25] David S and Lacroix S. Molecular approaches to spinal cord repair. *AR Reviews in Advance.* 19(21), 441-440. 2003.

[26] Diers-Fenger M, Kirchhoff F, Kettenmann H, Levine JM, and Trotter J. AN2/NG2 protein-expressing glial progenitor cells in the murine CNS: isolation, differentiation, and association with radial glia. *Glia.* 34, 213-228. 2001.

[27] Doetsch F, Garcia-Verdugo JM, and Alvarez-Buylla A. Regeneration of a germinal layer in the adult mammalian brain. *Proceedings of the National Academy of Science USA.* 96, 11619-11624. 1999.

[28] Draper JS, Smith K, Gokhale P, Moore HD, Maltby E, Johnson J, Meisner L, Zwaka TP, Thomson JA, and Andrews PW. Recurrent gain of chromosomes 17q and 12 in cultured human embryonic stem cells. *Nature Biotechnology.* 22(1), 53-54. 2004.

[29] Draper JS, Smith K, Gokhale P, Moore HD, Maltby E, Johnson J, Meisner L, Zwaka TP, Thomson JA, and Andrews PW. Recurrent gain of chromosomes 17q and 12 in cultured human embryonic stem cells. *Nature Biotechnology.* 22(1), 53-54. 2004.

[30] Ekdahl CT, Claasen J, Bonde S, Kokaia Z, and Lindvall O. Inflammation is detrimental for neurogenesis in adult brain. *Proc. Natl. Acad. Sci. U S A.* 100(23), 13632-13637. 2003.

[31] Emsley JG, Mitchell BD, Kempermann G, and Macklis JD. Adult neurogenesis and repair of the adult CNS with neural progenitors, precursors, and stem cells. *Progress in Neurobiology.* 75, 321-341. 2005.

[32] Fawcett JW and Asher RA. The glial scar and central nervous system repair. *Brain Research Bulletin.* 49(6), 377-391. 1999.

[33] Fehlings MG, Sekhon LHS, and Tator C. The role and timing of decompression in acute spinal cord injury. *Spine.* 26(24S), S101-S110. 2001.

[34] Fitch MT, Doller C, COmbs CK, Landreth GE, and Silver J. Cellular and molecular mechanisms of glial scarring and progressive cavitation: in vivo and in vitro analysis of inflammation-induced secondary injury after CNS trauma. *The Journal of Neuroscience.* 19(19), 8182-8198. 1999.

[35] Freed CR, Greene PE, Breeze RE, Tsai WY, DuMouchel W, Kao R, Dillon S, Winfield H, Culver S, Trojanowski JQ, Eidelberg D, and Fahn S. Transplantation of embryonic dopamine neurons for severe Parkinson's disease. *New England Journal of Medicine.* 344(10), 710-719. 2001.

[36] Fricker-Gates RA, Winkler C, Kirik D, Rosenblad C, Carpenter MK, and Bjorklund A. EGF infusion stimulates the proliferation and migration of embryonic progenitor cells transplanted in the adult rat striatum. *Experimental Neurology.* 165, 237-247. 2000.

[37] Friedrich G and Soriano P. Promoter traps in embryonic stem cells: a genetic screen to identify and mutate developmental genes in mice. Genes Dev. 5(9), 1513-1523. 1991.

[38] Gage FH, Ray J, and Fisher LJ. Isolation, characterization, and use of stem cells from the CNS. *Annual Review of Neuroscience.* 18, 159-192. 1995.

[39] Garcia-Alias G, Lopez-Vales R, Fores J, Navarro X, and Verdu E. Acute transplantation of olfactory ensheathing cells or Schwann cells promotes recovery after spinal cord injury in the rat. *Journal of Neuroscience Research.* 75(5), 632-641. 2004.

[40] Goldman SA and Windrem MS. Cell replacement therapy in neurological disease. *Phil. Trans. R. Sco. B.* 361, 1463-1475. 2006.

[41] Grothe C and Nikkah G. The role of basic fibroblast growth factor in peripheral nerve regeneration. *Anatomical Embryology,* 171-177. 2001.

[42] Gruner JA. A monitored contusion model of spinal cord injury in the rat. *Journal of Neurotrauma.* 9(2), 123-126. 1992.

[43] Haque NSK, Inokuma NS, Gold JS, Rao MS, and Carpenter MK. Transplantation of pluripotent human embryonic stem cells and their derivatives into the mammalian brain. *Social Neuroscience Abstract.* 327, 8. 2005.

[44] Haughey NJ, Liu D, Nath A, Borchard AC, and Mattson MP. Disruption of neurogeneis in the subventricular zone of adult mice, and in human cortical neuronal precursor cells in culture, by amyloid beta-peptide: implications for the pathogenesis of Alzheimer's disease. *Neuromolecular Medicine.* 1(2), 125-135. 2002.

[45] Hofstetter CP, Schwarz EJ, Hess D, Widenfalk J, Manira AE, Prockop DJ, and Olson L. Marrow stromal cells form guiding strands in the injured spinal cord and promote recovery. *Proceedings of the National Academy of Science USA.* 99(4), 2199-2204. 2002.

[46] Jiang Y, Jahagirdar BN, Reinhardt RL, Schwartz RE, Keene CD, Ortiz-Gonzalez XR, Reyes M, Lenvik T, Lund T, Du J, Lisberg A, Low WC, Largaespada DA, and Verfaille CM. Pluripotency of mesenchymal stem cells derived from adult marrow. *Nature.* 418, 41-49. 2002.

[47] Johann V, Schiefer J, Sass C, Mey J, Brook G, Kruttgen A, Schlangen C, Bernreuther C, Schachner M, Dihne M, and Kosinski CM. Time of transplantation and cell preparation determine neural stem cell survival in a mouse model of Huntington's disease. *Experimental Brain Research Epub:* Sept 30. 2006.

[48] Jomura S, Uy M, Mitchell K, Dallasen R, Bode C, and Xu Y. Potential treatment of cerebral global ischemia with Oct-4+ umbilical cord matrix cells. *Stem Cells Epub:* Sept 7. 2006.

[49] Jones LL, Yamaguchi Y, Stallcup WB, and Tuszynski MH. NG2 is a major chondroitin sulfate proteoglycan produced after spinal cord injury and is expressed by macrophges and oligodendrocyte progenitors. The Journal of Neuroscience 22(7), 2792-2803. 2002.

[50] Kempermann G and Neumann H. Microglia: The enemy within? *Science.* 302, 1689-1690. 2003.

[51] Keyoung HM, Roy NS, Benraiss A, Louissaint A, Suzuki A, Hashimoto M, Rashbaum WK, Okano H, and Goldman SA. High-yield selection and extraction of two promoter-defined phenotypes of neural stem cells from the fetal human brain. *Nature Biotechnology.* 19, 843-850. 2001.

[52] Kordower JH, Freeman TB, Snow BJ, Vingerhoets FJ, Mufson EJ, Sanberg PR, Hauser RA, Nauert GM, and e. al. Perl DP. Neuropathological evidence of graft survival and

striatal reinnervation after the transplantation of fetal mesencephalic tisue in a patient with Parkinson's disease. *New England Journal of Medicine.* 332(17), 1118-1124. 1995.

[53] Kuhn HG and Svendsen CN. Origins, functions, and potential of adult neural stem cells. *BioEssays.* 21(8), 625-630. 1999.

[54] Kuhn HG, Winkler J, Kempermann G, Thal LJ, and Gage FH. Epidermal growth factor and fibroblast growth factor-2 have different effects on neural progenitors in the adult rat brain. *The Journal of Neuroscience.* 17(15), 5820-5829. 1997.

[55] Kwak YD, Brannen CL, Ou T, Kim HM, Dong X, Soba P, Majumdar A, Kaplan A, Bevreuther K, and Sugaya K. Amyloid precursor protein regulates differentiation of human neural stem cells. *Stem Cells Development.* 15(3), 381-389. 2006.

[56] Laywell ED, Kukekov VG, and Steindler DA. Multipotent neurospheres can be derived from forebrain subependymal zone and spinal cord of adult mice after protracted postmortem intervals. *Experimental Neurology.* 156, 430-433. 1999.

[57] Levine JM, Reynolds R, and Fawcett JW. The oligodendrocyte precursor cell in health and disease. *Trends in Neuroscience.* 24, 39-47. 2001.

[58] Li S, Mealing GAR, Morley P, and Stys PK. Novel injury mechanism in anoxia and trauma of spinal cord white matter: glutamate release via reverse Na-dependent glutamate transport. *The Journal of Neuroscience.* 19, 1-9. 1999.

[59] Lindvall O and Hagell P. Clinical observations after neural tranplantation in Parkinson's disease. *Progress in Brain Research.* 127, 299-320. 2000.

[60] Lindvall O and Kokaia Z. Stem cell therapy for human brain disorders. *Kidney International.* 68, 1937-1939. 2005.

[61] Liu J, Solway K, Messing RO, and Sharp FR. Increased neurogenesis in the dentate gyrus after transient global ischemia in gerbils. *The Journal of Neuroscience.* 18(19), 7768-7778. 1998.

[62] Liu S, Qu Y, Stewart TJ, HOward MJ, Chakrabortty S, Holekamp TF, and McDonald JW. Embryonic stem cells differentiate into oligodendrocytes and myelinate in culture and after spinal cord transplantation. *Proceedings of the National Academy of Science USA.* 97(11), 6126-6131. 2000.

[63] Liu XZ, Xu XM, HuR, DuC, Zhang SX, McDonald JW, Dong HX, Wu YJ, Fan GS, Jacquin MF, Hsu CY, and Choi DW. *Neuronal and glial apoptosis after traumatic spinal cord injury.* 17 (14), 5395-5406. 1997.

[64] Liu Y, Han SSW, Wu Y, Tuohy T, Xue H, Cai J, Back SA, Sherman LS, Fischer I, and Rao MS. CD44 expression identifies astrocyte-restricted precursor cells. *Developmental Biology.* 276, 31-46. 2004.

[65] Lobo MVT, Alonso FJM, Redondo C, Lopez-Toledano MA, Caso E, Herranz AS, Paino CL, Reimers D, and Bazan E. Cellular characterization of epidermal growth factor-expanded free-floating neurospheres. *The Journal of Histochemistry and Cytochemistry.* 51(1), 89-103. 2003.

[66] Lu P, Jones LL, Snyder EY, and Tuszynski MH. Neural stem cells constitutively secrete neurotrophic factors and promote extensive host axonal growth after spinal cord injury. *Experimental Neurology.* 181, 115-129. 2003.

[67] Lucas PA, Calcutt AF, Southerland SS, Wilson JA, Harvey RL, and Young HE. A population of cells resident within embryonic and newbornrat skeletal muscle is capable of differentiating into multiple mesodermal phenotypes. *Wound Repair and Regeneration.* 3, 449-460. 1995.

[68] Magavi SS, Leavitt BR, and Macklis JD. Induction of neurogenesis in the neocortex of adult mice. *Nature.* 405, 951-955. 2000.

[69] Malouf NN, Coleman WB, Grisham JW, Lininger RA, Madden VJ, Sproul M, and Anderson PA. Adult-derived stem cells from the liver become myocytes in the heart in vivo. *American Journal of Pathology.* 158(6), 1929-1935. 2001.

[70] Martens DJ, Tropepe V, and van der Kooy D. Separate proliferation kinetics of fibroblast growth factor-responsive and epidermal growth factor-responsive neural stem cells within the embryonic forebrain germinal zone. *Journal of Neuroscience.* 20(3), 1085-1095. 2000.

[71] Martin JB and Longo FM. 1998. Molecular Diagnosis of Neurologic Disorders *In* Fauci AS, Braunwald E, Isselbacher KJ, Wilson JD, Martin JB, Kasper DJ, Hauser SL, and Longo DL (ed.), *Harrison's Priniciples of Internal Medicine.* McGraw Hill Health Profession Division, New York.

[72] Martin MJ, Muotri A, Gage F, and et al. Human embryonic stem cells express an immunogenic nonhuman sialic acid. *Nature Medicine.* 11, 228-232. 2005.

[73] Matsuoka N, Nozaki K, Takagi Y, Nishimura M, Hayashi J, Miyatake S, and Hashimoto N. Adenovirus-mediated gene transfer of fibroblast growth factor-2 increases BrdU-positive cells after forebrain ischemia in gerbils. *Stroke.* 34, 1519-1525. 2002.

[74] McDonald JW, Liu X, Qu Y, Liu S, Mickey SK, Turetsky D, Gottlieb DI, and Choi DW. Transplanted embryonic stem cells survive, differentiate, and promote recovery in injured rat spinal cord. *Nature Medicine.* 5(12), 1410-1412. 1999.

[75] McDonald JW and the Research Consortium of the Christopher Reeve Paralysis Foundation. Repairing the damaged spinal cord. Scientific American , 65-73. 1999.

[76] McKay R. Stem cells in the central nervous system. *Science.* 276, 66-71. 1997.

[77] Mehler MF and Gokhan S. Postnatal cerebral cortical multipotent progenitors: regulatory mechanisms and potential role in the development of novel neural regenerative strategies. *Brain Pathology.* 9, 515-526. 1999.

[78] Merkle FT, Tramontin AD, Garcia-Verdugo JM, and Alvarez-Buylla A. Radial glia give rise to adult neural stem cells in the subventricular zone. *Proceedings of the National Academy of Science USA.* 101(50), 17528-17532. 2004.

[79] Mezey E and Chandross KJ. Bone marrow: a possible alternative source of cells in the adult nervous system. *European Journal of Pharmacology.* 405(1-3), 297-302. 2000.

[80] Milosevic A and Goldman JE. Progenitors in the postnatal cerebellar white matter are antigenically heterogeneous. *The Journal of Comparative Neurology.* 452, 192-203. 2002.

[81] Monje ML, Mizumatsu S, Fike JR, and Palmer TD. *Nature Medicine.* 8, 955. 2002.

[82] Moore KA and Lemischka IR. Stem cells and their niches. *Science.* 311, 1880-1885. 2006.

[83]   Moyer MP, Johnson RA, Zompa EA, Cain L, Morshed T, and Hulsebosch CE. Culture, expansion, and transplantation of human fetal neural progenitor cells. *Transplantation Proceedings.* 29, 2040-2041. 1997.

[84]   Ohta M, Suzuki Y, Noda T, Ejiri Y, Dezawa M, Kataoka K, Chou H, Ishikawa N, Matsumoto N, Iwashita Y, Mizuta E, Kuno S, and Ide C. Bone marrow stromal cells infused into the cerebrospinal fluid promote functional recovery of the injured rat spinal cord with reduced cavity formation. *Experimental Neurology.* 187, 266-278. 2004.

[85]   Palmer TD, Ray J, and Gage FH. FGF-2-responsive neuronal progenitors reside in proliferative and quiescent regions of the adult rodent brain. *Molecular and Cellular Neuroscience.* 6(5), 474-486. 1995.

[86]   Pankratz N and Foroud T. Genetics of Parkinson Disease. NeuroRx: *The Journal of the American Society for Experimental NeuroTherapeutics.* 1, 235-242. 2004.

[87]   Perrier AL, Tabar V, Barberi T, Rubio ME, Bruses J, Topf N, Harrison NL, and Studer L. Derivation of midbrain dopamine neurons from human embryonic stem cells. *Proc. Natl. Acad. Sci. U S A.* 101(34), 12543-12548. 2004.

[88]   Picard-Riera N, Nait-Oumesmar B, and Baron-Van Evercooren A. Endogenous adult neural stem cells: limits and potential to repair the injured central nervous system. *Journal of Neuroscience Research.* 76(2), 223-231. 2004.

[89]   Piccini P, Brooks DJ, Bjorklund A, Gunn RN, Grasby PM, Rimoldi O, Brundi P, Hagell P, Rehncrona S, Widner H, and Lindvall O. Dopamine release from nigral transplants visualized in vivo in a Parkinson's patient. *Nat. Neurosci.* 2(12), 1137-1140. 1999.

[90]   Pineda JR, Rubio N, Akerud P, Urban N, Badimon L, Arenas E, Alberch J, Blanco J, and Canals JM. Neuroprotection by GDNF-secreting stem cells in a Huntington's disease model: optical neuroimage tracking of brain-grafted cells. *Nature Gene Therapy.* (Epub: Aug 31), 1-11. 2006.

[91]   Polak JM and Bishop AE. Stem cells and tissue engineering: past, present, and future. *Annuals of New York Academy of Science.* 1068, 352-366. 2006.

[92]   Polgar S, Borlongan CV, Koutouzis TK, Todd SL, Cahill DW, and Sanberg PR. Implications of neurological rehabilitation for advancing intracerebral transplantation. *Brain Research Bulletin.* 44(3), 229-232. 1997.

[93]   Ramon-Cueto A, Cordero MI, Santos-Benito F, and Avila J. Functional recovery of paraplegic rats and motor axon regeneration in their spinal cords by olfactory ensheathing glia. *Neuron.* 25, 425-435. 2000.

[94]   Reh TA. Neural stem cells: form and function. *Nature Neuroscience.* 5(5), 392-394. 2002.

[95]   Reier PJ, Perlow MJ, and Guth L. Development of embryonic spinal cord transplants in the rat. *Brain Research.* 312(2), 201-219. 1983.

[96]   Reubinoff BE, Pera MF, Fong CY, Trouson A, and Bongso A. Embryonic stem cell lines from human blastocysts: somatic differentiation in vivo. *Nature Biotechnology.* 18, 399-404. 2000.

[97]   Rohwedel J, Guan K, and Wobus AM. Induction of cellular differentiation by retinoic acid in vitro. *Cells Tissues Organs.* 165, 190-202. 1999.

[98] Romero-Ramos M, Vourc'h P, Young HE, Lucas PA, Wu Y, Chivatakarn O, Zaman R, Dunkelman N, El-Kalay MA, and Chesselet M. Neuronal differentiation of stem cells isolated from adult muscle. *Journal of Neuroscience Research.* 69, 894-907. 2002.

[99] Roy NS, Cleren C, Singh SK, Yang L, Beal MF, and Goldman SA. Functional engraftment of human ES cell-derived dopaminergic neurons enriched by coculture with telomerase-immortalized midbrain astrocytes. *Nature Medicine.* 6(3), 271-277. 2006.

[100] Roy NS, Wang S, Jiang L, Kang J, Benraiss A, Harrison-Restelli C, Fraser RA, Couldwell WT, Kawaguchi A, Okano H, Nedergaard M, and Goldman A. In vitro neurogenesis by progenitor cells isolated from the adult human hippocampus. *Nature Medicine.* 6(3), 271-277. 2000.

[101] Sattler R, Xiong Z, Lu W, MacDonald JF, and Tymianski M. Distinct rolse of synaptic and extrasynaptic NMDA receptors in excitotoxicity. *The Journal of Neuroscience.* 20(1), 22-33. 2000.

[102] Schmidt W and Reymann KG. Proliferating cells differentiate into neurons in the hippocampal CA1 region of gerbils after global cerebral ischemia. *Neuroscience Letters.* 334(3), 153-156. 2002.

[103] Schuller BW, Binns PJ, Riley KJ, Ma L, Hawthorne MF, and Coderre JA. Selective irradiation of the vascular endothelium has no effect on the survival of murine intestinal crypt stem cells. *Proc. Natl. Acad. Sci. U S A.* 103(10), 3787-3792. 2006.

[104] Schultz SS. Adult stem cells application in spinal cord injury. *Current Drug Targets.* 6(1), 63-73. 2005.

[105] Schultz SS, Abraham S, and Lucas PA. Stem cells isolated from adult rat muscle differentiate across all three dermal lineages. *Wound Repair and Regeneration.* 14(2), 224-231. 2006.

[106] Schultz SS and Lucas PA. Human stem cells isolated from adult skeletal muscle differentiate into neural phenotypes. *Journal of Neuroscience Methods.* 152(1-2), 144-155. 2006.

[107] Schwab ME. Differing views on spinal cord repair. *Science.* 296, 1400. 2002.

[108] Schwatz M and Hauben E. Differing views on spinal cord repair. *Science.* 296, 1400. 2002.

[109] Sharp FR, Liu J, and Bernabeu R. Neurogenesis following brain ischemia. *Developmental Brain Research.* 134, 23-30. 2002.

[110] Shen Y, Chow J, Wang Z, and Fan G. Abnormal CpG island methylation occurs during in vitro differentiation of human embryonic stem cells. *Hum. Mol. Genet.* 15(17), 2623-2635. 2006.

[111] Shihabuddin LS, Ray J, and Gage FH. FGF-2 is sufficient to isolate progenitors found in the audlt mammalian spinal cord. *Experimental Neurology.* 148(2), 577-586. 1997.

[112] Singec I, Knoth R, Meyer RP, Maciaczyk J, Volk B, Nikkhah G, Frotscher M, and Snyder EY. Defining the actual sensitivity and specificity of the neurosphere assay in stem cell biology. *Nature Methods.* 3(10), 801-806. 2006.

[113] Singh SK, Clarke ID, Hide T, and Dirks PB. Cancer stem cells in nervous system tumors. *Oncogene.* 23, 7267-7273. 2004.

[114] Singh SK, Clarke ID, Terasaki M, Bonn VE, Hawkins C, Squire J, and Dirks PB. Identification of a cancer stem cell in human brain tumors. *Cancer Research.* 63, 5821-5828. 2003.

[115] Steiner B, Kronenberg G, Jessberger S, Brandt MD, Reuter K, and Kempermann G. Differential regulation of gliogenesis in the context of adult hippocampal neurogenesis in mice. *Glia.* 46, 41-52. 2004.

[116] Stewart R, Christie VB, and Przyborski SA. Manipulation of human pluripotent embryonal carcinoma stem cells and the development of neural subtypes. *Stem Cells.* 21, 248-256. 2003.

[117] Strubing C, Ahnert-Hilger G, Shan J, Wiedenmann B, Hescheler J, and Wobus AM. Differentiation of pluripotent embryonic stem cells into the neuronal lineage in vitro gives rise to mature inhibitory and excitatory neurons. *Mechanisms of Development?* 53, 275-287. 1995.

[118] Studer L, Csete M, Lees SH, Kabbani N, Walikonis B, Wold B, and McKay R. Enhanced proliferation, survival, and dopaminergic differentiation of CNS precursors in lowered oxygen. *Journal of Neuroscience.* 20, 7377-7383. 2000.

[119] Sugava K. Possible use of autologous stem cell therapies for Alzheimer's disease. *Current Alzheimer Research.* 2(3), 367-376. 2005.

[120] Svendsen CN, ter Borg MG, Armstrong RJE, Rosser AE, Chandran S, Ostenfeld T, and Caldwell MA. A new method for the rapid and long term growth of human neural precursor cells. *Journal of Neuroscience Methods.* 85, 141-152. 1998.

[121] Tator CH. Strategies for recovery and regeneration after brain and spinal cord injury. *Injury Prevention.* 8, iv33-iv36. 2002.

[122] Tend YD, Lavik EB, Qu X, Park KI, Ourednik J, Zurakowski D, Langer R, and Snyder EY. Functional recovery following traumatic spinal cord injury mediated by a unique polymer scaffold seeded with neural stem cells. *Proceedings of the National Academy of Science USA.* 99(5), 3024-3029. 2002.

[123] Theriault E, Frankenstein UN, Hertzberg EL, and Nagy JI. Connexin43 and astrocytic gap junctions in the rat spinal cord after acute compression injury. *The Journal of Comparative Neurology.* 382, 199-214. 1997.

[124] van Praag H, Schinder AF, Christie BR, Toni N, Palmer TD, and Gage FH. Functional neurogenesis in the adult hippocampus. *Nature.* 415(6875), 1030-1034. 2002.

[125] Villa A, Rubio FJ, Navarro B, Bueno C, and Martinez-Serrano A. Human neural stem cells in vitro. A focus on their isolation and perpetuation. *Biomedical Pharmacotherapy.* 55, 91-95. 2001.

[126] Vroemen M, Aigner L, WInkler J, and Weidner N. Adult neural progenitor cell grafts survive after acute spinal cord injury and integrate along axonal pathways. *European Journal of Neuroscience.* 18, 743-751. 2003.

[127] Wachs F, Couillard-Despres S, Engelhardt M, Wilhelm D, Ploetz S, Vroemen M, Kaesbauer J, Uyanik G, Klucken J, Karl C, Tebbing J, Svendsen C, Weidner N, Kuhn H, WInkler J, and Aigner L. High efficacy of clonal growth and expansion of adult neural stem cells. *Laboratory Investigation.* 83(7), 949-962. 2003.

[128] Wang K, Wang J, Wang Y, He Q, Wang X, and Wang X. Infusion of epidermal growth factor and basic fibroblast growth factor into the striatum of parkinsonian rats leads to

in vitro proliferation and differentiation of adult neural progenitor cells. *Neuroscience Letters.* 364, 154-158. 2004.

[129] Wang TY, Sen A, Behie LA, and Kallos MS. Dynamic behavior of cells within neurospheres in expanding pupulations of neural precursors. *Brain Research.* 1107, 82-96. 2006.

[130] Warejcka DJ, Harvey R, Taylor BJ, Young HE, and Lucas PA. A population of cells isolated from rat heart capable of differentiating into several mesodermal phenotypes. *Journal of Surgical Research.* 62, 233-242. 1996.

[131] Weidner S, Blesch A, and Tuszynski MH. Nerve growth factor-hypersecreting schwann cell grafts augment and guide spinal cord axonal growth and remyelinate central nervous system axons in a phenotypically appropriate manner that correlates with expression of L1. *The Journal of Comparative Neurology.* 413, 495-506. 1999.

[132] Weiss S, Dunne C, Hewson J, Wohl C, Wheatley M, Peterson AC, and Reynolds BA. Multipotent CNS stem cells are present in the adult mammalian spinal cord and ventricular neuroaxis. *The Journal of Neuroscience.* 16(23), 7599-7609. 1996.

[133] Wichterle H, Lieberam I, Porter JA, and Jessell TM. Directed differentiation of embryonic stem cells into motor neurons. *Cell.* 110, 385-397. 2002.

[134] Winner B, Geyer M, Couillard-Despres S, Aigner R, Bogdahn U, Aigner L, Kuhn G, and WInkler J. Striatal deafferentation increases dopaminergic neurogenesis in the adult olfactory bulb. *Exp. Neurol.* 197(1), 113-121. 2006.

[135] Wobus AM and Boheler KR. Embryonic stem cells: prospects for developmental biology and cell therapy. *Physiology Review.* 85, 635-678. 2005.

[136] Woodbury D, Reynolds K, and Black IB. Adult bone marrow stromal stem cells express germline, ectodermal, endodermal, and mesodermal genes prior to neurogenesis. *The Journal of Neuroscience.* 69(6), 908-917. 2002.

[137] Woodbury D, Schwarz EJ, Prockop DJ, and Black IB. Adult rat and human bone marrow stromal cells differentiate into neurons. *Journal of Neuroscience Research.* 61, 364-370. 2000.

[138] Wu S, Suzuki Y, Noda T, Bai H, Kitada M, Kataoka K, Nishimura Y, and Ide C. Immunohistochemical and electron microscopic study of invasion and differentiation in spinal cord lesion of neural stem cells grafted through cerebrospinal fluid in rat. *Journal of Neuroscience Research.* 69, 940-945. 2002.

[139] Yamamoto S, Yamamoto N, Kitamura T, Nakamura K, and Nakafuku M. Proliferation of parenchymal neural progenitors in response to injury in the adult rat spinal cord. *Experimental Neurology.* 172, 115-127. 2001.

[140] Yang Z and Levinson SW. Hypoxia/ischemia expands the regenerative capacity of progenitors in the perinatal subventricular zone. *Neuroscience.* 139(2), 555-564. 2006.

[141] Yokoyama A, Yang L, Itoh S, Mori K, and Tanaka J. Microglia, a potential source of neurons, astrocytes, and oligodendrocytes. *Glia.* 45, 96-104. 2004.

[142] Young HE, Steele TA, Bray RA, Hudson J, Floyd JA, Hawkins K, Thomas K, Austin T, Edwards C, Cuzzourt J, Duenzl M, Lucas PA, and Black ASAC. Human reserve pluripotent mesenchymal stem cells are present in the connective tissues of skeletal muscle and dermis derived from fetal, adult, and geriatric donors. *The Anatomical Record.* 264, 51-62. 2001.

[143] Zhou L, Del Villar K, Dong Z, and Miller CA. Neurogenesis response to hypoxia-induced cell death: map kinase signal transduction mechanisms. *Brain Research.* 1021, 8-19. 2004.

[144] Zuk PA, Benhaim P, and Hedrick MH. 2004. Stem cells from adipose tissue., p. 425-447. *In* Lanza R, Blau H, Melton D, Moore M, Thomas ED, Verfaille C, Weissman I, and West M (ed.), *Handbook of Stem Cells: Adult and Fetal Stem Cells.* Elsevier Academic Press, Burlington, MA.

[145] Zukin RS, Jover T, Yokota H, Calderone A, Simionescu M, and Lau CG. 2004. Molecular and cellular mechanisms of ischemia-induced neuronal death, p. 829-849. *Stroke.*

In: Stem Cell Research Developments
Editor: Calvin A. Fong, pp. 161-186

ISBN: 978-1-60021-601-5
© 2007 Nova Science Publishers, Inc.

Chapter V

Fibrocytes, Mesenchymal Stem Cells and Monocytes: Who Is Who in Circulating Stem Cells ?

Pablo Gomez-Ochoa[1], Francisco Gomez[2], Javier Miana[3], Maria Jesus Munoz[4], Manuel Gascon[5], Juan Antonio Castillo[6], Ignacio Gomez[7], Luis Larrad[8], Maria Jose Martinez[9], C. Guillermo Couto[10],

[1] Department of Animal Pathology
Veterinary Faculty University of Zaragoza, Spain.
[2] Department of Medicine. Medicine Faculty, University of Zaragoza, Spain.
[3] Department of Pharmacology and Physiology.
Medicine Faculty, University of Zaragoza, Spain.
[4] Department of Pharmacology and Physiology.
Veterinary Faculty, University of Zaragoza, Spain.
[5] Department of Animal Pathology. Veterinary Faculty,
University of Zaragoza, Spain.
[6] Department of Animal Pathology.
Veterinary Faculty, University of Zaragoza, Spain.
[7] Department of Medicine. Medicine Faculty,
University of Zaragoza, Spain.
[8] Department of Medicine. Medicine Faculty,
University of Zaragoza, Spain.
[9] Department of Medicine. Medicine Faculty,
University of Zaragoza, Spain.
[10] Department of Veterinary Clinical Sciences. College of Veterinary
Medicine, The Ohio State University, Columbus, USA.

ABSTRACT

The main purposes of this chapter are to serve as a compilation of all contradictory data on circulating stem cells, and to describe new methods for their isolation and differentiation in animal models.

A population of round cells and spindle cells, morphologically similar to fibroblasts, isolated from the peripheral blood mononuclear cell Buffy coat in a liquid culture medium without any stimulating factors was described in the eighties. In 1997 Bucala called them fibrocytes, and they were immunophenotyped as CD34+, Collagen I+, and Vimentin+. These are powerful antigen-presenting cells -more even than monocytes and dendritic cells- and play an important role in wound repair.

In the last few years, due to the fact that research using human embryonic stem cells raises serious ethical issues, mesenchymal stem cells (MSC) have become the center of attention, even more so when regenerative medicine became a reality. Their presence among bone marrow stromal cells was know, but they were recently found as circulating MSC. These round to elongated cells were first typified as CD14-, CD45-, and CD34-, although there is little consensus because other research teams were unable to repeat these results. However, it is widely accepted that MSCs, also known as mesenchymal progenitor cells, can differentiate into osteocytes, chondrocytes, or adipocytes, and are CD34-, CD45-, CD14-, CD44+, CD13+, CD29+ and CD90+.

In 2003 a monocyte-derived subset of CD45+, CD14+, and CD34+ was isolated from human peripheral blood; hence, monocytes became relevant in stem cell research. These cells were differentiated into mature macrophages, epithelial cells, endothelial cells, hepatocytes, and neurons by Zhao and cols.

Our studies in several animal species using liquid media without stimulating factors, and semisolid media enriched with recombinant human cytokines show growth patterns very similar to those obtained in human beings, with a preponderant CD34+ fibroblast-like cell population. Another relevant finding in these assays that has to be highlighted is the stimulation achieved using only recombinant human cytokines (CSF,IL-3,IL-6, G-CSF, GM-CSF, EPO).

Even though there is a wealth of emerging new data, it clear that starting with the same fibroblastic population different immunophenotypes (pertaining to CD45/CD14/CD34) could be obtained, and completely different tissues could be generated. Despite cursory knowledge in identification and differentiation of these circulating stem cells, several results of ongoing clinical trials will yield advances in regenerative medicine.

SOME PRIOR QUESTIONS

Few findings of cellular exploration are as expressive of "A Store of Inspiration and Effort" [1] as the birth of the concept of the Stem Cell (SC) in the early years of the 20th Century; until then no one had asked whether blood cells were everlasting or if they needed replacing and when, in 1868, Ernst Neumann and Giulio Bizzozero proposed the blood marrow as the seed bed of the blood a great polemic arose.

The first attempt to find the common progenitor of the blood cells was made by Artur Pappenheim with the description of the *Lymphoidozyt*. This was a theoretical creation which linked the morphology of the extensions stained following the Romanowsky method to philosophical speculations, but had the merit of proposing a unitary concept to define the SC. Just a few years later, his disciple Adolfo Ferrata - "a clear thinking, practical Latin" [1] - coined the term *Hemocytoblast* to delimit the second version of the SC concept. This was also based on morphology but added a functional focus which permitted the development of a simple scheme of hematopoiesis which is, to a great extent, still valid today. On a theoretical level it certainly made the concept very clear of a pluripotent SC from which each cell type was derived. However, methodological reality did not yet permit the identification of the individual cell or the observation of its differentiation: it was the moment of the clear concept and the confused cell.

In the 50s and 60s three steps were taken which demonstrated the authenticity of the SC concept. The pioneers were Eugene P. Cronkite, George Brecher y Fredrick Stohlman Jr. who performed the first transfusions of leucocytes in irradiated dogs to protect them from infection. The second step was taken simultaneously by the group of Donald Metcalf and Thomas Ray Bradley in Australia and that of Dov H. Pluznik and Leo Sachs in Israel. In 1966, both groups set up an *in vitro* cloning system for granulocytes and macrophages which marked the route of cell cultures already initiated by Thomas Michael Dexter with the long-term marrow culture system.

The decisive third step was made by Ernest Armstrong McCulloch, James E. Till and L. Simonovich, when they discovered that CFU-S was the SC which was able to reconstitute the complete hematopoiesis when lethally irradiated mice received bone marrow transfusions. This finding closed the circle with the proof of the functionality of the individual stem cell, but there were still insufficient morphological data to identify it and therefore the SC remained unrecognizable.

This initiated a long race to find reliable SC markers and some, such as CD34, remained firmly associated to HSC and clinical use. This third, and current, version of the SC could now allow the proposal of "A new concept of stem cell disorders and their new therapy" [2], although the morphology continues to be an important source of conceptual conflicts.

All the early development of the SC concept was bound to hematopoiesis and the target organ of the methodology was naturally bone marrow. In recent years the proof of the circulation of SCs and their increasing involvement in regenerative medicine moved the focus of attention of research to the circulating SCs. New questions arose to be added to the old ones; some of them have been answered but others still remain when certain prior issues are raised about circulating SCs...

- Is there a single Pluripotent Circulating SC?
- Are Fibroblasts / CFU-F / Fibroblast-like / Fibrocytes the same SC ?
- Do Fibrocytes derive from the HSC ?
- Do MSCs and Fibrocytes share precursors ?
- Are immunophenotypes conclusive for identifying circulation SCs?
- Are Monocytes the true "hidden" SCs of the circulating SCs?
- Is the CD34+ present in all the circulating SCs?
- Do SCs circulate in peripheral blood in appreciable quantities or do they "appear" according to necessity? ...and, at present, "the answer is blowing in the wind".

THE ENCOUNTER WITH THE FIRST CIRCULATING FIBROBLAST-LIKE ... MORE THAN A HUNDRED YEARS LATER

Until the 1980s the F-CFC were only found in bone marrow and connective tissue... although a hundred years ago their peripheral circulation had been suspected.

Fibroblasts are old buddies; they originate in the mesenchyma of the embryo and later repair lesions in the adult connective tissue. The implantation of wound chambers into the subcutaneous tissues of mice showed the rapid appearance of peripheral blood cells and later of other long cells with a fibroblastic morphology, which was always attributed to the recruitment produced in the connective tissue adjacent to the lesion. However, as early as 1902, Maximow described monocyte-to-fibroblast metaplasia in sterile exudates in rabbits, although even he recognised that this was a contribution that more orthodox hematologists would find difficult to accept. Around the same time, Alexis Carrel also reported the finding of fibroblasts from monocyte cultures, but the methodology was not clear and in 1935 JK Moen, using the same Carrel Flasks, observed some "typical fibroblast colonies" when following the growth of mononuclear cells obtained by irritating the guinea pig pleura. In the 1930s and 40s, lymphocytes, previously transformed into Monocytes, were proposed as possible fibroblast precursors, a claim that did not go beyond a mere lucubration (reviewed in Ref. [3]). The consideration of the fibroblast as a circulating cell was a concept that met strong opposition and was left very much in the background in the following years with some exceptions such as the observation of Petrakis [4]. He foun them on human buffy coats placed in diffusion chambers implanted in human volunteers, reporting the presence of a "mesenchymal progenitor cell pool" in the peripheral blood mononuclear cells and the presence of India ink particles first in the macrophages and later in the fibroblasts. Unfortunately, these findings were not given the adequate relevance and the concept of the fibroblast originating in peripheral blood continued to be ignored.

Although their name reflects the characteristic fusiform morphology (*fiber-blastos*) rounded forms were also identified with some cytoplasmatic prolongation and other variants attributable to age which distinguish between the young fibroblast and the old fibroblast or Fibrocyte. The truth is that the morphology of the fibrocytes seems to be highly variable, as are its functions, and the names have been repeatedly changed to adjust to the findings. In 1957, Theodore T. Puck introduced the term Fibroblast-like in a study [5] on "Clonal growth in vitro of human cells with fibroblastic morphology" to integrate the morphological variations of the fibroblasts and to differentiate them from the Epithelioid cells. The name found favour and has been used since then to refer to the fibroblastic forms with stem cell functions [6].

Certainly, the breakthrough in the understanding of the fibroblast physiology came about with the introduction of the methods of long-term tissue cultures of human bone marrow [7] with three typical growth phases (myeloid phase, round-cell phase and fibroblastic) and their systematization on glass substrates [8] in the 1950s. However, nearly another thirty years had to pass for the bone marrow fibroblastoid colony-forming cells (F-CFC) to be characterized in liquid medium cultures, with immunofluorescent staining using monospecific antibodies for the presence and distribution of fibronectin and collagen types[9, 10]. Comparative morphological studies in bone marrow cultures obtained from humans, dogs, and mice were also performed [11] and descriptions were made of the relationships of the medullar fibroblasts with the activation of the CSF and the growth of CFU-GM in medullar aphasia patients [12], their influence on the regulation of canine lymphopoiesis [13] and the possibility that fibroblast-like mouse embryo has the capacity to undergo nonterminal differentiation into macrophages [14].

The identification of the fibroblast-like/F-CFC in cultures of bone marrow and of different tissues in humans and animals contrasted with the absence of these same findings in peripheral blood and in none of the liquid medium cultures of humans [15], dogs [16], or mice [17],could the presence of fibroblastic cells be demonstrated.

The Fibroblast-like were still invisible in peripheral blood.

The Fibroblasts/Fibroblast-Like Appear in Peripheral Blood Mononuclear Cell Cultures

In 1987, when culturing adherent peripheral blood cells of human origin, Gómez-Casal et al. [18] reported the presence of fibroblastic cells on the 5th day of culture, observing the formation of F-CFC colonies on the 15th day of incubation. A modification of the methodology of Kaneko et al. [15] was used and an attempt was made for cytochemical (peroxidise, alkaline phosphatise, sterases and NBT test) and immunological (OKT3, OKT9,OKT10, OKT11....) characterization which did not register any differences between circulating F-CFC and the fibroblasts cultured from bone marrow. Moreover circulating ones demonstrated positivity to the NBT test, to the monoclonal antibody D-Macrophage and to the sterases thus suggesting the existence of phagocytic activity. A study was also performed dealing with the impact of several drugs ans some diseases in the behaviour of the culture and it was demonstrated that sodium dichlophenac and mepivacaine inhibited their growth while hydrocortisone at doses of 0.05mg/ml increased fibroblastic proliferation. Also some hemopathies such as chronic myeloid leukaemia and the non Hodgkin lymphomas or prior cytostatic treatments also modified their behaviour in culture [19].

In 1994 Bucala [20] reported "a New Leukocyte Subpopulation that mediates Tissue Repair" formed by Blood-Borne Fibrocytes in cultures of human and mouse adherent peripheral blood cells. He followed the usual methodology, including the addition of 20% fetal bovine serum and the depletion of nonadherent cells by aspiration and at weekly intervals the cultures were replenished with fresh medium. The morphological studies were performed after 6 weeks of culture and included immunofluorescence and FACS analysis and Light/Electron Microscopy. The proliferant cells had a spindle-shaped morphology which was very similar to that of the fibroblast-like and since then have been called Fibrocytes. The analysis with FACS required the collection of the cells by gentle scraping and trituration and direct incubation with antibodies. The observation of the results identified the Fibrocytes as follows:.

- **Positive** : Collagen I and III, Vimentine, Fibronectine,
CD11,CD18,CD34,CD45,CD71

- **Negative :** Sterases, Cytokeratine, F. Von Willebrand, Desmin
CD14,CD33,CD38,CD25,CD54,CD56

From the analysis of these data, and especially of the positivity to CD34 and to Vimentine and Collagen I, the hypothesis was formulated that attributes to the Fibrocyte the identity of a circulation population of uncommitted or incompletely differentiated fibroblastic precursors which would probably have a medullar origin.

For the first time the Fibroblasts/Fibroblast-like were visible in peripheral blood with the name of Fibrocytes.

The Identifying Fingerprints of the Fibrocyte

The expression of surface markers on fibrocytes was gradually completed in the ten years following its discovery until a very specific profile was achieved. Pilling et al. in 2003 [21] from PBMC depleted of T-cells with anti-CD3, B-cells with anti-CD19, monocytes with anti-CD14 or all APCs with anti-HLA class II, and then cultured in serum-free conditions. They demonstrated that Fibrocytes grew at 72 hours when the Monocytes and the APC had not been excluded. The determination of surface markers was performed on the 5th day of culture, with immunohistochemistry on glass microscope slides – in the previous studies this had been performed after six weeks and with FACS, and increasing the markers from 31 to 58. The results were equivalent with the exception of α-smoot muscle actin and CD11a which, in the initial studies, were negative. The new identity profile of the Fibrocytes, which extended the phenotype to the chemokine receptors and to the integrin family was now established as follows:

- **Positive**: CD11a;CD11b;CD45;CD80;CD86;MHC   class   II;   collagen   I; fibronectine; Chemokine receptors (CCR3;CCR5;CCR7;CXCR4 and α-smooth muscle actin). Integrins (CD49a,CD49b,CD49e,CD29,CD61 and CD18)
- **Negative**: CD1a;CD3;CD19,CD38. Integrins (α3, α4, α6, α4β7, αE and cutaneous lymphocyte-associated Ag)

Although the identification criteria of the Fibrocytes are more and more specific, the mechanisms envolved in their differentiation are still, to a great extent, unknown.

Some plasmatic factors have been reported which inhibit the differentiation of the Fibrocytes and, in the same study, the role of Serum Amyloid P (SAP) in the differentiation of the fibrocytes was evaluated. It was seen that the presence in plasma of SAP levels of between 10 and 0.1% produced a significant decrease of the fibroblasts which proliferated rapidaly again at a plasma concentration of 0.01% or when the serum was heated to 95°C. It was also observed that the aggregated IgG were able to inhibit fibroblast differentiation, suggesting the hypothesis that the activation of the Fc receptors of IgG, the same site where the SAP joins, might be a specific signal for the fibrocytic differentiation, because these facts did not occur with the aggregates of IgA, IgE or IgM [22].

At the same time, the conditions have been highlighted which favour the differentiation of fibrocytes in humans and mice, underlining the relevant role of T-cells and of TGF-β1 [23]. Certainly, the T lymphocytes are necessary for fibrocytic differentiation and it can be seen that the optimum CD14+/T-cell proportion is 3:1; it was also observed that the addition of TGF-β1 (1-10 ng/ml) in the cultures, between days 3 and 10, produces a great accumulation of Collagen I in a dose-dependent manner. The role of TGF-β1 extends to promoting morphological and functional differentation of the Myofibroblast [24] and to increasing the contractility and expression of α-smooth muscle actin in a dose dependent manner, as can be seen in the cultures with collagen which it can contract by 20%, in contrast to those with PBMC.

The identity of the fibrocytes also includes their capacity to segregate inflammatory cytokines, and the study of mRNAs by cells isolated from bound chambers implanted into mice are able to express IL-1β, IL-10, TNF-α, MIP-1α, MIP-β, MIP-2, PDGF-A, TGF-β1 y M-CSF [25], or several proangiogenic factors including VEGF, bFGF, IL-8, PDGF and hematopoietic growth factors that promote endothelial proliferation [26].

The Involvement of the Fibrocyte in Immunity and Some Diseases is Discovered

The proof provided by means of flow cytometry that fibrocytes express surface markers involved in antigen presentation such as the class II HCM molecules (HLA-DP, DQ and DR), coestimulatory molecules (CD80,CD86) and the adhesion molecules (CD11a,CD45,CD58), suggested the involvement of fibrocytes in immunity. To verify the capacity of fibrocytes to activate allogenic T cells in a mixed leukocyte reaction a comparison was made with the antigen-presenting capacity of the Monocytes and that of the dendritic cells. The results, measured by the relative flourescence intensity with phycoerythrin-conjugated or fluorescein isothiocyanate-conjugated mABs, showed that the fibrocytes induced a higher response than the Monocytes and lower than that of the dendritic cells. The functional response in vivo with purified mouse fibrocytes was also studied and 5% of the marked fibrocytes were detected in the popliteal lymph node [27]. These data included the fibrocytes as a potent antigen-presenting cell.

The relation with the inflammatory response and the localization of the fibrocytes in fibrotic tissues led to the suspicion that they were involved in the pathogeny of a great number of diseases [28] and, in recent years, we have seen their spectacular growth in burn patients, in direct relation to the level of TGF-β1 and the burnt surface (greater than 30%) [29], their activity in a new disease entity called nephrogenic fibrosing dermophaty [30], and they have been allotted a relevant role in leihmaniasis [31]. The role of fibrocytes in disease continues to increase and they are now associated to cutaneous lesions, pulmonary fibrosis, tumors, keloids and, in general, to all the processes which include pathologic fibrosis [32]. Recently they were also credited with the regeneration of lung tissue, including them in the pathogeny of idiopathic interstitial pneumonia [33].

The Search for the Mesenchymal Stem Cell (MSC)

The Mesechymal Cells and the Menchymal Stem Cells

The "Mesenchyme", the origin of the mesenchymal cells, should not exist in the adult, as was claimed in the 1960s, because it is a embrionyc tissue derived from the mesoderm and, in a broad sense, gives rise to the connective tissue. However, rather than a tissue it is more an extensive concept which includes other tissues such as the bone, the cartilage, fat, the tendons, the muscles and even the nervous tissue, which means there is practically nowhere in the anatomy without connective tissue. This great variety of cells in such different structures, which are generally attributed functions of support and, at most, local repair, has its most genuine representative in bone marrow. Thus, when in 1985 Owen described the stromal cell system (reviewed in Ref.[34]), he reported bone marrow to be the most significant deposit of mesenchymal cells in the adult. Underlining their obvious influence in the regulation and control of hematopoiesis, he attributed four cellular components: macrophages, adipocytes, osteogenic cells and alkaline phosphatase positive reticular cells, in contrast to the the in vitro adherent layer derived from long-term in vitro bone marrow culture which also included fibroblasts, endothelial cells and smooth muscle cells. The stromal cell system is the morphological concretion which regulates hematopoiesis, via direct cellular relations or by means of cytokines. Previously it had been proposed when the hematopoeitic inductive micrienvironment (HIM) had been created as a structural arrangement poorly characterized, but suspected of having great influence in the regulation and differentiation of hematopoiesis [35]. The data which underlined the fundamental role of the stroma cells in hematopoiesis, and certainly the fundamental motive of their study, are overwhelming [36] and, moreover, are confirmed in culture and in vivo on verifying the reestablishment of hematopoiesis with the infusion of the stroma cells and the hematopoietic stem cells [37].

A more controversial aspect was the determination of the Stem Cell character of the mesenchymal cells, for which three conditions would have to be fulfilled: self-renewal capacity, multilinear differentiation from a single cell and functional reconstitution of the originating tissues. Certainly, there was already some proof of the presence of committed precursors of the MSCs in local regeneration but Friedenstein in 1976 [38] verified the differentiation in bone, fat and cartilage of the fibroblast-like obtained in the culture of human and mouse adherent medullar cells. In 1991, Caplan [39] reported that this same medullar population of adherent cells capable of differentiation in vitro and in vivo into bone, cartilage and fat and he called them mesenchymal stem cells (MSC). This demonstration of an Uncommitted Precursor of the MSCs was also verified in the culture of stellate cells of the adult skeletal muscle – able to transform into muscle, bone, cartilage and fat – [40] and in that of bone cell lines able to produce bone and fat [41]; however, these data collected from cultures of heterogeneous cells did not definitively demonstrate the presence of pluripotent MSCs, and only allowed the confirmation that some MCs were capable of differentiation and that, at most, could be committed or uncommitted progenitors with bi- or tri-lineal differentiation, but they did not fulfil the requirements of Stem Cells.

In 1999, Pittenger [42] demonstrated the carácter of the Pluripotent Stem Cell of the MSCs by achieving differentiation into several cell lines from the colonies obtained from the culture of a single cell. This finding was complemented with the implantation of these cells in various organs of preimmune sheep, which demonstrated their functionality [43]. In the stromal cell system and in the other compartments of the connective tissue, heterogeneous mesenchymal populations are certain to be found, with a mixture of precursors among which there is a small compartment of Pluripotent Mesenchymal Stem Cells.

Surface Markers...

If there is one characteristic which complicates the concept of MSC, it is the absence of unanimity in the description of the phenotype of the stroma cells and especially of the MSCs. It was first suggested that there was a common progenitor between the hematopoietic line and the MSCs with characteristics CD34+, CD38- y HLA-DR [44] and some years later the expression of CD50 was reported as the criterion of separation between the hematopoietic– positive – and the mesenchymal – negative – lines in the bone marrow of the human fetus [45]. However, Pittenger [42] did not find the expression of CD34 in the extended MSC culture, a fact in agreement with its low expression when associated with Stro-1. The phenotypic characteristics which have been described in MSC cultures demonstrate the level of complexity and the difficulty of identification: the list collected by Deans et al. in 2000 [34] includes more than 60 markers. Some of the most significant findings in the search for the MSC phenotype may be grouped following the review by Barry et al. [46]:

- Markers which attempted to be specific but were later verified as being expressed in other cells: Stro-1, SB-10 (CD166), SH-2 (CD105), SH-3 and SH-4 (CD73).
- Adhesion molecules: with high expression, $\alpha1, \alpha5, \beta1$; with low expression, $\alpha2, \alpha3, \alpha6, \beta2$ and $\beta4$; lack of expression, $\alpha4, \alpha L$.
- MHC: expression of HLA-A,B,C, and negativity for HLA-DR

Although they cannot be considered to be definitive, and the controversy still persists as to the suitability of CD34 for differentiating MSC from hematopoietic lines, the current phenotypic model for the MSC is that obtained by Le Blanc [47] in 18 cultures of extended MSC, in which he defined, by means of flow cytometry, the same phenotype in more than 97% of the cells:

- Positive : CD29, CD44, CD 105, CD106, CD166, CD13 y HLA class I
- Negative: CD45, CD34, CD80, CD86 y HLA-DR

... And the Possibilities of Differentiation

The contradictions in the adjudication of surface markers are compensated by the proof of differentiation and the most conclusive test for the identification of the MSCs is the development in culture of diverse cell lines. This path is at present the focus of research attention because of the benefits it contributes to regenerative medicine and the approach of the conditioning factors of this differentiation in culture is essential. Some of these are already well established [46] such as those relative to bone production - β-glycerol-phosphate, ascorbic acid, dexametasone and fetal bovine serum -, chondrogenic differentiation – serum free medium and added with TGF-β -, obtaining the adipose tissue – nuclear receptor and transcription factor, peroxisome proliferator-activated receptor-gamma -, and the induction of myogenesis – 5-azacytidine -, of nerve tissue – brain-derived neurotrophic factor -, or of cardiomyocytes and endothelial phenotypes.

The Mesenchymal Stem Cells Are Also Immunomodulators

The interaction of the MSCs with the immune system, modulating the CD4+ response, is widely documented and is of great relevance. Highly relevant clinical observations demonstrate that the infusion of MSCs expanded in culture reduces the incidence and severity of the GVHD in the hematopoietic transplant [48]. The extent of the role of MSCs in the immune system is still unknown and there are controversies as to the mechanisms used. Previous studies in vitro had already documented the effect of adding MSCs in the alloreactivity of T lymphocytes, which ranged from a small inhibition to the stimulation of the proliferation of the mixed lymphocyte reaction (MLR). It was seen that the action of these MSCs from the bone marrow of healthy individuals has an inhibitory effect with regard to the number of MSCs used: between 10 and 100 cells achieved a light suppression and between 10,000 and 40,000 cells achieved total inhibition. It was also observed that the stimulation of the MLC with phytohaemagglutinin, Concavalin A or protein A led to a low number of MSCs being able to stimulate proliferation, while a high number continued producing inhibition [47].

In order to explain the suppression of T-cell reactivity to alloantigens, a dependent mechanism of cell-to-cell contacts was initially proposed [49]; however, recently one or various soluble molecules have been considered to be responsible for this suppression which are capable of acting through a membrane and are not influenced by previous treatment of the MSCa with INF-α, or with the addition to the culture of IL-1α, IL-1β y TNF-α [50]. So as to extend the study of the immunoregulating role of the MSCs, especially in the field of hematopoietic transplants, a study was designed with human bone marrow MSCs expanded ex vivo, which, in contrast to other studies, were not irradiated so that no variables which might affect cell survival or their differentiation might be introduced [51]. The immune response was evaluated in primary and secondary mixed lymphocyte culture (MLC), quantifying the differentiation of the Dendritic cells (DC), the expansion of the T-cells and NK-lymphocytes and the cytotoxic activity. The results showed the strong inhibition of the differentiation of the DC1 over the DC2 (more than 80% of the DC co-expressed CD11/CD123), a dose-dependenet decrease of the NK cells and of the T lymphocytes, especially of CD8, and a decrease of the cytotoxic activity mediated by cytotoxic-antigen lymphocytes A4 (CTLA-4). The use of 1/3 allogenic MSCs with 100% autologic MSCs was also contrasted, verifying that the allogenic ones of an non-related subject are more efficient that the autologous ones, which might be of evident use in the prevention of immune complications in transplants.

Humoral immunity is also being explored with regard to the immunomodulators role of MSC and recently [52] it has been seen that the MSC of medullar origin inhibit the proliferation and differentiation of peripheral blood B lymphocytes, annulling the synthesis of the immunoglobulins. It is suggested that the main mechanism of this suppression is a soluble factor (hMSC) able to cross membranes.

It seems to be clear that there is ever more proof attributing a highly significant role as immunomodulator to the MSCs and the more recent contributions show that the targets are very diverse both in cellular as in humoral immunity.

From Bone Marrow to Peripheral Blood: A Controversial Leap

The first attempts to find the circulating MSCs were made in collections of peripheral blood precursor cells (PBPC) which had been mobilized with GM-CSF, and the results were certainly contradictory because sometimes they were not detected and when they were found, they were attributed to a "leap" of the Mobilized medullar MSCs. In 1997, Fernández et al. [53] described stroma cells in the PBPC of 14 patients with breast cancer, mobilized with G-CSF and GM-CSF; however, Lazarus et al. were not able to reproduce these results [54] and neither Wexler et al. [55] nor Koc and Lazarus [56] managed to demonstrate the presence of MSCs in peripheral blood or in the umbilical cord. Recently, da Silva Meirelles et al. [57], in long-term adult rat cultures, succeeded in generating MSCs in almost all the organs and in the great blood vessels but were not able to detect them in peripheral blood.

In contrast to these findings, the hematopoietic transplants of peripherical progenitors have produced the first proofs of the presence of circulating MSCs. Villaron et al. [58] demonstrated the graft of peripheral blood allogenic MSCs in the bone marrow of 2 patients with transplanted myeloma and also detected them in mobilized PBPC. Dickhut et al (Dickhut, 2005 #111), demonstrated using transplanting products of leukapheresis, that all the circulating MSCs of the receptor were from the donor; similar results were registered by Poloni et al. [59] 60 days post-transplant.

Various methods have also been tried to improve the selection of these circulating MSCs. Tondreau et al [60] compared various methods of separation which included the adhesion to plastic, alone and supplemented with fetal bovine serum, and the selection with monoclonal antibodies of CD135-positive cells. They observed that the fraction of CD135 cells contained more mesenchymal cells and with a greater proliferative potential than those obtained from adherence to plastic. The use of fibrin microbeads also seems to produce a good performance in the selection, especially when there are few cells[61].

In recent years evidence has been growing that clearly suggests the presence of MSCs in peripheral blood although we still do not possess a unanimous identifying profile and cannot explain the mechanisms implied in their mobilization and differentiation.

Monocytes and Fibrocytes: The Rebellion of Plasticity Against the Hierarchy

The presence of circulating stem cells is a fact which has been clearly established in recent years with the finding of different candidates which started with the Fibroblast-like and continued with the Fibrocytes and the Mesechymal Stem Cells. There are certainly significant differences between them regarding the surface markers as there are also in the method of isolation and identification of the markers, however, the "fibroblastoid" morphology is homogeneous and the possibilities of differentiation to other cell lines are becoming more and more homogeneous. It is probably a question of the same cell type in different precursor states, suggesting that they might have a common origin in the hematopoietic stem cells. Recently [62] it has been seen in mice how the fibroblasts and their precursors derive from a single hematopoietic cell marked with enhanced green fluorescent protein (EGFP) which was later identified in the fibroblast-like adherent cells of the bone marrow.

In peripheral blood, surprisingly, the monocyte seems to be the origin of the circulating stem cells. In 1995 Reuter [63] made an attempt to reproduce the proliferative vitreoretinopathy, culturing together during 17 days fresh calf vitreous with monocytes from peripheral blood, checking their differentiation into fibroblast-like that expressed CD11c from the 3rd day, the CD18 from the 7th day and the CD68 from the 15th day of culturing. In 2003 the presence of circulating CD14 monocytes were firstly demonstrated in human peripheral blood [64] and they were cultured with fibronectin and fetal bovine serum being differentiated into mesenchymal cells CD12, CD45, CD34 and type I collagen positives. These cells called monocyte-derived mesechymal progenitors (MOMPs) were able to turn into cardiomyocytes when co-cultured with rat cardiomyocytes [65]. Evidences stablishing links between monocytes and fibroblast-like with stem cell functions are growing, both cellullar type share markers like CD68 considered before as monocyte specific [66], and recently phagocytic abilities similar to those exhibit by macrophages have been demonstrated in the embryonic stem cells [67] . Also endothelial markers (KDR+) were experessed by monocytes stimulated with G-CSF and GM-CSF [68]. The missing piece of the puzzle was set by Zhao [6], confirming the pluripotent stem cell ability of the monocytes and their derivates the fibroblast-like cells: the peripheral blood mononuclear cells differentiate into fibroblastoid cells CD14+, CD34+ y CD45+, can be induced to turn into macrophages if stimulated with lipopolysaccharide, to limphocytes if stimulated with IL-2, to epithelial cells if stimulated with the epidermal growth factor, to neuronal cells if stimulated with nerve growth factor and to hepathocytes if stimulated with growth factor.

The orthodox concept of Stem Cell that implies self renewal and hierarchy of the differentiation till the mature cell, and the end of this by apoptosis or another mechanisms, is being defied by a wealth of new findings. In fact a lot of voices against the functional behavior of the Stem Cell are growing, requiring a change in this classic approach.

New emerging data like the pluripotent function of the peripheral stem cells are growing, but nowadays there are still a lot of basic questions dealing with the identity markers, with the differentiation control mechanisms, with the variability between species, or even with the real value of the results obtained using cultures or its interpretation as a mere experimental artifact [69]. The implications of this "postmodern biology" [70] lead to a new conception of the Stem Cell like a continuum of transcriptional opportunity [71] characterized as an ability in forming diverse cells different from the original tissue in a process called plasticity [72]. In fact it has been hypothesized a continous change in the fenotype of the SC depending on the microenvironmental stimuli which can lead to a differentiation toward a mature cell or can lead to come back to a SC consition. This approach is a challenge against the hierarchized classic model [73], setting up a kinetic model in which the SC is able to return to G_0 in the presence of a microenvironmental stimuliy witout expressing the CD34 marker [74].

In november 2006 Dov Zipori [75] analyzes the weak points of the actual concept of the SC, he focuses on the presence of pluripotent SCs everywhere, on the autorenewal of mature cells such as limphocytes and on the evidence of the differentiation in the HCS into cells derived from endoderm, mesoderm ans ectoderm. He also concluded that the autorenewal and the hierarchy are optional characteristics associated with a phenotype in a specific SC, taking its position as the essential properties the Plasticity and the Pluripotent ability. The new Stem Cell concept is the result of an state in the cellular cycle called Stem State characterizad by the Plasticity as the fundamental quality.

The Stem State Plasticity [76] implies the capability of showing new identities of certain cellular types; however transformation from mature cells into fibroblast-like with SC function also has been observed. These facts have been described in mamary gland epithelial cells as a response to TGFβ [77], in murine hepatocytes with TGFβ1 [78], or in the adult intestinal epithilium cultures in an "artificial niche" with mouse embryonic fibroblasts [79]. This turning back into Stem Cell from the mature state in the presence os specific stimuli involve a "inverse plasticity" completely antagonic with the hierarchized conception currently accepted of the SC.

PLURIPOTENT CELLS FROM PERIPHERAL BLOOD IN ANIMAL MODELS

Cellular Cultures Added to Plasticity Showed by the PSC Represent a New Tool in the Workfield of Drug Testing and in the Animal Models for Human Diseases

Since Zhao was able to isolate, culture and differentiate into several human tissues stem cells from peripheral blood [6] the beginning of a lot of studies dealing with animal models was heralded. Prior to that, in the last few years, it has been demonstrated that Pluripotent Stem Cells can be found in numerous adult tissues such as skeletal muscle[80], liver[81], bone-marrow[82] and the central nervous system[83], but all of them were unpractical related to peripheral blood.

There are a wealth of contradictory data on that point that have been tunned down above, but the main objective of this subchapter is to review the animal models and to explain our methodology in culturing and differentiating the fibroblast-like cell population isolated from the peripheral blood. There are a lot of examples of animal models for human diseases in wich these cultures could be a useful tool are listed as follow:

- Mouse: Alzheimer[84], Parkinson[85], diabetes[86], Amiotrophic Lateral Sclerosis[87], Lisosomal diseases[88], Duchenne muscular dystrophy[89], Hemophilia[90].
- Rat: Parkinson[91], Spinal cord injury[92].
- Pig: Ischemic heart disease[93].
- Dog: diabetes[94], Hemophilia[95].

The first step is the standardisation of the cultures for every specie. The description of the methodology to isolate fibroblast-like cells and round cells from peripheral blood and one example of differentiation into myeloid and erythroid precursors are described.

Firstly a blood sample was taken, the plasce and the volume obtained depended on the specie. Each sample was diluted in 0.9% sterile saline solution (1:1) (v/v). After dilution was completed, 5 ml of the mix was added to 5 ml of Ficoll-Paque® PLUS (1.077 g/ml.; #07907, StemCell Technologies) in an other sterile tube and centrifuged at 400g for 30 minutes at room temperature. Using a sterile Pasteur pipette the plasma layer on top was removed and discarded; care being taken to prevent any disturbance of the mononuclear cell layer. A small number of PBMNCs from this layer was removed and transferred into a sterile 17 x 100 mm polystyrene tube. Then the PBMNCs were washed three times with 10 ml of McCoy's 5A culture media, centrifuging at 400g for 5 minutes each time. A cell count was then performed using an automatic cell counter in order to detrmine the number of nucleated cells in the culture plate. This methodology for cells separation was the same in all the species, rat, mouse, hamster, rabbit, dog, cat, cow, horse, sheep, goat and pig.

Liquid Medium

Using this sample, 1x10^6 PBMNCs were cultured in 35 mm Petri dishes in 3 ml of McCoy's 5A medium. Half of the medium was renewed weekly.

Several parameters were checked on day 21. Total cellular growth was classified by a trained observer with the following four subjective scoring system: 0 points if no growth, 1 point if low growth, 2 points if medium growth and 3 points if an intense or very intense growth was found. In the same way, confluence degree was classified from 0 if very sparse to 3 if confluent. The last parameter observed was macrophage : fibroblast-like cell ratio. Cell morphology was examined by means of optical microscopy after May Grünwald-Giemsa staining.

In addition, immunostaining was performed in order to demonstrate the stem cell nature of fibroblast-like cells found. We used the streptavidin conjugated alkaline phosphatase-anti alkaline phosphatase technique (Biogenex HK330-59K), with a primary mouse anti-CD34 antibody (PeliCluster CD34, CLB. Menarini Diagnosticos S.A., Barcelona), and a rabbit anti-mouse antibody (Biogenex HK340-9K) as the secondary antibody. Moreover vimentine and sterases immunostain was performed, finding positivity for both in macrophages and fibroblast-like. After that to check this fagocytic capability of the fibroblast-like cells we used the NBT test showing as well positive results in all the species.

Semisolid Culture Media

In order to check the ability of this cells for differentiation into myeloid and erythroid precursos semisolid media was used. To study the number and colony type, erythroid-burst forming unit (E-BFU), colony erythroid-forming unit (E-CFU), granulomacrophagic-colony forming unit (GM-CFU), mixed-colony forming unit, (Mix-CFU) 1.5×10^4 PBMNCs were plated in 2 ml of 4 standardized semisolid media with recombinant human cytokines:

- *Medium A (MethoCult™ GF$^+$ H4435.* StemCell Technologies, Vancouver, Canada*):* 1% methylcellulose in Iscove's MDM, 30% foetal bovine serum (FBS), 1% BSA, 10^{-4}M 2-mercaptoethanol, 2mM L-glutamine, 50ng/ml rh stem cell factor, 20ng/ml rh granulomacrophagic-colony stimulating factor (GM-CSF), 20ng/ml rh IL-3, 20ng/ml rh IL-6, 20ng/ml rh G-CSF, 3 units/ml rh erythropoietin (Epo). This was been used used in assays of very primitive human clonogenic haematopoietic progenitor cells in purified populations[96, 97].

- *Medium B (MethoCult™ GF H4534.* StemCell Technologies, Vancouver, Canada*):* 1% methylcellulose in Iscove's MDM, 30% FBS, 1% BSA, 10^{-4}M 2-mercaptoethanol, 2mM L-glutamine, 50ng/ml rh stem cell factor, 10ng/ml rh GM-CSF, 10ng/ml rh IL-3 (without Epo). This medium is recommended by the manufacturer for use in assays of human clonogenic haematopoietic progenitor cells from human bone marrow, peripheral blood, cord blood, leukopheresis products and purified CD34$^+$ cells[97, 98], and supports the growth of GM-CFU, granulocyte-colony forming unit (CFU-G) and macrophage-colony forming unit (M-CFU).

- *Medium C (MethoCult™ GF$^+$ H4535.* StemCell Technologies, Vancouver, Canada*):* 1% methylcellulose in Iscove's MDM, 30% FBS, 1% BSA, 10^{-4}M 2-mercaptoethanol, 2mM L-glutamine, 50ng/ml rh stem cell factor, 20ng/ml rh GM-CSF, 20ng/ml rh IL-3, 20ng/ml rh IL-6 and 20ng/ml rh G-CSF (without Epo). Constituents were selected to support optimal growth of human GM-CFU, G-CFUand M-CFU. H4535 medium is used in assays of purified populations of very primitive human clonogenic haematopoietic progenitor cells [99].

- *Control mediumD (MethoCult™ SF^{BIT} H4236.* StemCell Technologies, Vancouver, Canada*):* 1% methylcellulose in Iscove's MDM, 1% BSA, 10μg/ml human recombinant insulin, 200μg/ml human transferrin (Iron-saturated), 10^{-4}M 2-mercaptoethanol, 2mM L-glutamine. This medium does not contain FBS, Epo or recombinant cytokines.

Cultures were placed on a level tray at 37°C in a humidified incubator that maintained an internal atmosphere of 5% CO_2. After 21 days of incubation, the culture plates were removed, colonies and clusters were scored in situ using an inverted microscope.

Throughout our studies, the existence of circulating progenitor cells in peripheral blood of several species frequently used as human disease models has been demonstrated. In addition these cells can be easily isolated and cultivated. These cells, previously described in human beings, can be differentiated with the presence of different growth factors into macrophages, T-lymphocytes, epithelial cells, endothelial cells, neuronal cells and hepatocytes[6]. In our study, different cellular subgroups were observed such as macrophages, erythroid cells and fibroblast-like cells, which exhibit the CD34 haematopoietic stem cell marker[100]. Indeed these cells are those which [6] indicated as being precursor cells of mature tissues[6].

In preceding studies[101, 102] the fusion of these cells with pre-existing tissue in the culture was shown to be the possible origin for the mature tissue, however in our assays this possibility is completely discarded due to the only use of commercial media without cells.

Another important point, in agreement with [6], is the presence of erythroid cells in some culture media in the absence of Epo, which could indicate that there are certain cytokines stimulating those precursor cells towards the erythroid cell family, or that the original cells are in a very primitive stage. At this stage, cells do not need to be stimulated by Epo to be differentiated into erythroid cells[103, 104]. We would therefore agree that cells can be differentiated into several cell lines as was demonstrated in human medicine[6].

We found differences in growth depending on the specie. This could imply that these species have a greater number of circulating precursor cells or the culture media used may be more suitable for hamster and murine cells. It is important to highlight that specific cytokine are not required for precursor cell growth, representing a reliable method, the commercial and standardized media with recombinant human cytokines.

The semisolid culture media represent a good tool to obtain and differentiate haematopoietic precursor cells. Medium A *(MethoCult™ GF⁺ H4435.* StemCell Technologies, Vancouver, Canada*)* can be used to culture erytroid lines, whereas media B *(MethoCult™ GF H4534.* StemCell Technologies, Vancouver, Canada*)* and C *(MethoCult™ GF⁺ H4535.* StemCell Technologies, Vancouver, Canada*)* can be used to culture myeloid lines.

The presence of these cells in the peripheral blood of experimental animals, and the case with which they can be obtained makes them ideal for a number of applications including the study of toxicity or drug effects, or the study of cellular therapy applied to animal models of different human diseases.

REFERENCES

[1]   Wintrobe, M.M., Hematology, the Blossoming of a Science: A Story of Inspiration and Effort, ed. L. Febiger. 1985, Philadelphia.

[2]   Ikehara, S., A new concept of stem cell disorders and their new therapy. *J. Hematother. Stem Cell Res,* 2003. 12(6): p. 643-53.

[3]   Majno, G., Chronic inflammation: links with angiogenesis and wound healing. *Am. J. Pathol,* 1998. 153(4): p. 1035-9.

[4]   Petrakis, N.L., M. Davis, and S.P. Lucia, The in vivo differentiation of human leukocytes into histiocytes, fibroblasts and fat cells in subcutaneous diffusion chambers. *Blood,* 1961. 17: p. 109-18.

[5]   Puck TT, C.S., Fisher HW, Clonal grow in vitro of human cells with fibroblastic morphology. *J. Exp. Med,* 1957. 106: p. 145-58.

[6]   Zhao, Y., D. Glesne, and E. Huberman, A human peripheral blood monocyte-derived subset acts as pluripotent stem cells. *Proc. Natl. Acad. Sci. U S A,* 2003. 100(5): p. 2426-31.

[7]   Berman L , S.C., Ruddle FH ,Cunningham N, Long-Term Tissue Culture of Human
       Bone Marrow. I. Report of Isolation of a Strain of Cells Resembling Epithelial Cells
       from Bone Marrow of a Patient with Carcinoma of the Lung. *Blood,* 1955. 10(9): p.
       896-911.

[8]   Woodliff, H., Glass substrate cultures of human blood and bone marrow cells. *Exp. Cell
       Res,* 1958. 14(2): p. 368-377.

[9]   Castro-Malaspina, H., et al., Characterization of human bone marrow fibroblast colony-
       forming cells (CFU-F) and their progeny. *Blood,* 1980. 56(2): p. 289-301.

[10]   Castro-Malaspina, H., et al., Characteristics of bone marrow fibroblast colony-forming
       cells (CFU-F) and their progeny in patients with myeloproliferative disorders. *Blood,*
       1982. 59(5): p. 1046-54.

[11]   Wilson, F.D., et al., Morphological studies on 'adherent cells' in bone marrow cultures
       from humans, dogs, and mice. *Stem Cells,* 1981. 1(1): p. 15-29.

[12]   Gordon, M.Y. and E.C. Gordon-Smith, Bone marrow fibroblast function in relation to
       granulopoiesis in aplastic anaemia. *Br. J. Haematol,* 1983. 53(3): p. 483-9.

[13]   Klein, A.K., et al., The influence of fibroblast-like cells derived from canine fetal
       hematopoietic tissues on the regulation of lymphohematopoiesis. *Int. J. Cell Cloning,*
       1984. 2(1): p. 20-33.

[14]   Krawisz, B.R., D.L. Florine, and R.E. Scott, Differentiation of fibroblast-like cells into
       macrophages. *Cancer Res,* 1981. 41(7): p. 2891-9.

[15]   Kaneko, S., S. Motomura, and H. Ibayashi, Differentiation of human bone marrow-
       derived fibroblastoid colony forming cells (CFU-F) and their roles in haemopoiesis in
       vitro. *Br. J. Haematol,* 1982. 51(2): p. 217-25.

[16]   Klinnert, V., W. Nothdurft, and T.M. Fliedner, CFU-F from dog marrow: a colony
       assay and its significance. *Blut,* 1985. 50(2): p. 81-7.

[17]   Piersma, A.H., R.E. Ploemacher, and K.G. Brockbank, Transplantation of bone marrow
       fibroblastoid stromal cells in mice via the intravenous route. *Br. J. Haematol,* 1983.
       54(2): p. 285-90.

[18]   Gomez-Casal F, V.C., Moneva J, Miguelena M, Yoldi N, Isolation and culture of
       Fibroblast-like (F-CFU)from peripheral blood. *Sangre,* 1987. 32(5): p. 505.

[19]   Yoldi, N., Fibroblast-like cells (F-CFU) from peripheral blood: An in vitro assay to
       check the influence of several drugs over the cultura, in Faculty of Medicine. 1990,
       University of Zaragoza: Zaragoza (Spain). p. 184.

[20]   Bucala, R., et al., Circulating fibrocytes define a new leukocyte subpopulation that
       mediates tissue repair. *Mol. Med,* 1994. 1(1): p. 71-81.

[21]   Pilling, D., et al., Inhibition of fibrocyte differentiation by serum amyloid P. *J.
       Immunol,* 2003. 171(10): p. 5537-46.

[22]   Pilling, D., N.M. Tucker, and R.H. Gomer, Aggregated IgG inhibits the differentiation
       of human fibrocytes. *J. Leukoc. Biol,* 2006. 79(6): p. 1242-51.

[23]   Abe, R., et al., Peripheral blood fibrocytes: differentiation pathway and migration to
       wound sites. *J. Immunol,* 2001. 166(12): p. 7556-62.

[24]   Vaughan, M.B., E.W. Howard, and J.J. Tomasek, Transforming growth factor-beta1
       promotes the morphological and functional differentiation of the myofibroblast. *Exp.
       Cell Res,* 2000. 257(1): p. 180-9.

[25] Chesney, J., et al., Regulated production of type I collagen and inflammatory cytokines by peripheral blood fibrocytes. *J. Immunol,* 1998. 160(1): p. 419-25.

[26] Hartlapp, I., et al., Fibrocytes induce an angiogenic phenotype in cultured endothelial cells and promote angiogenesis in vivo. *Faseb J,* 2001. 15(12): p. 2215-24.

[27] Chesney, J., et al., The peripheral blood fibrocyte is a potent antigen-presenting cell capable of priming naive T cells in situ. *Proc. Natl. Acad. Sci. U S A,* 1997. 94(12): p. 6307-12.

[28] Chesney, J. and R. Bucala, Peripheral blood fibrocytes: mesenchymal precursor cells and the pathogenesis of fibrosis. *Curr. Rheumatol. Rep,* 2000. 2(6): p. 501-5.

[29] Yang, L., et al., Peripheral blood fibrocytes from burn patients: identification and quantification of fibrocytes in adherent cells cultured from peripheral blood mononuclear cells. *Lab. Invest,* 2002. 82(9): p. 1183-92.

[30] Quan, T.E., et al., Circulating fibrocytes: collagen-secreting cells of the peripheral blood. *Int. J. Biochem. Cell Biol,* 2004. 36(4): p. 598-606.

[31] Grab DJ, S.M., Dumler JS, Bucala R, A role for the peripheral blood fibrocyte in leishmaniasis? *Trends Parasitol,* 2004. 20(1).

[32] Quan, T.E., S.E. Cowper, and R. Bucala, The role of circulating fibrocytes in fibrosis. *Curr. Rheumatol. Rep,* 2006. 8(2): p. 145-50.

[33] Lama, V.N. and S.H. Phan, The extrapulmonary origin of fibroblasts: stem/progenitor cells and beyond. *Proc. Am. Thorac. Soc,* 2006. 3(4): p. 373-6.

[34] Deans, R.J. and A.B. Moseley, Mesenchymal stem cells: biology and potential clinical uses. *Exp. Hematol,* 2000. 28(8): p. 875-84.

[35] Trentin, J.J., Determination of bone marrow stem cell differentiation by stromal hemopoietic inductive microenvironments (HIM). *Am. J. Pathol,* 1971. 65(3): p. 621-8.

[36] Cherry, et al., Production of hematopoietic stem cell-chemotactic factor by bone marrow stromal cells. *Blood,* 1994. 83(4): p. 964-71.

[37] Almeida-Porada, G., et al., Cotransplantation of human stromal cell progenitors into preimmune fetal sheep results in early appearance of human donor cells in circulation and boosts cell levels in bone marrow at later time points after transplantation. *Blood,* 2000. 95(11): p. 3620-7.

[38] Friedenstein, A.J., J.F. Gorskaja, and N.N. Kulagina, Fibroblast precursors in normal and irradiated mouse hematopoietic organs. *Exp. Hematol,* 1976. 4(5): p. 267-74.

[39] Caplan, A.I., Mesenchymal stem cells. *J. Orthop. Res,* 1991. 9(5): p. 641-50.

[40] Williams, J.T., et al., Cells isolated from adult human skeletal muscle capable of differentiating into multiple mesodermal phenotypes. *Am. Surg,* 1999. 65(1): p. 22-6.

[41] Nuttall, M.E., et al., Human trabecular bone cells are able to express both osteoblastic and adipocytic phenotype: implications for osteopenic disorders. *J. Bone Miner Res,* 1998. 13(3): p. 371-82.

[42] Pittenger, M.F., et al., Multilineage potential of adult human mesenchymal stem cells. *Science,* 1999. 284(5411): p. 143-7.

[43] Liechty, K.W., et al., Human mesenchymal stem cells engraft and demonstrate site-specific differentiation after in utero transplantation in sheep. *Nat. Med,* 2000. 6(11): p. 1282-6.

[44] Huang, S. and L.W. Terstappen, Formation of haematopoietic microenvironment and haematopoietic stem cells from single human bone marrow stem cells. *Nature,* 1992. 360(6406): p. 745-9.

[45] Waller, E.K., et al., The "common stem cell" hypothesis reevaluated: human fetal bone marrow contains separate populations of hematopoietic and stromal progenitors. *Blood,* 1995. 85(9): p. 2422-35.

[46] Barry, F.P. and J.M. Murphy, Mesenchymal stem cells: clinical applications and biological characterization. *Int. J. Biochem. Cell Biol,* 2004. 36(4): p. 568-84.

[47] Le Blanc, K., et al., Mesenchymal stem cells inhibit and stimulate mixed lymphocyte cultures and mitogenic responses independently of the major histocompatibility complex. *Scand. J. Immunol,* 2003. 57(1): p. 11-20.

[48] Le Blanc, K., et al., Treatment of severe acute graft-versus-host disease with third party haploidentical mesenchymal stem cells. *Lancet,* 2004. 363(9419): p. 1439-41.

[49] Di Nicola, M., et al., Human bone marrow stromal cells suppress T-lymphocyte proliferation induced by cellular or nonspecific mitogenic stimuli. *Blood,* 2002. 99(10): p. 3838-43.

[50] Klyushnenkova, E., et al., T cell responses to allogeneic human mesenchymal stem cells: immunogenicity, tolerance, and suppression. *J. Biomed. Sci,* 2005. 12(1): p. 47-57.

[51] Maccario, R., et al., Interaction of human mesenchymal stem cells with cells involved in alloantigen-specific immune response favors the differentiation of CD4+ T-cell subsets expressing a regulatory/suppressive phenotype. *Haematologica,* 2005. 90(4): p. 516-25.

[52] Corcione, A., et al., Human mesenchymal stem cells modulate B-cell functions. *Blood,* 2006. 107(1): p. 367-72.

[53] Fernandez, M., et al., Detection of stromal cells in peripheral blood progenitor cell collections from breast cancer patients. *Bone Marrow Transplant,* 1997. 20(4): p. 265-71.

[54] Lazarus, H.M., et al., Human bone marrow-derived mesenchymal (stromal) progenitor cells (MPCs) cannot be recovered from peripheral blood progenitor cell collections. *J. Hematother,* 1997. 6(5): p. 447-55.

[55] Wexler SA, D.C., Denning-Kendall P, Rice C,Bradley B, Hows JM, Adult bone marrow is a rich source of human mesenchymal "stem" cells but umbilical cord and mobilized adult blood are not. *British Journal Haematology,* 2003. 121(2): p. 368-374.

[56] Koc, O.N. and H.M. Lazarus, Mesenchymal stem cells: heading into the clinic. *Bone Marrow Transplant,* 2001. 27(3): p. 235-9.

[57] da Silva Meirelles, L., P.C. Chagastelles, and N.B. Nardi, Mesenchymal stem cells reside in virtually all post-natal organs and tissues. *J. Cell Sci,* 2006. 119(Pt 11): p. 2204-13.

[58] Villaron, E.M., et al., Mesenchymal stem cells are present in peripheral blood and can engraft after allogeneic hematopoietic stem cell transplantation. *Haematologica,* 2004. 89(12): p. 1421-7.

[59] Poloni, A., et al., Engraftment capacity of mesenchymal cells following hematopoietic stem cell transplantation in patients receiving reduced-intensity conditioning regimen. *Leukemia,* 2006. 20(2): p. 329-35.

[60] Tondreau, T., et al., Mesenchymal stem cells derived from CD133-positive cells in mobilized peripheral blood and cord blood: proliferation, Oct4 expression, and plasticity. *Stem Cells,* 2005. 23(8): p. 1105-12.

[61] Kassis, I., et al., Isolation of mesenchymal stem cells from G-CSF-mobilized human peripheral blood using fibrin microbeads. *Bone Marrow Transplant,* 2006. 37(10): p. 967-76.

[62] Ebihara, Y., et al., Hematopoietic origins of fibroblasts: II. In vitro studies of fibroblasts, CFU-F, and fibrocytes. *Exp. Hematol,* 2006. 34(2): p. 219-29.

[63] Reuter, U., C. Champion, and H.L. Kain, Transdifferentiation of human monocytes into fibroblast-like cells in vitro. *Ger. J. Ophthalmol,* 1995. 4(3): p. 182-7.

[64] Kuwana, M., et al., Human circulating CD14+ monocytes as a source of progenitors that exhibit mesenchymal cell differentiation. *J. Leukoc. Biol,* 2003. 74(5): p. 833-45.

[65] Kodama, H., et al., Cardiomyogenic potential of mesenchymal progenitors derived from human circulating CD14+ monocytes. *Stem Cells Dev,* 2005. 14(6): p. 676-86.

[66] Kunz-Schughart, L.A., et al., [The "classical" macrophage marker CD68 is strongly expressed in primary human fibroblasts]. *Verh. Dtsch. Ges. Pathol,* 2003. 87: p. 215-23.

[67] Charriere, G.M., et al., Macrophage characteristics of stem cells revealed by transcriptome profiling. *Exp. Cell Res,* 2006. 312(17): p. 3205-14.

[68] Bruno, S., et al., Combined administration of G-CSF and GM-CSF stimulates monocyte-derived pro-angiogenic cells in patients with acute myocardial infarction. *Cytokine,* 2006. 34(1-2): p. 56-65.

[69] Gokhale, P.J. and P.W. Andrews, A prospective on stem cell research. *Semin. Reprod. Med,* 2006. 24(5): p. 289-97.

[70] Theise, N.D., Implications of 'postmodern biology' for pathology: the Cell Doctrine. *Lab. Invest,* 2006. 86(4): p. 335-44.

[71] Colvin, G.A., P.J. Quesenberry, and M.S. Dooner, The stem cell continuum: a new model of stem cell regulation. *Handb. Exp. Pharmacol,* 2006(174): p. 169-83.

[72] Serafini, M. and C.M. Verfaillie, Pluripotency in adult stem cells: state of the art. *Semin. Reprod. Med,* 2006. 24(5): p. 379-88.

[73] Quesenberry, P.J., G.A. Colvin, and J.F. Lambert, The chiaroscuro stem cell: a unified stem cell theory. *Blood,* 2002. 100(13): p. 4266-71.

[74] Lemoli, R.M., et al., Stem cell plasticity: time for a reappraisal? *Haematologica,* 2005. 90(3): p. 360-81.

[75] Zipori, D., The stem state: plasticity is essential, whereas self-renewal and hierarchy are optional. *Stem Cells,* 2005. 23(6): p. 719-26.

[76] Filip, S., D. English, and J. Mokry, Issues in stem cell plasticity. *J. Cell Mol. Med,* 2004. 8(4): p. 572-7.

[77] Hosobuchi, M. and M.R. Stampfer, Effects of transforming growth factor beta on growth of human mammary epithelial cells in culture. *In Vitro Cell Dev. Biol,* 1989. 25(8): p. 705-13.

[78] Gotzmann, J., et al., Hepatocytes convert to a fibroblastoid phenotype through the cooperation of TGF-beta1 and Ha-Ras: steps towards invasiveness. *J. Cell Sci,* 2002. 115(Pt 6): p. 1189-202.

[79] Wiese, C., et al., Signals from embryonic fibroblasts induce adult intestinal epithelial cells to form nestin-positive cells with proliferation and multilineage differentiation capacity in vitro. *Stem Cells,* 2006. 24(9): p. 2085-97.

[80] Asakura, A., Stem cells in adult skeletal muscle. *Trends Cardiovasc. Med,* 2003. 13(3): p. 123-8.

[81] Zhang, Y., X.F. Bai, and C.X. Huang, Hepatic stem cells: existence and origin. *World J. Gastroenterol,* 2003. 9(2): p. 201-4.

[82] Tocci, A. and L. Forte, Mesenchymal stem cell: use and perspectives. *Hematol. J,* 2003. 4(2): p. 92-6.

[83] Bottai, D., Neural stem cells: plasticity and therapeutic potential. *J. Neurochem,* 2003. 85(Suppl 2): p. 13.

[84] Mucke, L., et al., High-level neuronal expression of abeta 1-42 in wild-type human amyloid protein precursor transgenic mice: synaptotoxicity without plaque formation. *J. Neurosci,* 2000. 20(11): p. 4050-8.

[85] Sotnikova, T.D., M.G. Caron, and R.R. Gainetdinov, DDD mice, a novel acute mouse model of Parkinson's disease. *Neurology,* 2006. 67(7 Suppl 2): p. S12-7.

[86] Didion, S.P., C.M. Lynch, and F.M. Faraci, Cerebral Vascular Dysfunction in TallyHo Mice: A New Model of Type II Diabetes. *Am. J. Physiol. Heart Circ. Physiol,* 2006.

[87] Miana-Mena, F.J., et al., Optimal methods to characterize the G93A mouse model of ALS. *Amyotroph. Lateral Scler. Other Motor Neuron Disord,* 2005. 6(1): p. 55-62.

[88] Fukuda, T., et al., Dysfunction of endocytic and autophagic pathways in a lysosomal storage disease. *Ann. Neurol,* 2006. 59(4): p. 700-8.

[89] Hodgetts, S., et al., Reduced necrosis of dystrophic muscle by depletion of host neutrophils, or blocking TNFalpha function with Etanercept in mdx mice. *Neuromuscul. Disord,* 2006. 16(9-10): p. 591-602.

[90] Lillicrap, D., T. VandenDriessche, and K. High, Cellular and genetic therapies for haemophilia. *Haemophilia,* 2006. 12 Suppl 3: p. 36-41.

[91] Ravindran, G. and H.S. Rao, Enriched NCAM-positive cells form functional dopaminergic neurons in the rat model of Parkinson's disease. *Stem Cells Dev,* 2006. 15(4): p. 575-82.

[92] Yoshihara, H., et al., Combining motor training with transplantation of rat bone marrow stromal cells does not improve repair or recovery in rats with thoracic contusion injuries. *Brain Res,* 2006. 1119(1): p. 65-75.

[93] Choi, J.S., et al., Efficacy of therapeutic angiogenesis by intramyocardial injection of pCK-VEGF165 in pigs. *Ann. Thorac. Surg,* 2006. 82(2): p. 679-86.

[94] Gupta, N., et al., Direct and indirect effects of insulin on hepatic glucose production in diabetic depancreatized dogs during euglycemia. *J. Endocrinol,* 2006. 190(3): p. 695-702.

[95] Sarkar, R., et al., Long-term efficacy of adeno-associated virus serotypes 8 and 9 in hemophilia a dogs and mice. *Hum. Gene Ther,* 2006. 17(4): p. 427-39.

[96]   Wang, Z., et al., Receptor tyrosine kinase, EphB4 (HTK), accelerates differentiation of select human hematopoietic cells. *Blood,* 2002. 99: p. 2740-2747.

[97]   Gribaldo, L., et al., Inhibition of CFU-E/BFU-E by 3'-azido-3'-deoxythymidine, chlorpropamide, and protoporphirin IX Zinc (II): A comparison between direct exposure of progenitor cells and long-term exposure of bone marrow cultures. *Toxicol. Sci,* 2000. 58: p. 96-101.

[98]   LaRosee, P., et al., In vitro studies of the combination of imatinib mesylate (Gleevec) and arsenic trioxide (Trisenox) in chronic myelogenous leukemia. *Exp. Hematol,* 2002. 30: p. 729-737.

[99]   Keir, M., et al., Sensitivity of c-erbB positive cells to a ligant toxin and its utility in purging breast cancer cells from peripheral blood stem cell (PBSC) collections. *Stem Cells,* 2000. 18: p. 422-427.

[100] Abbas, A.K., A.H. Lichtman, and J.S. Pober, *Cellular and Molecular Immunology.* 2003: Elsevier Science.

[101] Ying, Q.L., et al., Changing potency by spontaneous fusion. *Nature,* 2002. 416(6880): p. 545-8.

[102] Terada, N., et al., Bone marrow cells adopt the phenotype of other cells by spontaneous cell fusion. *Nature,* 2002. 416(6880): p. 542-5.

[103] Ghaffari, S., et al., BCR-ABL and v-SRC tyrosine kinase oncoproteins support normal erythroid development in erythropoietin receptor-deficient progenitor cells. *Proc. Natl. Acad. Sci. U S A,* 1999. 96(23): p. 13186-13190.

[104] Akela, S., et al., Neutralization of Autocrine Transforming Growth Factor-ß in Human Cord Blood CD34+CD38-Lin- Cells Promotes Stem-Cell-Factor-Mediated Erythropoietin-Independent Early Erythroid Progenitor Development and Reduces Terminal Differentiation. *Stem Cells,* 2003. 21: p. 557-567.

APPENDIX - FIGURES

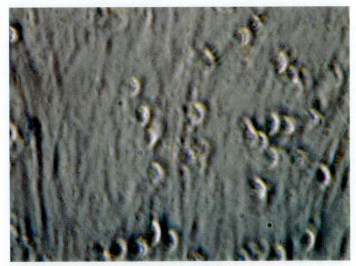

Figure 1. In vivo fibroblast-like net from peripheral blood of pig.

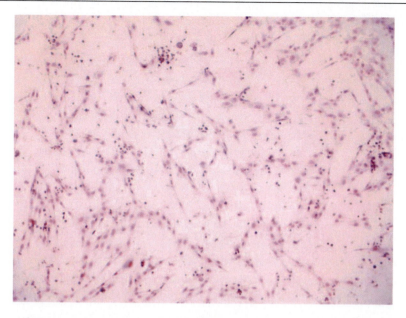

Figure 2. Stained fibroblast-like and monocytes from dog, medium confluence degree is seen.

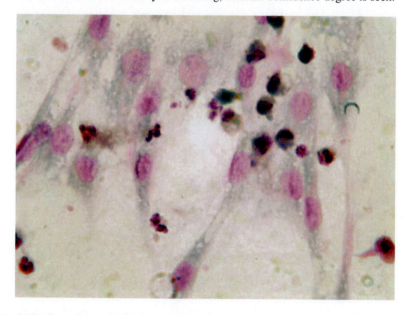

Figure 3. Stained fibroblast-like cells from peripheral blood of mouse, after 21 days of culture.

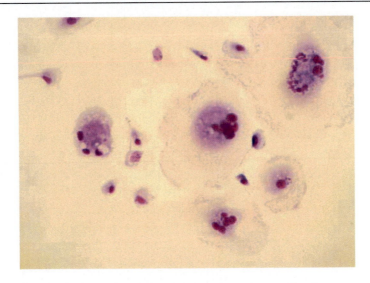

Figure 4. Stained monocytes from peripheral blood of goat, after 21 days of culture.

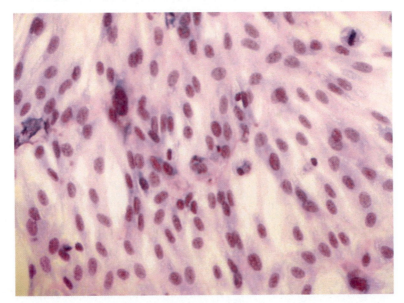

Figure 5. Stained fibroblast-like cells from peripheral blood of cow, after 21 days of culture.

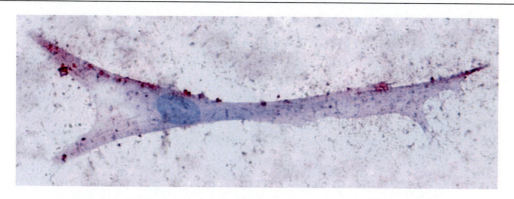

Figure 6. CD34+ fibroblast like cell from peripheral blood of mouse, after 21 days of culture.

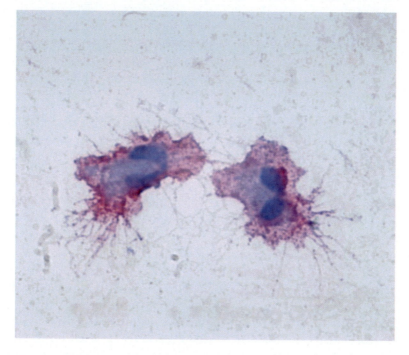

Figure 7. Vimentine + cells (fibroblast-like and monocytes) from peripheral blood of mouse, after 15 days of culture.

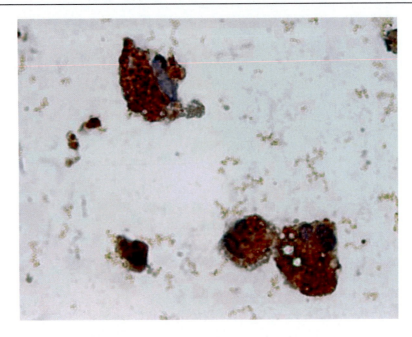

Figure 8. Sterase + monocytes from peripheral blood of dog, after 15 days of culture.

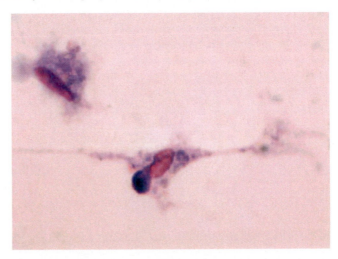

Figure 9. NBT + fibroblast and monocyte cells from peripheral blood of dog, after 21 days of culture.

In: Stem Cell Research Developments
Editor: Calvin A. Fong, pp. 187-201

ISBN: 978-1-60021-601-5
© 2007 Nova Science Publishers, Inc.

Chapter VI

Neural Stem Cell Niche-Dependency: A Theoretical Model of Spatially Restricted Responses to the Activation of Multiple Receptors

Lia Scotti Campos[*]
Wellcome Trust Sanger Institute, Hinxton, Cambridge, CB10 1SA, UK
Department of Pathology, Addenbrookes Hospital,
Hills Road, Cambridge, CB2 2QQ, UK.

ABSTRACT

Neural stem cells (NSC) are present in the embryonic and adult vertebrate brain. The study of the role of extra cellular factors in the generation, maintenance and differentiation of NSC is complex because: 1) Although embryonic NSC belong to a glial lineage their morphology, proliferation potential, multi potentiality and membrane markers expression evolve during embryogenesis and differ from the adult NSC. 2) The extra cellular environment that surrounds NSC is not static and changes throughout development. 3) A number of proteins expressed at multiple stages of central nervous system (CNS) development appear to function in a "context-dependent" manner. In the light of this complexity it is not surprising that the definition of the NSC niche poses a difficult problem. Here a qualitative theoretical model is proposed to explain how expression of specific proteins that alter the signalling responses of activated receptors, which themselves may not be spatially restricted to the putative NSC niche area (the ventricular zone, VZ) may help define a functional rather than an architectural niche. Such a model may be applied or extended to proteins that are involved in the internalization, processing and degradation of receptors not restricted to the VZ, thereby affecting their signalling in a spatially controlled manner, which compartmentalizes the signalling output rather than the receptor expression pattern. Experimental data on

[*] Lia Scotti Campos: Email-1: lsc@sanger.ac.uk, Email-2: lslbc2@cam.ac.uk

Caveolin1 will be discussed as an example of a possible functionally defining niche protein.

THE FORMATION OF THE VENTRICULAR ZONE (VZ) AND THE DEVELOPMENT OF NEURO-EPITHELIAL PROGENITORS (NE) AND NEURAL STEM CELLS (NSC)

The vertebrate Central Nervous System (CNS) develops from a simple hollow structure lined by neuroepithelium, originated from the invagination and closure of the neural plate. At early stages the neural tube contains Neuro-Epithelial Progenitors (NEP) that express markers such as the intermediate filament Nestin [1] and Prominin1 (CD133, at the apical plasma membrane) [2]. NEPs have the potential to generate neural cells and between embryonic days 10 and 12.5 they give rise to Radial Glial Cells (RGCs) [3], which express glial/astroglial markers such as glycogen granules, astrocyte specific glutamate transporter (GLAST), S100β, Vimentin, Brain Lipid Binding Protein (BLBP) and Glial Fibrillary Acidic Protein (GFAP). Although the RGCs were believed to serve mainly as "rail tracks" for the newly formed neural cells to migrate and reach a final cortical position, it is now accepted that they can divide and they are considered to be fully-fledged stem cells. RGCs are more fate restricted than the NEPs, and the former give rise to most of the neuronal populations of the developing CNS. Therefore NEPs and RGCs are both thought to be neural stem cells (NSC) that belong to the same lineage and are generated sequentially although they differ in their differentiation potential, the former having a wider differentiation range than the later. NEPs and RGCs share some (but not) all markers. At the onset of neurogenesis another type of mitotic cell can be found on the basal side of the VZ, the so-called basal progenitor cells (BPC): these cells are NEP- and RGC-daughter cells that have lost contact with the apical surface, and are still considered to be NSC in spite of a very limited (mono lineage) differentiation potential [2]. Towards the end of neurogenesis the RGCs give rise to a GFAP-positive population [4, 5] and in the adult brain a group of GFAP-expressing cells that reside in the lateral ventricle sub ventricular zone (SVZ) and in the hippocampus are believed to be the descendants of the RGC and to constitute the adult NSC pool [6-8]. The adult NSCs do not share the bipolar morphology of the NEPs and RGCs and express fewer markers. Nevertheless they can re-enter the cell cycle [9] and generate progenitors that migrate to the olfactory bulb, where they differentiate as interneurons.

COMMON CHARACTERISTICS BETWEEN NEPs AND NSC

As previously discussed NSCs are believed to belong to a glial lineage [10], which comprises the RGCs that develop in the vertebrate developing Central Nervous System from the NEPs, just prior to the onset of neurogenesis. Both NEP and NSC share multiple characteristics and derive from a common epithelial precursor. In particular both types of cells are *polarised* and show an *apical-basal orientation* in the neural tube wall and later in the ventricular zone (VZ) area of the developing CNS, respectively. Both are *adherent* to the apical, luminal surface. Both may be subject to *concentration gradients of soluble molecules* diffusing from the neural tube lumen into the neuroepithelial layer and, later, from the ventricle lumen into the VZ. Both are embedded in *specialized extra cellular matrix components*, which are strictly confined spatially and appear to define architectural areas [11] (figure 1). These characteristics distinguish the NEPs and NSCs from the basal progenitor cells (BPC), which arise from divisions of either NEPs or RGCs, are located just basal to the VZ and generate only neurons. Although still considered a NSC by some authors (although an unusual, unipotent one [2]) polarity may not be a key feature of BCPs (when compared to NEPs and RGCs) and the role of the axis of division in cell fate determination is less clear. More importantly, the basal progenitor cells (BPC) do not *adhere* to the apical surface. Theoretically, they may be exposed to lower concentrations of soluble molecules diffusing from the ventricle (or they may not exposed at all to such gradients) and their position, lack of anchoring and presumed increased motility may result in their exclusion from the influence area of a particular group of ventricular zone ECM molecules and their extrusion into a different ECM micro-environment [11]. It is interesting to note that the SVZ GFAP-positive adult NSC appears to retain a contact with the apical surface of the ventricular wall, through a cytoplasmic and membranar extension [12].

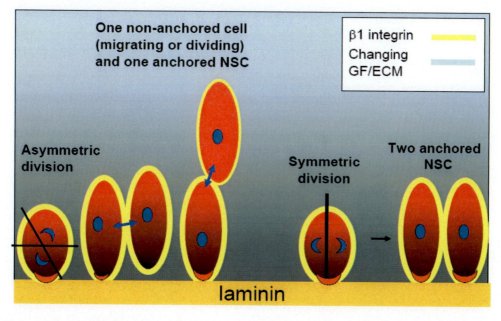

Figure 1. Asymmetric divisions in the VZ (with axis of division parallel to apical surface or with an axis that divides apical domains unequally) can give rise to a cell anchored to the apical ECM (extra cellular matrix) and a second non-anchored cell. Perfectly symmetric divisions will originate two anchored cells, both of which will have elements belonging to the apical adhesion region (shown as a red semi lunar apical structure in the diagram). The cells at different distances from the ventricle and from the apical surface may also be subject to different concentrations of growth factors (GF), represented by the blue gradient (lighter blue: low concentrations, darker blue: high concentrations of GF).

In the restricted (but complex) space defined by the VZ environment where NSCs reside, remain as stem cells or evolve into different types of cells we need to account for: 1) the possible existence and effects of ligand gradients; 2) the spatially defined expression of multiple receptors and/or ligands on the surface of the VZ cells; 3) the concurrent context-dependent signalling of specific receptors, cross-talks and synergistic/antagonistic effects between different pathways; 4) the spatially defined distribution of proteins that are involved in the activation (for example through proteolysis, internalization) or de-activation (for example through degradation) of receptors and ligands.

The role of ligand gradients in the VZ has been suggested [11] but evidence remains scarce. The spatially defined expression of multiple receptors will not be explored in this review and has been discussed elsewhere [11]. In this chapter the focus will be on 3) the context-dependent signalling of receptors (including localized cross-talk and synergistic/antagonistic effects between different signalling pathways) and on 4) the role of proteins that are involved in the activation (for example through internalization or other processes such as proteolysis) or de-activation (for example through degradation) of receptors and ligands. The emphasis will be on the extra layer of complexity added to NSC control in the niche when we take into account: A) the context-dependent receptor signalling and B) the spatially organized activation and de-activation of signalling mechanisms. The context-dependent signalling of Notch1 will be used to illustrate A. The role of Caveolin1 in NSC will be discussed as an example of B to show that proteins active in endocytic pathways and trafficking mechanisms may affect signalling and ultimately cell fate determination. This exercise will highlight the fact that a clear-cut definition of the neural stem cell niche in vertebrate systems may present a formidable challenge.

CELL DIVISIONS IN THE VZ: ROLE OF LOCATION AND CONTEXT-DEPENDENCY

The role of symmetric and asymmetric divisions in the sequential cell fate restriction of NEPs and NSCs during neural development has been investigated and debated. It has long been believed that *asymmetric* divisions of stem cells in the VZ (defined by a plane of division that is parallel to the apical VZ surface) give rise to a new apical NSC and a basal daughter cell that is committed to differentiate, while *symmetric* divisions (defined by a plane of division that is perpendicular to the apical VZ surface) will give rise to two daughter cells that share the apically distributed cell surface determinants equally and generate two equivalent NSCs. The plane of division of cells in the VZ has been extensively studied, with conflicting results [13, 14], until the role of apical domain distribution amongst daughter cells was described and highlighted [15]. These authors observed that the apical membrane region needs to be transected and inherited equally by the two daughter cells to insure pluripotency and stem cell maintenance through the generation of two new NSCs. A detailed analysis demonstrated that even when the axis was almost perpendicular (and would have appeared to generate a symmetric VZ division) the asymmetric distribution of a small portion of the apical membrane had a significant effect on cell fate determination [15]. Interestingly, a role for the plane of division of the basal progenitor cells (the ones that have *left the VZ and divide basally to enlarge the pool of committed progenitors* prior to terminal differentiation) is poorly known, although there is evidence that these cells may be asymmetrically distributing receptors such as the EGFR [16]. Therefore, rather than the plane of division itself it is the location (and context-dependency) of the division (*in the VZ/out of the VZ*) together with the adherence to the apical surface, and the distribution of specific apical membrane domains (perhaps related to localized internalization and activation of receptors) that appear to play a crucial role in NSC cell fate determination in the developing CNS (figure 1). The importance of the cell location at the time of division highlights the role of the micro-environmental structure of the VZ in the control of cell behavior (for example the presence of Laminin in the VZ versus Fibronectin in more basal locations). The role of adherence of NSC to the apical surface may reflect the local activation of signalling pathways through this adhesion area and/or the controlled exposure to ventricular molecules.

LOCATION-DEPENDENT AND CONTEXT-DEPENDENT RECEPTOR SIGNALLING

One of the indications that location dependent and context-dependent cell signalling may play an important role in NSC biology comes from the study of the $\beta1$-integrin expression and its ligands in NSCs and in the VZ micro environment. *In vivo* NSCs express high levels of $\beta1$-integrins and they are located within a Laminin-rich and well defined apical VZ area [17]. NSC require both $\beta1$-integrins and EGFR activation for survival and maintenance [17, 18]. Likewise, human neural precursor cells are regulated by Laminin and Integrins [19] and in other NSC, such as the neural crest cells, $\alpha1\beta1$-integrin interaction with distinct Laminin1 domains affects spreading, migration and survival through independent signalling pathways [20]. The expression of Integrins and their ligands can affect location dependent and context-dependent signalling in a number of ways: for example location dependency may be due to a pure mechanical anchorage of cells (expressing the adequate Integrin) to a specific substrate. This appears to be the case in the VZ, where adherence to the apical surface (through Integrins) could insure that only *anchored* apical cells are exposed to the adequate factors that allow them to remain as stem cells. Alternatively, adherence may play more active roles (figure 2) by either 1) localizing asymmetrically membrane components that are essential for cell fate determination 2) or by *focally* activating pathways that may be, directly or indirectly, involved in cell fate determination, in the retention of "stem cell ness", in cell survival or for cell migration 3) by insuring that receptor cross-talk occurs only at anchored/activated sites 4) by providing focal internalization of receptors. An example of the first mechanism (figure 2 A) is given by Numb, whose role as an asymmetric cell fate determinant has been extensively reviewed. Interestingly, Numb can interact with $\beta1$-integrin [21]. Examples of the second mechanism (figure 2 B) are less well known. Some receptors that are generously distributed in the cell membrane of the VZ cells may be preferentially activated in apical areas of the cell, where these cells are strongly attached to the ependymal surface. For example, $\beta1$-integrin rich VZ cells [17] are surrounded by Laminin [11, 17] but there appears to be an "asymmetric activation" of these receptors, as seen by the polarized distribution of Actin filaments detected with phalloidin [11]. Such focal activation could have more general repercussions in the small, restricted space of the VZ where a few adherent and physically constrained NSC are dividing: for example it could affect the cell cycle. Recently it was shown that a mutation in the $\beta1$-integrin cytoplasmic tail (that suppresses $\beta1$-integrin activation) allows the cells to enter mitosis but inhibits the assembly of microtubules from the centrosome and disrupts cytokinesis, by preventing the formation of a normal bipolar spindle [22]. Therefore, local (*focal*) activation of β1-integrin on a particular area of the NSC surface could play an important role in spindle positioning and contribute to the differential distribution of specific membrane domains, with a final effect on cell fate.

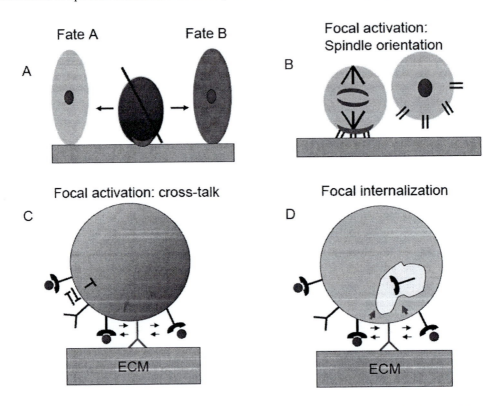

Figure 2. The adherence of neuroprogenitors/neural stem cells to molecules located apically in the VZ could: a) affect cell fate determination, by asymmetrically distributing molecules involved in this process (example: Numb); b) affect spindle orientation (example β1-integrin); c) lead to focal activation of surface signalling receptors and/or focal cross-talk between different pathways; d) lead to focal internalization of receptors and focal modulation of signalling pathways.

Cross-talk and/or protein-protein interaction could preferentially occur at anchored activated sites (figure 2 C). For example, Notch1 is another highly expressed VZ protein whose *focal activation* in the VZ could affect NSC behavior. Notch1 is a large transmembrane protein involved in cell fate choices during development [23]. It promotes neural stem cell maintenance [24], and sequential glial and neural differentiation [25]. Interestingly, in NSCs Notch1 signals in a context-dependent manner [11] which depends, at least partially, on a β1-integrin dependent modulation of the amount of Notch intracellular domain (NICD) fragments that are freely available to reach the nucleus. In NSC the β1-integrin cytoplasmic tail appears to sequester the Notch intracellular domain (NICD) and to retain this active fragment in the cytoplasmic and cell membrane fractions of the neural progenitors [26] (See figure 3). This suggested sequestration mechanism adds a subtle control to the Notch function, which could be important at crucial times such as during cell division to ensure that the available NICD is "tied up" during the whole mitosis and cytokinesis sequence and is dutifully released in the daughter cell only after completion of cytokinesis, to act in the nucleus and stop differentiation of the newly formed VZ cell.

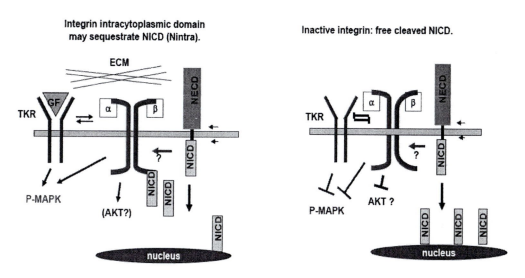

Figure 3. Context-dependent receptor signalling of the Notch receptor. The diagram depicts one possible mechanism to explain how cross-talk occurs between Notch, Integrins and TKR signalling pathways at the level of the cellular membrane. In this hypothetical model the presence of ECM (extra cellular matrix) and GF (growth factors) (A) modulates the levels of Notch intracellular domain (NICD) that reaches the nucleus through sequestration of the NICD by the intra cytoplasmic tail of the β1-integrin. In the absence of NICD sequestration (B) the levels of the NICD fragments that reach the nucleus are higher. These interactions may require the presence of other proteins.

Furthermore, this sequestration mechanism may also localize Notch to adequate sites on the cell surface and be required for Notch internalization, a process that may partially depend on both Caveolin1 and on β1-integrins [26] (figure 2 D). Interestingly, recent studies suggest that endocytosis may be involved in the S3 cleavage of Notch [27]. In this scenario only the surface of the cell where β1-integrin is actively engaged (the apical surface) could adequately traffic Notch, therefore conferring to the anchored cell a "stem cell ness advantage". If both β1-integrin and Caveolin1 are required (and possibly other cooperating proteins) the whole process may depend on the Integrin activation state, which in turn may require the surrounding Laminin and/or cross-talk with the EGFR or other TKRs. There is some evidence that location-dependent cell fate determination could involve the differential processing and/or internalization of TKR receptors by cells expressing different groups of specific adhesion surface molecules (figure 2 D). For example, the Vascular Endothelial Cadherin (VEC) has recently been shown to limit cell proliferation in endothelial cells by retaining vascular endothelial growth factor receptor 2 (VEGFR-2) at the membrane and preventing its internalization into signalling compartments [28]. A similar mechanism could exist in the VZ/SVZ, where both N-cadherin [29] and E-cadherin are expressed [11]. It is noteworthy that N-cadherin is ubiquitous throughout the brain between E12 and E16 but its expression is most prominent in the proliferative neuroepithelium [30]. Interestingly, the combinatorial expression of Cadherins subdivides the embryonic brain into functional units and Cadherins are seen as modulators of cellular phenotypes [31]. This could occur through a number of mechanisms. For example, E-Cadherin-mediated adhesion inhibits ligand-dependent activation of TKRs by decreasing the receptor mobility and the ligand-binding affinity [32]. An interesting hypothesis is that differential Cadherin expression may affect the response to diverse growth factors (GF) by controlling the GF receptors internalization at the membrane. In fact there is evidence showing that FGF induces the internalization, through a common endocytic machinery, of FGFR1 and E-Cadherin into early endosomes, followed by the nuclear translocation of the FGFR1 [33]. Other cell surface receptors may explore similar mechanisms. For example, extra cellular matrix proteins modulate the endocytosis of the insulin receptor (IR) [34]. In this case the Actin organization (but not the microtubules) is critical for IR internalization after Integrin-mediated signalling pathways are activated by cell adhesion to Fibronectin, highlighting the importance of the surrounding matrix for receptor function.

CELL MEMBRANE SPECIALIZATION IN THE VZ NSC

The unequal activation of receptors throughout the membrane of the same cell could occur if these receptors were preferentially located in special membrane micro domains. Such "signalling platforms" have been described: lipid rafts are heterogeneous domains of the cell membrane, which play a role in signal transduction, membrane and protein sorting and in several human diseases [35, 36]. Lipid rafts are specialized cholesterol-rich membrane micro domains that act as receptor signalling platforms and contain resident proteins such as Flottilin and Caveolin1 [37, 38]. Caveolin1 is required for the formation of the cell plasma membrane invaginations (named caveolae) that are involved in Clathrin-independent membrane transport. Interestingly, the polarized VZ cells have apical plasma membranes that contain proteins such as Prominin1, also known to be associated with cholesterol-based membrane micro domains. It is therefore not surprising to find that lipid raft resident proteins such as Caveolin1 are expressed on VZ cells [11], on primary NSC neurosphere cultures [11] and on embryonic stem cell derived NSC (*unpublished data*). Interestingly, around E12.5 when the NEPs are generating RGCs, the mouse VZ cells express abundant Caveolin1 (figure 4 A) and the expression is later down-regulated. Caveolin-stabilized membrane domains are used as multi-functional transport and sorting devices in endocytic membrane traffic [39]. Furthermore, Caveolin1 is required for signalling and membrane targeting of EphB1 receptor tyrosine kinases [40] and BMP receptors co-localize with Caveolin1 on the cell surface [41]. Recently, Caveolin was found to be necessary for Wnt-3a-dependent internalization of the Wnt receptor low-density lipoprotein receptor-related protein 6 (LRP6) [42]. Caveolin also suppresses the expression of Survivin, and controls cell proliferation and cell death in culture lines [43]. Therefore Caveolin1 plays crucial roles for multiple signalling pathways and its roles in NSC may be equally multiple and important.

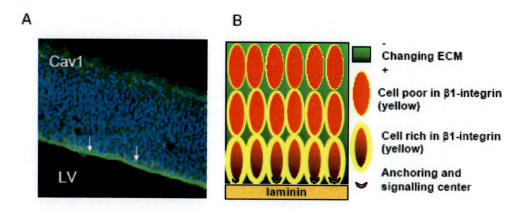

Figure 4. Differential expression of Caveolin1 in the E12.5 mouse embryonic VZ as seen by immunofluorescence (A, caveolin in green. Nuclei counterstained with DAPI in blue) and comparison with the model of variable ECM/GF expression in the mouse developing cortex (Laminin is shown at the apical surface of the model as an orange bar). The different levels of β1-integrin expression between the VZ and the pial surface are diagrammatically depicted by the thickness of the yellow rim surrounding the cells (B). Caveolin1 is clearly enriched in apical cells only. These cells are the ones in contact with Laminin (presumably activating Integrin receptors) and closer to GF sources from the lateral ventricles (e.g., choroid plexus).

Further suggestions of potential roles for Caveolin in NSC arise from the study of glioblastomas where Caveolin1 is known to be involved in EGFR signalling. In these glial tumors Caveolin1 interacts directly with EGFR and dissociates from the receptor upon ligand-induced tyrosine phosphorylation of the EGFR [44]. In turn, EGFR has been shown to be present in the VZ and SVZ neural stem cells [16] and the proliferation of β1-integrin deficient NSC can be rescued by exposing the cells to higher levels of EGF in culture [18]. An interaction between EGFR and Caveolin1 (or between Caveolin and other TKRs) in NSC remains to be evaluated, but is likely to occur as Caveolin1 is known to affect EGFR function in other systems. Interestingly, our results (*unpublished data*) show that the absence of Caveolin1 on NSCs causes MAPK hyper-phosphorylation (a result that recalls the observations made on the Caveolin1 and 3 null animals, where there is hyper-phosphorylation of MAPK [45, 46]), suggesting that signalling through receptors like TKRs and Integrins, both of which rely on downstream ERK/MAPK signalling [47], may be modulated by the presence or absence of Caveolin1 at the cell surface. The distribution of Caveolin1 we have observed *in vivo* (figure 4) may therefore contribute to "compartmentalize" signalling through receptors commonly found on the surface of NSC and neural progenitors in the VZ. A model can be proposed where the VZ *Caveolin1-rich* cells react to receptor X activation in one way and SVZ *Caveolin1-poor* cells react to the same receptor X activation in a different manner (figure 5). This could provide a fine *spatial control of signalling*, where the activation of the same receptor leads to a different end result, depending on its location and on the partnerships at the cell membrane. The presence or absence of Caveolin1 may also alter the quality of the signaling from a pulse-like transient type to a continuous sustained type. This may be important to control cell cycle length which, in turn, has been associated to cell fate determination as discussed below.

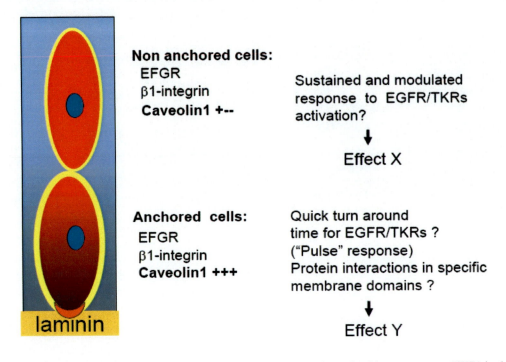

Figure 5. Model of differential spatial modulation of the activation of tyrosine kinase receptors (TKR) in the presence or absence of Caveolin1. Cells with high Caveolin1 levels will respond to TKR activation differently than cells with low levels of Caveolin1. This may be due, for example, to changes in the turn-around time of the receptor at the membrane and/or changes in protein interactions dependent on the presence of Caveolin1.

CELL CYCLE LENGTH AND SIGNALLING IN NEP AND RGC

During CNS development the lengthening of the cell cycle time appears to be associated with the transition from proliferative symmetric divisions to neurogenic asymmetric divisions [48]. How this happens is not clear, but it is assumed that extrinsic or intrinsic factors may lead to a cell fate change depending on the amount of time they are allowed to act upon the cells. In the VZ this may be achieved by controlling the duration of cell signaling (either by limiting or extending the activation of receptors effects) through specific receptors such as TKRs or Integrins, generating either a sustained or a pulse-like downstream signaling event. Some of the receptors involved in NSC maintenance, survival, differentiation and migration include β1-integrins [17] and the EGFR [16], both of which activate downstream the ERK1/2 (MAPK) pathways [17, 47]. Interestingly, continuous (but not transient) ERK activation is known to down regulate anti proliferative genes throughout the G1 phase of the cell cycle, thus allowing cell-cycle progression [49]. Sustained ERK activation elevates the levels of Cyclin D1, which is important for S-phase entry [50] [51]. The mode of ERK activation (sustained versus transient) can be controlled in several ways by "regulators" which can alter the duration, magnitude, and/or compartmentalization of the ERK phosphorylation after stimulation [52]. In the VZ some of these mechanisms may be at work to control the EGFR, β1-integrin and perhaps other receptors activation levels. In particular, the presence of

Caveolin1 in the VZ and its absence more basally may significantly affect receptor internalization, activation and/or degradation, creating a spatially defined differential ERK response to the same receptor activation, such as the EGFR. Receptor activation could be, for example, transient in the presence of Caveolin1 on the cell surface or sustained in its absence. Furthermore, the magnitude of response may hypothetically be controlled by a diffusion gradient of molecules from the lateral ventricle, causing a more intense (but transient) response from the Caveolin1-rich apical cells (exposed to higher GF concentrations) and a weaker response (although sustained) from the more basal Caveolin1-poor cells (exposed to lower GF concentrations). Finally we can not ignore the regulatory effects that the growth factors can have on the Caveolin1 expression levels. For example, HGF (hepatocyte growth factor) causes down regulation of Caveolin1 in satellite cells during muscle regeneration. This down regulation of Caveolin1 leads to activation of ERK, which in turn stimulates proliferation and migration [53]. More importantly, the down regulating effect of the growth factor on Caveolin1 expression levels has also been described for EGF in tumor cells [54] and the down regulation of Caveolin1 we observe at E14.5 and E15.5 (at the time when a switch from bFGF to EGF exposure occurs in the neuroepithelium [55]) could represent a similar phenomenon (*unpublished data*).

Cyclical changes may be important to understand the biology of the VZ, and may be responsible for the alternating waves of VZ proliferation and migration of post-mitotic cells away from the VZ, which are required for the proper development of a multi layered cortex. Therefore, changes in cell cycle length could be related to the differential responses to mitogenic stimuli, partly controlled by the endocytic mechanisms available on the cells. In this hypothesis Caveolin1 could be acting as a VZ "ERK-activation regulator" [52] by affecting the downstream signalling of NSC receptors that are activated by the local ECM and/or GF environment. Ultimately, this simple mechanism may affect cell fate determination and/or migration of post mitotic neural progenitor cells.

CONCLUSIONS

The embryonic vertebrate murine NSC niche is defined architecturally by a stratified epithelium where highly polarized, elongated, anchored cells divide (under the control of growth factors, extra cellular matrix molecules and other proteins) to generate NSC and committed neural progenitors that will give rise to differentiated neural cells. The VZ cells contain a large number of receptors that can cross-talk extensively and/or signal in a context-dependent manner. The activated cell surface signalling pathways in the VZ can also interact (and can be controlled) at multiple levels including: 1) on the anchored polarized cell surface that faces the specialized VZ extra cellular matrix environment and where focal activation an/or internalization of receptors may occur; 2) in the specific membrane micro domains that partition receptors and cell fate determinants; 3) in the endocytic compartments (caveolae, clathrin pits) that internalize receptors for recycling or degradation. In this chapter we discussed how context-dependent receptor signalling, focal activation of cell surface receptors and the specialized expression of caveolar proteins such as Caveolin1 may spatially change the final effect of activated receptors expressed throughout the neuroepithelium. The importance of the compartmentalization of the signalling output (rather than the role of the receptors expression patterns) highlights the functional nature of the NSC niche. The cell anchorage status and the shape of the NSC also appear to be important for the functional definition of the niche.

REFERENCES

[1]   Dahlstrand, J., Zimmerman, L.B., McKay, R.D., and Lendahl, U. (1992). Characterization of the human nestin gene reveals a close evolutionary relationship to neurofilaments. *J. Cell Sci. 103*, 589-597.

[2]   Gotz, M., and Huttner, W.B. (2005). The cell biology of neurogenesis. *Nat. Rev. Mol. Cell Biol. 6*, 777-788.

[3]   Gotz, M., and Barde, Y.A. (2005). Radial Glial Cells Defined and MajorIntermediates between EmbryonicStem Cells and CNS Neurons. *Neuron. 46*, 369-372.

[4]   Voigt, T. (1989). Development of glial cells in the cerebral wall of ferrets: direct tracing of their transformation from radial glia into astrocytes. *J. Comp. Neurol. 289*, 74-88.

[5]   Culican, S.M., Baumrind, N.L., Yamamoto, M., and Pearlman, A.L. (1990). Cortical radial glia: identification in tissue culture and evidence for their transformation to astrocytes. *J. Neurosci. 10*, 684-692.

[6]   Doetsch, F., Caille, I., Lim, D.A., Garcia-Verdugo, J.M., and Alvarez-Buylla, A. (1999). Subventricular zone astrocytes are neural stem cells in the adult mammalian brain. *Cell. 97*, 703-716.

[7]   Alvarez-Buylla, A., and Lim, D.A. (2004). For the long run: maintaining germinal niches in the adult brain. *Neuron. 41*, 683-686.

[8]   Alvarez-Buylla, A., and Garcia-Verdugo, J.M. (2002). Neurogenesis in adult subventricular zone. *J. Neurosci. 22*, 629-634.

[9]   Doetsch, F., Petreanu, L., Caille, I., Garcia-Verdugo, J.M., and Alvarez-Buylla, A. (2002). EGF converts transit-amplifying neurogenic precursors in the adult brain into multipotent stem cells. *Neuron. 36*, 1021-1034.

[10]   Doetsch, F. (2003). The glial identity of neural stem cells. *Nat. Neurosci. 6*, 1127-1134.

[11]   Campos, L.S. (2005). ß1 integrins and neural stem cells: making sense of the extra cellular environment. *BioEssays. 27*.

[12]   Mercier, F., Kitasako, J.T., and Hatton, G.I. (2003). Fractones and other basal laminae in the hypothalamus. *J. Comp. Neurol. 455*, 324-340.

[13]   Cayouette, M., and Raff, M. (2003). The orientation of cell division influences cell-fate choice in the developing mammalian retina. *Development. 130*, 2329-2339.

[14]   Lyons, D.A., Guy, A.T., and Clarke, J.D. (2003). Monitoring neural progenitor fate through multiple rounds of division in an intact vertebrate brain. *Development. 130*, 3427-3436.

[15]   Kosodo, Y., Roper, K., Haubensak, W., Marzesco, A.M., Corbeil, D., and Huttner, W.B. (2004). Asymmetric distribution of the apical plasma membrane during neurogenic divisions of mammalian neuroepithelial cells. *Embo J. 23*, 2314-2324.

[16] Sun, Y., Goderie, S.K., and Temple, S. (2005). Asymmetric distribution of EGFR receptor during mitosis generates diverse CNS progenitor cells. *Neuron. 45*, 873-886.

[17] Campos, L.S., Leone, D.P., Relvas, J.B., Brakebusch, C., Fassler, R., Suter, U., and ffrench-Constant, C. (2004). beta1 integrins activate a MAPK signalling pathway in neural stem cells that contributes to their maintenance. *Development. 131*, 3433-3444.

[18] Leone, D.P., Relvas, J.B., Campos, L.S., Hemmi, S., Brakebusch, C., Fassler, R., Ffrench-Constant, C., and Suter, U. (2005). Regulation of neural progenitor proliferation and survival by beta1 integrins. *J. Cell Sci. 118*, 2589-2599.

[19] Flanagan, L.A., Rebaza, L.M., Derzic, S., Schwartz, P.H., and Monuki, E.S. (2006). Regulation of human neural precursor cells by laminin and integrins. *J. Neurosci. Res. 83*, 845-856.

[20] Desban, N., Lissitzky, J.C., Rousselle, P., and Duband, J.L. (2006). {alpha}1{beta}1-integrin engagement to distinct laminin-1 domains orchestrates spreading, migration and survival of neural crest cells through independent signaling pathways. *J. Cell Sci. 119*, 3206-3218.

[21] Calderwood, D.A., Fujioka, Y., de Pereda, J.M., Garcia-Alvarez, B., Nakamoto, T., Margolis, B., McGlade, C.J., Liddington, R.C., and Ginsberg, M.H. (2003). Integrin beta cytoplasmic domain interactions with phosphotyrosine-binding domains: A structural prototype for diversity in integrin signaling. *PNAS. 100*, 2272-2277.

[22] Reverte, C.G., Benware, A., Jones, C.W., and Laflamme, S.E. (2006). Perturbing integrin function inhibits microtubule growth from centrosomes, spindle assembly, and cytokinesis. *J. Cell Biol. 174*, 491-497.

[23] Lewis, J. (1998). Notch signalling and the control of cell fate choices in vertebrates. *Semin. Cell Dev. Biol. 9*, 583-589.

[24] Hitoshi, S., Alexson, T., Tropepe, V., Donoviel, D., Elia, A.J., Nye, J.S., Conlon, R.A., Mak, T.W., Bernstein, A., and van der Kooy, D. (2002). Notch pathway molecules are essential for the maintenance, but not the generation, of mammalian neural stem cells. *Genes Dev. 16*, 846-858.

[25] Grandbarbe, L., Bouissac, J., Rand, M., Hrabe de Angelis, M., Artavanis-Tsakonas, S., and Mohier, E. (2003). Delta-Notch signaling controls the generation of neurons/glia from neural stem cells in a stepwise process. *Development. 130*, 1391-1402.

[26] Campos, L.S., Decker, L., Taylor, V., and Skarnes, W. (2006). Notch, epidermal growth factor receptor, and beta1-integrin pathways are coordinated in neural stem cells. *J. Biol. Chem. 281*, 5300-5309.

[27] Gupta-Rossi, N., Six, E., LeBail, O., Logeat, F., Chastagner, P., Olry, A., Israel, A., Brou, C., Storck, S., Griebel, P.J., Reynaud, C.A., Weill, J.C., and Dahan, A. (2004). Monoubiquitination and endocytosis direct gamma-secretase cleavage of activated Notch receptor. *J. Cell Biol. 166*, 73-83.

[28] Lampugnani, M.G., Orsenigo, F., Gagliani, M.C., Tacchetti, C., and Dejana, E. (2006). Vascular endothelial cadherin controls VEGFR-2 internalization and signaling from intracellular compartments. *J. Cell Biol. 174*, 593-604.

[29] Redies, C., Ast, M., Nakagawa, S., Takeichi, M., Martinez-de-la-Torre, M., and Puelles, L. (2000). Morphologic fate of diencephalic prosomeres and their subdivisions revealed by mapping cadherin expression. *J. Comp. Neurol. 421*, 481-514.

[30] Redies, C., and Takeichi, M. (1993). Expression of N-cadherin mRNA during development of the mouse brain. *Dev. Dyn. 197*, 26-39.

[31] Wheelock, M.J., and Johnson, K.R. (2003). Cadherins as modulators of cellular phenotype. *Annu. Rev. Cell Dev. Biol. 19*, 207-235.

[32] Qian, X., Karpova, T., Sheppard, A.M., McNally, J., and Lowy, D.R. (2004). E-cadherin-mediated adhesion inhibits ligand-dependent activation of diverse receptor tyrosine kinases. *Embo J. 23*, 1739-1748.

[33] Bryant, D.M., Wylie, F.G., and Stow, J.L. (2005). Regulation of endocytosis, nuclear translocation, and signaling of fibroblast growth factor receptor 1 by E-cadherin. *Mol. Biol. Cell. 16*, 14-23.

[34] Boura-Halfon, S., Voliovitch, H., Feinstein, R., Paz, K., and Zick, Y. (2003). Extracellular matrix proteins modulate endocytosis of the insulin receptor. *J. Biol. Chem. 278*, 16397-16404.

[35] Lai, E.C. (2003). Lipid rafts make for slippery platforms. *J. Cell Biol. 162*, 365-370.

[36] Williams, T.M., and Lisanti, M.P. (2004). The Caveolin genes: from cell biology to medicine. *Ann. Med. 36*, 584-595.

[37] Drab, M., Verkade, P., Elger, M., Kasper, M., Lohn, M., Lauterbach, B., Menne, J., Lindschau, C., Mende, F., Luft, F.C., Schedl, A., Haller, H., and Kurzchalia, T.V. (2001). Loss of caveolae, vascular dysfunction, and pulmonary defects in caveolin-1 gene-disrupted mice. *Science. 293*, 2449-2452.

[38] Le Roy, C., and Wrana, J.L. (2005). Clathrin- and non-clathrin-mediated endocytic regulation of cell signalling. *Nat. Rev. Mol. Cell Biol. 6*, 112-126.

[39] Pelkmans, L., Burli, T., Zerial, M., and Helenius, A. (2004). Caveolin-stabilized membrane domains as multifunctional transport and sorting devices in endocytic membrane traffic. *Cell. 118*, 767-780.

[40] Vihanto, M.M., Vindis, C., Djonov, V., Cerretti, D.P., and Huynh-Do, U. (2006). Caveolin-1 is required for signaling and membrane targeting of EphB1 receptor tyrosine kinase. *J. Cell Sci. 119*, 2299-2309.

[41] Nohe, A., Keating, E., Underhill, T.M., Knaus, P., and Petersen, N.O. (2005). Dynamics and interaction of caveolin-1 isoforms with BMP-receptors. *J. Cell Sci. 118*, 643-650.

[42] Yamamoto, H., Komekado, H., and Kikuchi, A. (2006). Caveolin Is Necessary for Wnt-3a-Dependent Internalization of LRP6 and Accumulation of beta-Catenin. *Dev. Cell. 11*, 213-223.

[43] Torres, V.A., Tapia, J.C., Rodriguez, D.A., Parraga, M., Lisboa, P., Montoya, M., Leyton, L., and Quest, A.F. (2006). Caveolin-1 controls cell proliferation and cell death by suppressing expression of the inhibitor of apoptosis protein survivin. *J. Cell Sci. 119*, 1812-1823.

[44] Abulrob, A., Giuseppin, S., Andrade, M.F., McDermid, A., Moreno, M., and Stanimirovic, D. (2004). Interactions of EGFR and caveolin-1 in human glioblastoma cells: evidence that tyrosine phosphorylation regulates EGFR association with caveolae. *Oncogene. 23*, 6967-6979.

[45] Cohen, A.W., Park, D.S., Woodman, S.E., Williams, T.M., Chandra, M., Shirani, J., Pereira de Souza, A., Kitsis, R.N., Russell, R.G., Weiss, L.M., Tang, B., Jelicks, L.A.,

Factor, S.M., Shtutin, V., Tanowitz, H.B., and Lisanti, M.P. (2003). Caveolin-1 null mice develop cardiac hypertrophy with hyperactivation of p42/44 MAP kinase in cardiac fibroblasts. *Am. J. Physiol. Cell Physiol. 284*, C457-474.

[46] Woodman, S.E., Park, D.S., Cohen, A.W., Cheung, M.W., Chandra, M., Shirani, J., Tang, B., Jelicks, L.A., Kitsis, R.N., Christ, G.J., Factor, S.M., Tanowitz, H.B., and Lisanti, M.P. (2002). Caveolin-3 knock-out mice develop a progressive cardiomyopathy and show hyperactivation of the p42/44 MAPK cascade. *J. Biol. Chem. 277*, 38988-38997.

[47] Schlessinger, J. (2000). Cell signaling by receptor tyrosine kinases. *Cell. 103*, 211-225.

[48] Calegari, F., Haubensak, W., Haffner, C., and Huttner, W.B. (2005). Selective lengthening of the cell cycle in the neurogenic subpopulation of neural progenitor cells during mouse brain development. *J. Neurosci. 25*, 6533-6538.

[49] Yamamoto, T., Ebisuya, M., Ashida, F., Okamoto, K., Yonehara, S., and Nishida, E. (2006). Continuous ERK activation downregulates antiproliferative genes throughout G1 phase to allow cell-cycle progression. *Curr. Biol. 16*, 1171-1182.

[50] Weber, J.D., Raben, D.M., Phillips, P.J., and Baldassare, J.J. (1997). Sustained activation of extracellular-signal-regulated kinase 1 (ERK1) is required for the continued expression of cyclin D1 in G1 phase. *Biochem. J. 326 (Pt 1)*, 61-68.

[51] Balmanno, K., and Cook, S.J. (1999). Sustained MAP kinase activation is required for the expression of cyclin D1, p21Cip1 and a subset of AP-1 proteins in CCL39 cells. *Oncogene. 18*, 3085-3097.

[52] Ebisuya, M., Kondoh, K., and Nishida, E. (2005). The duration, magnitude and compartmentalization of ERK MAP kinase activity: mechanisms for providing signaling specificity. *J. Cell Sci. 118*, 2997-3002.

[53] Volonte, D., Liu, Y., and Galbiati, F. (2005). The modulation of caveolin-1 expression controls satellite cell activation during muscle repair. *Faseb J. 19*, 237-239.

[54] Lu, Z., Ghosh, S., Wang, Z., and Hunter, T. (2003). Downregulation of caveolin-1 function by EGF leads to the loss of E-cadherin, increased transcriptional activity of beta-catenin, and enhanced tumor cell invasion. *Cancer Cell. 4*, 499-515.

[55] Lillien, L., and Raphael, H. (2000). BMP and FGF regulate the development of EGF-responsive neural progenitor cells. *Development. 127*, 4993-5005.

In: Stem Cell Research Developments
Editor: Calvin A. Fong, pp. 203-227

ISBN: 978-1-60021-601-5
© 2007 Nova Science Publishers, Inc.

Chapter VII

Potential Application of Human Umbilical Cord Mesenchymal Stem Cells in Wharton's Jelly for the Treatment of Parkinsonism

Yu-Show Fu[1,], Yun-Chih Cheng[2] and Yu-Tsung Shih[2]*
[1] Department of Anatomy, School of Medicine,
National Yang-Ming University, Taipei, Taiwan ROC
[2] Institute of Anatomy and Cell Biology, School of Medicine,
National Yang-Ming University, Taipei, Taiwan, ROC

ABSTRACT

Neuronal transplantation has provided a direction for treating neurodegenerative diseases. Recent studies have started to induce various stem cells to transform into neurons in vitro. Here we have demonstrated human umbilical mesenchymal cells in Wharton's jelly behave as stem cells. Human umbilical mesenchymal cells are easily available and capable of rapid expansion in vitro. We are the first to differentiate a large quantity of neuronal-like cells derived from human umbilical mesenchymal cells in neuronal conditioned medium, which may be of great value in treating neurological diseases. Human umbilical mesenchymal cells started to express neuron-specific proteins, such as NeuN and neurofilament treatment with neuronal conditioned medium for 3 days. At the sixth day of culture in neuronal conditioned medium, the human umbilical mesenchymal cells have exhibited retraction of cell body, elaboration of process, clustering of cells and induction of functional mRNA and proteins, such as the subunits of kainate receptor and glutamate decarboxylase. At the ninth-twelfth days, the percentage of human umbilical mesenchymal cells expressed neurofilament could be as high as 87% and glutamate evoked an inward current. At this stage, cells were

---

* Correspondence should be addressed to Yu-Show Fu, Department of Anatomy, School of Medicine, National Yang-Ming University, No. 155, Sec. 2, Li-Nung Street, Taipei, Taiwan, 112, E-mail: ysfu@ym.edu.tw; Tel: 011-886-2-28267254; Fax: 011-886-2-28212884

differentiated into mature neurons with post-mitosis phase. These results have proven its application in clinical transplantation in future without a risk of being transformed to neuronal tumor.

Human umbilical mesenchymal stem cells in Wharton's jelly were induced to transform into dopaminergic neurons *in vitro* through stepwise culturing in neuron condition medium (NCM), SHH, and FGF8. The success rate was 12.7% as characterized by positive staining for tyrosine hydroxylase (TH), the rate limiting catecholaminergic synthesizing enzyme and dopamine being released into the culture medium. Transplantation of such cells into the striatum of rats previously made Parkinsonian by unilateral striatal lesioning with the dopaminergic neurotoxin 6-hydroxydopamine (6-OHDA) partially corrected the lesion-induced amphetamine-evoked rotation. Viability of the transplanted cells, at least 4 months after transplantation, was identified by positive TH staining and migration of 1.4 mm both rostrally and caudaully. The results suggest that human umbilical mesenchymal stem cells have the potential for treatment of Parkinson's disease.

INTRODUCTION

In clinical medicine, stroke, trauma or degenerative neuronal diseases is mainly due to ineffective prevention of degeneration of neurons. The degeneration or death of neurons may lead to malfunctions in the sensory and motor systems and then affect intelligence and life quality. Recent findings indicate that stem cells exist in the central nervous system [1, 2, 3, 4]. Under normal circumstances or when neurons are damaged, these neuron stem cells may proliferate and differentiate with a relative slow rate in vivo.

Stem cells are believed to possess certain characteristics including self-renewal, pluripotent, proliferation, longevity and differentiation. Stem cells are a valuable resource for neuronal transplantation. Fetuses [5, 6], umbilical cord blood [7] and bone marrow [8] are the most common sources of human stem cells. Transplantation of fetus tissues is hindered by disputes in the aspects of religion, law and ethic, and therefore not available to all. The conversion rate of umbilical cord blood into neurons is relatively low in vitro studies [9, 10], research and application of umbilical cord blood focus mainly on hematological diseases. Bone marrow mesenchymal stem cells are capable of differentiating into osteogenic, chondrogenic, adipogenic, and myogenic in vitro [8]. Direct transplantation of bone marrow mesenchymal cells, a relatively low percentage of cells differentiates into neurons with the majority differentiating into glia [11, 12] and thus cannot rescue the neurological diseases. Therefore, transplantation of postmitosis-neurons derived from stem cells has become an effective and direct treatment for the neurological diseases.

Parkinson's disease is a neurodegenerative disorder characterized by the progressive loss of striatal dopaminergic function [13-18] and affects >500,000 people in the United States [19]. Patients initially respond to treatment with dopaminergic enhancing medications such as levodopa (L-DOPA) [20]. However, the effectiveness of such treatments gradually diminishes because the conversion to dopamine within the brain is increasingly disrupted by the progressive degeneration of the dopaminergic terminals. As a result, after approximately ten years of dopamine-replacement treatment, most patients with Parkinson's disease suffer from disability that cannot be satisfactorily controlled [21].

An alternative approach for the restoration of the damaged dopaminergic system, considered to be an ultimate treatment for Parkinson's disease, is the transplantation of cells (or tissues) that synthesize catecholamines [22-26]. There is evidence both from animal studies and clinical investigations showing that fetal dopamine neurons can produce symptomatic relief [27-39]. However, technical and ethical difficulties in obtaining sufficient and appropriate graft tissues have limited the application of this therapy [40].

In this present studies, we showed that human umbilical mesenchymal stem cells in whartons' jelly (HUMSCs) cultured in neuronal conditioned medium (NCM) encourages and facilitates their transformation into neurons with good yield. The HUMSCs were then differentiated into dopaminergic neurons *in vitro*. These dopaminergic neurons were then transplanted into the striatum of rats previously made Parkinsonian by unilateral striatal lesioning with 6-OHDA. The results indicated that transplantation of *in vitro* differentiated HUMSCs alleviated the lesion-induced amphetamine evoked rotation in the Parkinsonian rats, demonstrating potential therapeutic values.

NEURONAL INDUCTION OF HUMSCs

Preparation of Human Umbilical Mesenchymal Stem Cells

Human umbilical cords were collected in HBSS (Biochrom L201-10) at 4 °C. The umbilical cord was soaked in 75% ethanol for 30 seconds for sanitization. The umbilical cord was placed in Ca^{2+}/Mg^{2+} free buffer (Gibco 14185-052), and cord vessels were detached. The mesenchymal tissue (Wharton's jelly) was diced into cubes of about 0.5 cm^3 and centrifuged at 250g for 5 minutes. The supernatant was removed, and the precipitate (mesenchymal tissue) was washed with serum-free DMEM (Gibco 12100-046) and centrifuging at 250g for 5 minutes. The mesenchymal tissue was treated with collagenase at 37 °C for 18 hours, washed, and then treated with 2.5% trypsin (Gibco 15090-046) at 37 °C for 30 minutes. FBS (Hyclone SH30071.03) was added to the mesenchymal tissue to quench the activity of trypsin. At this time, the mesenchymal tissue has become mesenchymal stem cells. The mesenchymal stem cells were treated with 10% FBS-DMEM to be dispersed and counted. The mesenchymal stem cells can now be directly used for culture, expansion or store in liquid nitrogen.

Preparation of Neuronal Conditioned Medium (NCM)

The P7 old Sprague-Dawley rats were anaesthetized by 10% chloride hydrate *i.p.* injection. The rat brain was removed and placed in Ca^{2+}/Mg^{2+} free buffer (Gibco 14185-052). The brain was centrifuged at 900 rpm for 5 minutes. The supernatant was removed, and 10% FBS-DMEM was added to the precipitate (brain tissue). The brain tissue was pipetted 15 times to be dispersed into single cells. The cells were mixed with the 10% FBS-DMEM and cultured in the 37 °C incubator. On the next day, final concentration 2 μM of AraC (Sigma, c-

6645) was added. On the fifth day of culture, the culture medium was removed to be used to culture umbilical mesenchymal cells. The human umbilical mesenchymal cells were cultured in NCM alone. The NCM has to be replaced very other day.

Morphological Indentification

About 10^6 of human umbilical mesenchymal cells were collected from 20cm in length of umbilical cord. The number of umbilical mesenchymal cells has doubled (2×10^6) in 10% FBS DMEM for 3 days. The umbilical mesenchymal cells may be directly used to induce into neurons, or store in liquid nitrogen for later uses. The umbilical mesenchymal cells were mesenchymal-like shape with a flat and polygonal morphology treatment with 10% FBS DMEM for 3 days (figure 1A). With a continuous culture for 6 days, the mesenchymal cells were mostly a spindle shape and were closely attached to each other due to proliferation (figure 1B). Treatment of human umbilical mesenchymal cells with neuronal conditioned medium (NCM) caused umbilical mesenchymal cell to display a neuronal-like morphology. These cells had a smaller cell body and displayed neurite- and axon-like processes in NCM for 3 days (figure 1C). Prolonging the NCM treatment time, cell cluster and process elongation were observed. After 12 day, these processes were exceedingly long, formed cell-cell contacts and created the appearance of a network (figure 1D).

Time Course of Neuronal-Like and Glial-Like Differentiation

To determine whether human umbilical mesenchymal derived cells could express the neuronal markers, we tested the immunocytochemistry of NeuN and Neurofilament (NF). On the 6th day after NCM treatment, umbilical mesenchymal cells presented a characteristic of cluster and expressed of NeuN (figure 1E) and NF (figure 1F). Morphology patterns of cells expressing NeuN included bipolar, multipolar and mesenchymal-like shape (figure 1G, H, I). A 3 day NCM treatment induced 42.2±5.0% of umbilical mesenchymal cells to acquire immunostaining for the neuronal marker NeuN. The proportion of cells expressing NeuN reached the maximum, 58.2±4.2%, at 9 day but dropped to 36.3±5.9% at 12 day (figure 2A). Treatment of umbilical mesenchymal cells with NCM, the morphology of umbilical mesenchymal cells expressing NF could display bipolar, multipolar or mesenchymal-like shape (figure 1J, K, L). After 3 day of treatment, 59.4±1.3% of the cells displayed a robust immunostaining for NF. The ratio of NF-positive further increased to 87.4±5.5%, reached a plateau on the 6th day and persisted up to 12 day after treatment (figure 2B).

In order to examine the number of astrocyte and microglia, the immunocytochemistry of GFAP and OX42 were performed. Before NCM treatment, 0.64% of human umbilical mesenchymal cells expressed GFAP-positive. Treatment of NCM for 3 day caused 1.3% umbilical mesenchymal cells to display GFAP. Such ratio reached the maximum on the 9th day but declined back to 1.95% on the 12th day (figure 2C). 1.77±0.63% of untreated umbilical mesenchymal cells expressed OX42. Treatment of NCM for 3 day caused more microglia differentiation (3.00±0.26%), and the ratio kept consistent and persisted up to 12 day (figure 2D).

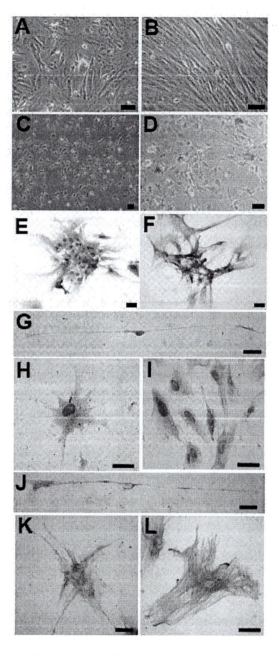

Figure 1. Photomicrographs showing the change of morphological pattern and the expression of neuronal specific protein NeuN and NF of human umbilical mesenchymal cells treatment with NCM. Umbilical mesenchymal cells treatment with 10% FBS DMEM for 3 days (A) and 6 days (B). (C) treatment with NCM for 3 days. (D) treatment with NCM for 12 days. Umbilical mesenchymal derived cells express neuronal specific protein NeuN (E) and NF (F) in NCM for 6 days. NeuN-positive cells with morphology of bipolar (G), multipolar (H) or mesenchymal-like (I) were shown. The morphology of NF-positive cells could be bipolar (J), multipolar (K) or mesenchymal (L). (Arrows indicate the positive-staining cells; arrow heads indicate the negative staining cells. Scale bar: 50 μm in A, B, E-L. 100 μm in C-D).

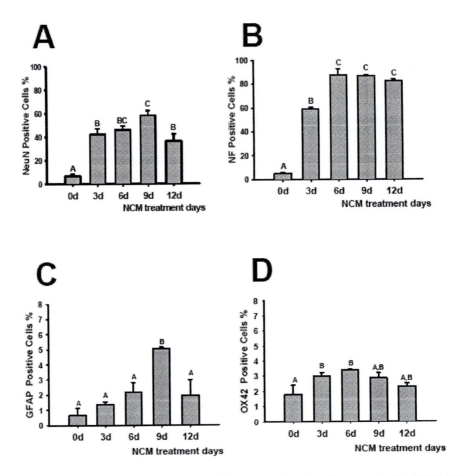

Figure 2. Histogram showing the ratio of human umbilical mesenchymal cells expressing NeuN (A), NF (B), GFAP (C), and OX42 (D) after NCM treatment (The results are the mean ± s.e. of six randomly selected microscopic fields each from three different experiments). In (A), * compare with 0 day. # compare with 3 day and 12 day. In (B), * compare with 0 day. # compare with 3 day. In (C) and (D), * compare with the other days. p<0.05.

Characterization of Functional Protein

In order to verify the expression of neuronal functional protein in human umbilical mesenchymal cells, the assay of subunits of kainate receptor were determined by western blots. As the results showed, the subunits of kainate receptor were not detected in human umbilical mesenchymal cells before treatment with NCM. We treated umbilical mesenchymal cells with NCM, the kainate receptor subunits, including GluR6, GluR7 and KA2 were observed at a small quantity at 6 day and then significantly labeled at 12 day (figure 3A). In order to eliminate the possibility of NCM contains glutamate receptor and GAD, RT-PCR experiments for GluR6, KA2 and GAD was performed. The results showed that the mRNA of GluR6, KA2 and GAD were found in human umbilical mesenchymal stem cells on the 12th day of NCM treatment (figure 3B).

In order to confirm the functionality of glutamate receptor, a whole cell record was made in neuronal-like human umbilical mesenchymal stem cells after they were cultured with NCM for 12 days (figure 3F). Bath application of 1 mM glutamate evoked an inward current with magnitude of (50.5±1.6) pA (n=13, two cells no response), with membrane voltage hold at –70 mV. The effect of glutamate was completely washed out in few minutes after the perfusion medium was change to normal Ringers solution (figure 3E). Taken together the electrophysiological result is consistent with results of western blot and RT-PCR, suggesting that the human umbilical mesenchymal cells do express functional glutamate receptor on the membrane after culture with NCM.

Further study was to identify the existence of calcium binding protein. Among various calcium binding proteins available in the nervous system, parvalbumin, calbindin-D28K and calretinin were the widest distribution in CNS [41]. Treatments with NCM for 9 days, some of human umbilical mesenchymal cells were induced to express several functional calcium binding proteins, including parvalbumin and calbindin (figure 3C, D).

In order to verify the capability for the synthesis of GABA neurotransmitters, immunostaining for GAD was employed. After a 6 day NCM incubation induced human umbilical mesenchymal cells to synthesize GAD and the GAD expression level was significantly increased on the 12th day (figure 3A).

In the present study we have identified, cultured, and propagated human umbilical mesenchymal cells that act as stem cells, similar result was provided by Kathy et al., [42]. The human umbilical mesenchymal cells were collected from Wharton's Jelly. Treatment with NCM, these cells can be induced to differentiate at 87% into neurons. Numerous studies have indicated that various growth factors, such as retinoic acid, bFGF, BDNF, GDNF, TGF-β, Insulin-like growth factor and EGF, are involved in the transformation of stem cells into neurons [43 - 47]. In addition, neurotransmitters could regulate the proliferation, growth, migration, differentiation and survival of neural precursor cells [48]. Moreover, we have tried to treat the umbilical mesenchymal cells cultured in 10%FBS DMEM with AraC, but no significant neurogenesis occurred. We therefore speculated that the NCM may contain some cytokines and neurotransmitters released from cultured neurons, so the NCM may urge stem cells to differentiate into neurons efficiently.

In the study of Woodbury et al., treatment of 1-10 mM β-mercaptoethanol for 5 hours induced 75% of bone marrow mesenchymal cells to transform into neurons [49]. However, β-mercaptoethanol is highly controversial. Some studies have indicated that β-mercaptoethanol posseses a toxic effect on organisms by breaking disulfide bonds [50]. In the other hand, β-mercaptoethanol exerted a positive effect by increasing the survival rate of neurons *in vitro* [51]. We have treated umbilical mesenchymal stem cells with 2~5mM β-mercaptoethanol for 3 days. This treatment induced umbilical mesenchymal stem cell to display damage (data not shown). We suggest the cause for such different tolerance may due to mesenchymal stem cells isolated from various adults. β-mercaptoethanol was not considered to be utilized in our present study.

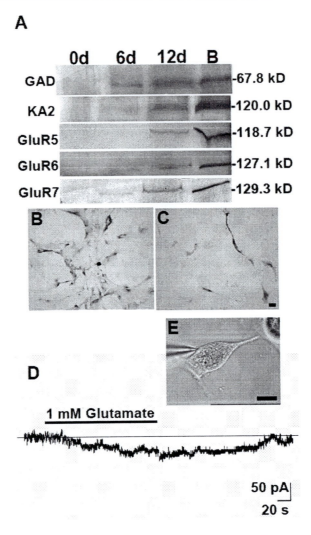

Figure 3. NCM induces the expressions of functional proteins of neuronal - like cells derived from human umbilical mesenchymal cells. (A) Western blot showing that the expression of the subunits of kainate receptor and neurotransmitter-GAD of human umbilical mesenchymal cells. B: adult rat brain. (B) RT-PCR showing mRNA expression of GluR6, KA2 and GAD on the 12th day after NCM treatment. These mRNAs were undetectable before NCM treatment. Photomicrograph shows the expressions of parvabulmin (C) and calbindin (D) of umbilical mesenchymal cells treatment with NCM for 9 days. Glutamate evoked inward current in human umbilical mesenchymal cell. (E) Whole cell patch records of the response to bath perfusion of 1 mM glutamate in human umbilical mesenchymal cell treatment with NCM for 12 days in response to glutamate. Glutamate elicits a 50pA current. (F) Photomicrograph of the recorded human umbilical mesenchymal cell. (Scale bar: 50 μm).

We found that NeuN and NF were expressed in untreated umbilical mesenchymal stem cells. While this result was somewhat surprising, it is consistent with results from Kathy et al. [42]. Similar results are found in the bone marrow stromal cells [49, 52]. *Woodbury et al.* [49] also found that NSE was expressed in untreated bone marrow stromal cells. In other work with bone marrow stromal cells, *Sanchez-Ramos et al.* [52] found that NeuN and GFAP, markers for early mature neurons and astrocytes, respectively, were expressed in uninduced bone marrow stromal cells. Likewise, we found that the glial cell markers, GFAP and OX42, were expressed in untreated umbilical mesenchymal cells. Our results, along with the studies described above, suggest that untreated umbilical mesenchymal stem cells express a low number of neural and glia proteins spontaneously and, perhaps, are primed to differentiate along a neural program.

In our study, the ratio of cell expressing NeuN reached a maximum at 9 day, decreased at 12 day. Such a drop in the number of NeuN positive cells on the 12th day could be due to the absence of NeuN expression in a part of mature neurons. Similar reports have revealed that neurons start to express NeuN in the early phase during development and the expression of NeuN of neurons in some brain areas may be decreased after maturation [53]. Numerous calcium binding proteins were found in the central nervous system with various calcium binding proteins being present on various types of neurons. Researches have indicated that PV and CB were expressed on approximately 5 - 10% of neurons; moreover, the expression of PV was confined in GABAergic neurons [54]. Therefore, PV and CB were only expressed on some of neurons derived from umbilical mesenchymal cells in our experiments. In our study show that NF positive neurons still posses the capability to proliferate at a 3 day treatment, however, no longer proliferated at the 9th day. As for what factors close the proliferation is an important issue and is worthy to be studied.

In the present study, less than 5% of umbilical mesenchymal cells were differentiated into astrocytes. We suggest that such low ratio of astrocytes had positive regulatory influence on neurons being differentiating or mature. Several studies have confirmed that astrocytes could secrete certain growth factors to affect the maturation of neurons. For example, the secretion of glial cell line-derived neurotrophic factor (GDNF) could effectively alleviate the damage of dopaminergic neuron [55]. In addition, tumor necrosis factor-α also could be secreted by astrocytes to regulate the formation of synapses on neurons and control the sensitivity of these synapses [56].

Concluding from our results, it is believed that the most suitable time point for performing the transplantation of human umbilical mesenchymal cells was at the 6 to 9 days NCM treatment, since in this stage, neurons have the lowest capability for proliferation and the highest ratio of neurons expressing NeuN and NF. In addition, a small quantity of astrocytes and microglia exist which may promote the neuronal survival and remodeling after transplantation. After being transplanted into individuals with neurological diseases, such neuronal-like cells derived from human umbilical mesenchymal cells can be expected to be able to substitute the functions of damaged neurons.

THE CHANGE OF CELL PROLIFERATION DURING NEURONAL INDUCTION

Although the treatment with NCM could induce human umbilical mesenchymal cells to express neuron-specific proteins and functional proteins, the capability for proliferation of these cells is still unclear. Therefore, proliferation assay was conducted. 4',6-diamidino-2-phenylindole dihydrocholoride (DAPI), a DNA binding fluorescence, is able to freely penetrate through cellular membranes and is used to count the total cell number. In order to count cell number exactly, the human umbilical mesenchymal cells were cultured with lower density (10^3/ml). After NCM treatment, the cell density on the 9th day was significantly higher than that on the day0 and 3rd days and consistent on the 12th day (figure 4A, B).

BrdU labeling is utilized to confirm the replication of cells. Double staining with BrdU and DAPI showed that most of umbilical mesenchymal cells were still able to proliferate in NCM for 3 days (figure 5A, B, C). NF and BrdU double labeling can identify the replication ability of neurons. These cells expressing NF were labeled by BrdU simultaneously (figure 5D, E, F). On the 9th day of treatment with NCM, cell proliferation was not observed in the majority of cells (figure 5G, H, I), furthermore, these BrdU-negative cells were neuronal-like cells expressing NF (figure 5J, K, L).

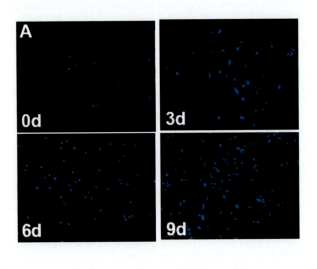

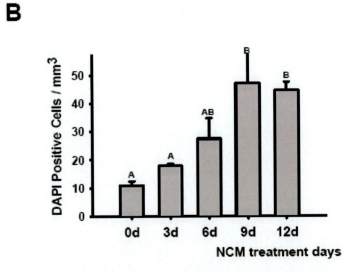

Figure 4. The altered cell density of human umbilical mesenchymal cells induced by NCM. (A) Photomicrograph showing the cell density, DAPI (blue) was performed to determine the number at the 0, 3rd, 6th, 9th and 12th day post-treatment. (B) Histogram indicating that cell density was significantly increased and reached a plateau at the 9th day, and persisted up to 12th days post-treatment (The results are the mean ± s.e. of six randomly selected microscopic fields each from three different experiments n=3, one way ANOVA followed by LSD test; * compare with 0 day and 3 day. P<0.01). Scale bar: 100 μm.

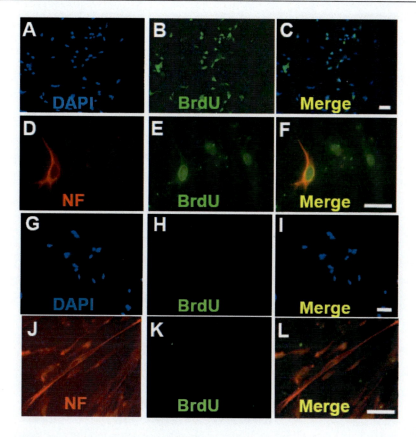

Figure 5. The proliferation assay of human umbilical mesenchymal cells. On the 3rd day after NCM treatment (A-F), the majority of the cells labeled with DAPI (blue in A) were presented BrdU-positive (green in B). (C) is the merged result of (A) and (B). Although these cells have been expressed NF (red in D), were still BrdU-positive (green in E). (F) is the merged result of (D) and (E). On the 9th after NCM Treatment (G-L), the cells labeled by DAPI (blue in G) were presented BrdU-negative (green in H). (I) is the merged result of (G) and (H). Moreover, these cells have been differentiated into mature neurons expressing NF (red in J) without BrdU labeling (green in K). (L) is the merged result of (J) and (K). (Scale bar: 100 μm).

ACQUISITION OF DOPAMINERGIC PHENOTYPE

The Protocol of Generation of Tyrosine Hydroxylase Positive Populations from Undifferentiated Human Umbilical Mesenchymal Stem Cells In Vitro

In vitro differentiation of HUMSCs into tyrosine hydroxylase positive (TH$^+$) neurons was carried out as previously described with modifications (figure 6) [57]. Stage 1: Expansion. Undifferentiated HUMSCs were dissociated into single cells and then cultured in 10% FBS DMEM for 3 - 6 days for expansion. Stage 2: Neuronal Induction. HUMSCs were cultured in NCM alone for 6-9 days, which was replaced every other day in order to induce neuron-like differentiation. Stage 3: Dopaminergic Neuron Differentiation. The cells were supplemented with NCM or 10% FBS DMEM in the presence of the murine N-terminal fragment of sonic hedgehog (SHH, 500 ng/ml, RandD 461-SH) and murine FGF8 isoform b (FGF8, 100 ng/ml, RandD 423-F8) for 3, 6, 9, or 12 days.

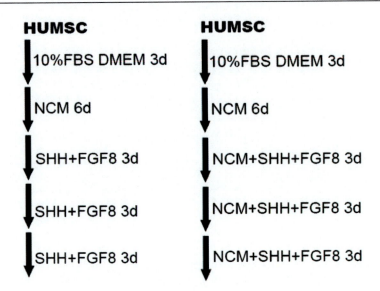

Figure 6. The grouping and scheme of *in vitro* incubation of HUMSCs. TH$^+$ populations were generated from undifferentiated HUMSCs by a three-step in vitro differentiation method.

Morphology Identification of Dopaminergic Neurons Differentiation of HUMSCs

Immunocytochemical staining for the catecholaminergic ratelimiting synthesizing enzyme TH showed that the HUMSCs were TH positive after incubation with NCM for 6 days and then SHH and FGF8 in 10% FBS-DMEM for 3, 6, or 9 days (figure 7A) or NCM for 6 days and then SHH and FGF8 in NCM for 3, 6, or 9 days (data not shown) but not after a 6-day NCM incubation only.

For the assessment of the possible differentiation of HUMSCs into subpopulations of dopaminergic, norepinephrine or GABAergic neurons, we applied double staining for human-specific nuclear antigen [58] and Tyrosine Hydroxylase (TH), dopamine-β-hydroxylase (DBH), and glutamate decarboxylase (GAD). Double staining of human-specific nuclear antigen and DBH and GAD indicated that the HUMSCs differentiated into, in addition to dopamine neurons, low yields of norepinephrine (figure 7B) and GABAergic neurons (figure 7C).

To facilitate counting cell number, the HUMSCs were cultured at a relatively low density (10^3 per ml). The proportion of cells expressing TH after treatment with NCM for 6 days followed by SHH and FGF8 for 3 days was 12.7% ± 2.1% ($p < 0.01$). No further increase in percentage of TH-containing cells was observed in cells treated with SHH and FGF8 for 6 or 9 days. No difference in the percentages of TH-expressing cells was observed between cells incubated in SHH and FGF8 in DMEM or NCM ($p < 0.05$) (figure 7D).

Human TH yields immunoreactive bands of 62 to 68 kD [59, 60], whereas that from the rat is estimated at 60 kD [61]. Our Western blot results showed that TH protein was not detected in HUMSCs treated with NCM only. The TH protein (68 kD) began to label significantly in the cells after treatment with NCM for 6 days and SHH and FGF8 for 3 or 6 days (figure 7E).

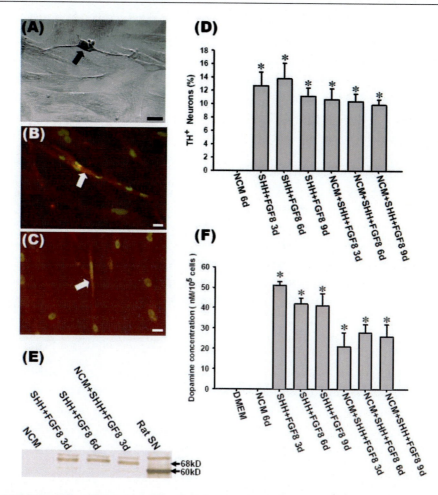

Figure 7. HUMSCs differentiation into dopaminergic, norepinephrine and GABAergic neurons *in vitro*. (A) Photomicrographs showing TH immunocytochemistry of cultured HUMSCs. The cells expressed TH after incubation with NCM for 6 days and then SHH and FGF8 in DMEM for 3 days. In addition to TH-positive neuron, DBH-positive (B) and GAD-positive (C) neurons were detected. Human-specific nuclear antigen are in green and DBH and GAD in red. Arrows indicate TH, DBH or GAD positively stained cells. Scale bar: 100 μm. (D) Histograms showing the percentage of TH positive cells after incubation with NCM, SHH, and FGF8. (Results represent the mean ± s.e. from three different experiments. At least 200 cells were counted from ten randomly selected microscopic fields in each experiment. Statistics consisted of one way ANOVA followed by the LSD test; * indicates statistical difference at p<0.05 compared with the NCM only group.) (E) TH expression in cultured cells by Western blotting. The molecular weight of rat and human THs were 60kDa and 68 kDa respectively. Rat SN (substantia nigra of rat) served as positive control. (F) Dopamine concentration in culture medium after HUMSCs treatment with NCM, SHH, and FGF8. (Results represent the mean ± s.e. from three different experiments, Statistics consisted of one way ANOVA followed by the LSD test; * indicates statistical significance at p<0.05 compared with the DMEM and NCM only groups).

Functional Assay of Dopaminergic Neurons Differentiation of HUMSCs

Dopamine was not detected in the medium of HUMSCs treated with DMEM or NCM. Dopamine concentration in the culture medium rose to a concentration of 51.0 ± 2.0 nM, as assayed by HPLC-ECD after a 6-day NCM and 3-day SHH and FGF8 culture of 10^5 cells in 10 ml of culture medium in a 100-mm-diameter culture dish (figure 7F) ($p < 0.01$).

The HUMSCs were induced to differentiate into TH^+ cells in vitro using a three-step protocol. The HUMSCs were expanded in 10% FBS DMEM for 3 - 6 days in stage 1. In a previous study similarly processed HUMSCs were found to express high levels of matrix receptors (CD44, CD105), integrin (CD29, CD51) and mesenchymal stem cell markers (SH2, SH3). Interestingly, these cells did not express hematopoietic lineage markers (CD34, CD45). These findings suggest that HUMSCs are similar to msenchymal stem cells [62].

In this study, the HUMSCs were transformed into non-dividing neurons after culturing in NCM alone for 6-9 days in stage 2. Our previous studies showed that 59.4±1.3% of the HUMSCs displayed robust immunostaining for neurofilament after 3 days of NCM treatment. The proportion of neurofilament-positive cells further increased to 87.4±5.5%, reached a plateau on the 6th day and persisted for up to 12 days after treatment. Double staining with BrdU and DAPI showed that most of HUMSCs were still able to proliferate in NCM for 3 days. On the 9th day of treatment with NCM, cell proliferation was no longer observed in the majority of cells. At this stage, HUMSCs differentiate into neurons in the post-mitosis phase [63]. In this study, the rats that received NCM+SHH+FGF8 cells did not develop any tumor in the brain, indicating the in-vitro-prepared grafts did not contain a population of proliferating cells.

In the present study, the HUMSCs differentiated into dopaminergic neurons in 10% FBS DMEM containing SHH (500 ng/ml and FGF8 (100 ng/ml) in stage 3. Previous studies have demonstrated that the increase of TH-positive neurons was even more pronounced when SHH and FGF8 were applied to mouse neural stem cell during in vitro differentiation. For the transformation of signaling molecules to neural stem cells in the mouse, the combined treatment of SHH and FGF8 was the most effective inducer of dopaminergic neurons [64].

As to the concentration of SHH and FGF8, Lee et al. used 500 ng/ml SHH and 100 ng/ml FGF8 in their study [57] whereas 200 ng/ml SHH and 100 ng/ml FGF8 were used by Perrier et al. [65]. The concentrations of SHH and FGF8 uesd in our system were the higher ones.

We used cells from a HUMSC-derived population as xenografts for unilaterally dopamine-denervated rats. Numerous studies have indicated that various growth factors, such as glial cell line-derived growth factor (GDNF), transforming growth factor-beta (TGF-β), interleukin-1 (IL-1) or bone morphogeneic protein (BMP) are involved in the differentiation of embryonic cells into dopaminergic neurons [66, 67, 68]. In addition, SHH and FGF8 simultaneously induce the expression of dopamine related proteins [57, 69]. Okabe et al. and Lee et al. reported a five-step in vitro differentiation method that yielded an efficient generation of dopamine neurons (33%) from undifferentiated mouse ES cells. We modified that protocol for the preparation of the graft cells used in the present study as the presence of dopamine neurons in the grafts and their subsequent production of dopamine are critical factors for the improvement of rotational behavior in Parkinsonian rats. We first examined whether the cells to be grafted expressed TH and produced dopamine. Bis-Benzidmide, used for tracking the cell movements, had no bearing on the percentage of TH-positive cells. Moreover, we detected TH protein production in the cells at stage 3 (figure 7A, D, E). Secreted dopamine was also detected by HPLC in the supernatant of cultured stage 3 cells (figure 7F). Therefore, we feel that differentiated cells from an undifferentiated HUMSCs population can be used as grafts for the treatment of Parkinsonian rats. Although TH$^+$ cells only amounted to for 12% of those in stage 3, we used whole fractions of the cells from that stage as grafts. Reasons that have been suggested to account for the difference in percentage yields include (1) the species of stem cells, (2) the different characteristics of embryonic stem cells and umbilical mesenchymal stem cells.

HUMSCs SURVIVED IN GRAFTED STRIATUM OF HEMIPARKINSONIAN RAT

Preparation of Parkinsonian Animals

Adult Sprague-Dawley rats (250-300g) were used in this study. Under chloride hydrate anesthesia (400 mg/kg i.p.), the rats were placed in a stereotaxic frame. The dopamine-innervated striatum were unilaterally lesioned by administering injections of 6-hydroxydopamine HCl (6-OHDA) into the median forebrain bundle AP: -4.3mm, R/L:+1.6mm, H:-8.2mm and AP:-4.0mm, R/L:+1.8mm, H:-8.0mm [70, 71]. Coordinates were set according to the atlas of Paxinos and Watson [72]. Each rat received 30 μg of 6-OHDA dissolved in 5 μl of physiological saline containing 0.02% ascorbic acid. Amphetamine-induced rotational behavior was assessed at 4, 8, 12, 16 and 20 weeks after 6-OHDA injection. For that the rats were placed in individual plastic hemispherical bowls and allowed to habituate for 10 min before being injected with a subcutaneous dose of Amphetamine (5 mg/kg). Left and right full-body turns were counted. Amphetamine-induced net rotation over a period of 60 min, starting 30 min after injection, was enumerated. Animals showing >360 turns/per hr ipsilaterally toward the lesioned side after a single dose of amphetamine were considered as successful Parkinsonian models and were selected for grafting [73-75]. All behavioral tests were performed in a closed room to avoid any environmental disturbance and assessed by an independent observer blind to the treatments.

Experimental Grouping

The Sprague-Dawley rats were divided into three groups of twelve animals each. One month after 6-OHDA injection, rats in group 1 received phosphate-buffered saline (PBS) into their dopamine-denervated striata. Rats in group 2 received a suspension of 1 x 10^5 graft cells that had been cultured in NCM only, and rats in the third group received a suspension of 1 x 10^5 graft cells that had been cultured in NCM, SHH and FGF8.

TH Positive Cell Bodies in Grafted Striatum

At 20 weeks after transplantation, bis-Benzimide–labeled cells were found in the striatum (figures 8A, 8B). Many cell somata staining positively for TH were clearly identified around the implantation site (figure 8C). Double-staining of human-specific nuclear antigen and TH indicated that the TH-positive cells were derived from HUMSCs (figure 8D). In contrast, no TH-positive soma was detected in the brains of rats that received grafted cells treated with NCM only (data not shown).

Cell migration patterns were followed by bis-Benzimide labeling in 30-μm serial sections. The labeled cells had migrated for approximately 1.4 mm in both directions of the rostrocaudal axis from the implantation site (Bregma +1.0). Most of the labeled cells were localized in the region of Bregma +2.0 to the region of Bregma -0.6, almost throughout the entire striatum (figure 9).

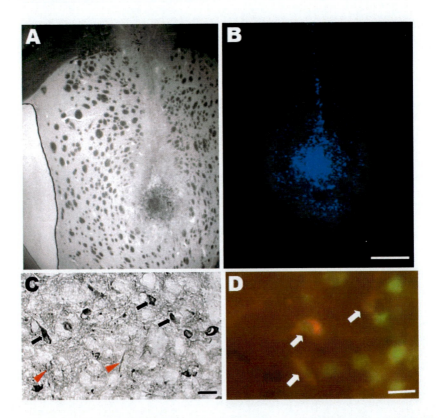

Figure 8. Photomicrographs showing the distribution of HUMSCs in rats 5 months after transplantation. The nuclei of HUMSCs were labeled with bis-Benzamide. The cells were microinjected into the striatum of Parkinsonian rats. The cells survived in the striatum 4 months after transplantation. (A) Phase contrast and (B) Same field fluorescence photomicrograph. (C) Existence of TH positive cell bodies in the gratfed striatum. Arrows indicate TH positively stained cell-bodies. Arrow-heads indicate TH positively stained processes. (D) TH-immunoreactive cells doubly stained with anti-human-specific nuclear antigen in grafted striatum. Arrows indicate TH and human-specific nuclear antigen positively doubly-stained cells. TH staining is in red and anti-human-specific nuclear antigen is in green. Scale bars: 1mm in B; 200 μm in C- D.

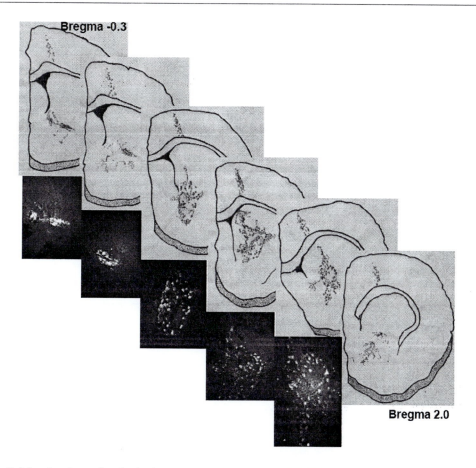

Figure 9. Line drawings of rat brain demonstrating the extent of HUMSCs migration after implantation in the striatum of the rat at the bregma level. •, cells of bis-Benzamide labeled HUMSCs.

Effect of Transplantation on Amphetamine-Induced Rotation

The effects of stem cell transplantation were examined in 6-OHDA–lesioned animals by quantification of rotations in response to amphetamine [71 –73]. Rotational scores were examined at 1, 2, 3, and 4 months after transplantation. One month after 6-OHDA lesioning, the number of amphetamine-induced rotations in all groups reached 381.0 ± 14.3 to 425.5 ± 19.7 rotations per hour with the control group ($n = 12$), which received injections of PBS in the dopamine-denervated striatum, showing a significant increase in numbers of rotation. Importantly, the increase in rotational scores was gradual over the months. No rats in the group that received grafted cells treated with NCM only ($n = 12$) showed any improvement ($p > 0$ .05). All of the rats receiving grafted cells treated by NCM, SHH, and FGF8 rotated significantly less than those in the control and NCM groups at the first observation time (1 mo.). Such rotation, which did not continue to get worse like the control group, was consistently observed in the NCM + SHH + FGF8 group throughout the experimental period (figure 10, table 1).

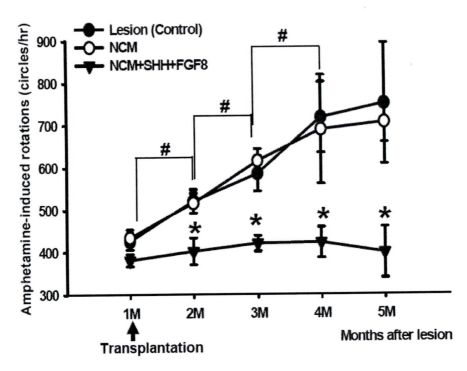

Figure 10. Rotation behavior in response to amphetamine tested at 1, 2, 3, 4, and 5 months post-lesion. A significant decrease in the number of amphetamine-induced turning was seen in animals with grafted cells treated with NCM+SHH+FGF8 (▼, n=6) compared with control (lesion only) animals (●, n=12) and lesioned animals that received grafted cells treated with NCM (○, n=12). Statistics consisted of two way ANOVA followed by the LSD test. (* indicates significant difference at $p<0.05$ between NCM+SHH+FGF8 treated group compared with the control and NCM groups at the same time point. # significant difference at $p<0.05$ between the control and NCM groups over one month intervals.)

In our study, no increase in rotation which didn't continue to get worse like the control (lesioned-only) group was observed 1 month after transplantation in all rats that received NCM+SHH+FGF8 treated cells. Subsequently for the next 3 months, neither significant further improvements (reduction) nor deteriorations (elevation) were observed. In contrast, the rotation behavior in group NCM was similar to that of the control (lesioned-only), which continued to deteriorate with time, suggesting that undifferentiated neuronal cells derived from HUMSCs did not improve rotation behavior in Parkinsonian rats. The rotation in group NCM+SHH+FGF8 was significantly decreased relative to the level of the control group, although not back to the normal level of intact rat. We suggest two possibilities. First of all, the number of dopaminergic neurons of implanted cells may have been relatively inadequate. Although it is difficult to determine the optimal number of dopamine neurons to be transplanted, we feel that the number of cells used in the present study (12% x 1 x 10^5 cells per rat) was not enough to completely alleviate the Parkinsonism symptoms in the afflicted rats, as was the case after 33% of dopaminergic neurons from mouse embryo stem cells treated with SHH+FGF8 were transplanted into the striata of the Parkinsonian rats. There was significant improvement in the rotational behavior in the transplanted group compared with that in the lesioned group although not to the extent of returning to the normal level, as in the case of transplantation of 80% of mouse embryo stem cells transfected with Nurr1 gene and treated with SHH and FGF8 for transformation into dopaminergic neurons [76]. We suggest that the number of dopaminergic neurons transplanted is an important factor in the treatment of Parkinson's disease. Similar results have been reported by Nishimura et al. [77].

Table 1. Rotations of individual rats in response to amphetamine tested at 1, 2, 3, 4, and 5 months post-lesioning

Month after Lesion / Grouping		1M	2M	3M	4M	5M
		Rotation Number				
Lesion	#1	404	516	603	632	897
	#2	397	528	616	789	854
	#3	401	479	655	666	689
	#4	386	459	503	799	876
	#5	432	563	613	785	879
	#6	442	511	546	713	736
	#7	440	496	589	705	Die
	#8	423	525	556	724	Die
	#9	438	513	598	764	Die
	#10	434	529	602	697	696
	#11	423	506	587	603	587
	#12	439	554	574	706	708
Lesion + NCM + SHH + FGF8	#1	364	420	450	443	446
	#2	403	433	401	351	339
	#3	374	330	419	470	420
	#4	404	432	421	409	411
	#5	398	398	429	420	412
	#6	392	421	405	422	352

Secondly, transplanted cells may take time to integrate in the host brain. The interaction time of donor cells may depend on the viability of transplanted cells and the species of the donor and the recipient. Studies have shown that symptomatic improvements can be observed by transplanting neurons from mouse, pig and human embryonic brains into the rat brain [78-80].

Two rats in group NCM+SHH+FGF8 survived for at least 8 months with amphetamine induced rotation behavior remaining similar to that 4 months after transplantation. The rest of the rats were sacrificed for other experiments before 8 months. We plan to examine the long term effects of transplantation.

Our findings may have a significant impact on the study of Parkinson's disease and potentially help to circumvent worrying ethical issues. Before human studies, firstly we should complete the observation of the effects and side-effects for more than one year following transplantation, including behavioral effects, secretion of transmitters, activation of microglia, release of cytokines (such as TNF_α and $IL1_\beta$), and possible development of brain tumor. Secondly, we should examine the toxicity included: growth factor (SHH and FGF8) and medium we used.

HUMSCs ARE GOOD DONOR CELLS

Ideal donor cells for Parkinson's disease therapy should be (i) easily available; (ii) capable of rapid expansion in culture; (iii) immunologically compatible; (iv) capable of long term survival and integration in the host brain, and (v) amenable to stable transfection and long-term expression of exogenous genes such as tyrosine hydroxylase [81]. HUMSCs in Wharton's jelly of the umbilical cord can be easily obtained and processed, compared to embryonic and bone marrow stem cells. In the present study, approximately 1×10^6 HUMSCs were collected from 20 cm of umbilical cord. The number of HUMSCs doubled (2×10^6) in 10% FBS DMEM in 3 days. We also found that the transformed HUMSCs in the striatum were still viable 4 months after transplantation without the need for immunological suppression, suggesting that HUMSCs might be a good stem cell source for transplantation.

ACKNOWLEDGMENT

We wish to thank Dr. Mu-Ming Poo has reviewed the paper and helped discussions. Dr. Yau-Chik Shum has helped for the English writing of the manuscript. Dr. Tsai's Obstetrical Clinic for providing human umbilical cord from patients.

REFERENCES

[1]   Beattie EC, Stellwagen D, Morishita W, Bresnahan JC, Ha B K, Von Zastrow M, Beattie MS, Malenka RC, Control of synaptic strength by glial TNFα. *Science.* 295: 2282-2285; 2002.

[2]   Kathy EM, Mark LW, Brianna MM, Phillip M, Duane D, Lois M, Bryan H, Mark B, Khalil AE, Tammi H, Deryl T, Matrix Cells from Wharton's Jelly Form Neurons and Glia. *Stem cells.* 21: 50-60; 2003.

[3]   Lois C, Alvarez-Buylla A, Proliferating subventricular zone cells in the adult mammalian forebrain can differentiate into neurons and glia. *Proc. Natl. Acad. Sci. USA.* 90: 2074-2077; 1993.

[4]   Markakis EA, Gage FH, Adult-generated neurons in the dentate gyrus send axonal projections to field CA3 and are surrounded by synaptic vesicles. *J. Comp. Neurol.* 406: 449- 460; 1999.

[5]   Cao QL, Zhang YP, Howard RM, Walters WM, Tsoulfas P, Whittemore SR, Pluripotent stem cells engrafted into the normal or lesioned adult rat spinal cord are restricted to a glial lineage. *Exp. Neurol.* 167: 48-58; 2001.

[6]   McDonald JW, Liu XZ, Qu Y, Liu S, Mickey SK, Turetsky D, Gottlieb DI, Choi DW, Transplanted embryonic stem cells survive, differentiate and promote recovery in injured rat spinal cord. *Nature Med.* 5: 1410-1412; 1999.

[7]   Forraz N, Pettengell R, McGuckin CP, Hematopoietic and neuroglial progenitors are promoted during cord blood ex vivo expansion. *British J. Haematology.* 119: 888; 2002.

[8]   Jiang Y, Jahagirdar BN, Lee-Reinhardt R, Schwartz RE, Keene CD, Ortiz-Gonzalez XR, Reyes M, Lenvik T, Lund T, Blackstad M, Du J, Aldrich S, Lisberg A, Low WC, Largaespada DA, Verfaillie CM, Pluripotency of mesenchymal stem cells derived from adult marrow. *Nature.* 418: 41-49; 2002.

[9]   Ha Y, Choi JU, Yoon DH, Yeon DS, Lee JJ, Kim HO, Cho YE, Neural phenotype expression of cultured human cord blood cells in vitro. *NeuroReport.* 12: 3523-3527; 2001.

[10]   Sanchez-Ramos JR, Song S, Kamath SG, Zigova T, Willing A, Cardozo-Pelaez F, Stedeford T, Chopp M, Sanberg PR, Expression of neural markers in human umbilical cord blood. *Exp. Neurol.* 171, 109-115; 2001.

[11]   Azizi SA, Stokes D, Augelli BJ, DiGirolamo C, Prockop DJ, Engraftment and migration of human bone marrow stromal cells implanted in the brains of albino rats-- similarities to astrocyte grafts. *Prco. Natl. Acad. Sci. USA.* 95: 3908-3913; 1998.

[12]   Kopen GC, Prockop DJ, Phinney DG, Marrow stromal cells migrate throughout forebrain and cerebellum, and they differentiate into astrocytes after injection into neonatal mouse brains. *Proc. Natl. Acad. Sci. USA.* 96: 10711-10716; 1999.

[13]   Hornykiewicz, O. Dopamine (3-hydroxytyramine) and brain function. *Pharmacol. Rev.* 1996; 18: 925–964.

[14]   Bernheimer H, Birkmayer W, Hornykiewicz O et al. Brain dopamine and the syndromes of Parkinson and Huntington: clinical, morphological and neurochemical correlations. *J. Neurol. Sci.* 1973; 20: 415–455.

[15]   Nagatsu T, Yamaguchi T, Rahman MK et al. Catecholamine-related enzymes and the biopterin cofactor in Parkinson's disease and related extrapyramidal diseases. *Adv. Neurol.* 1984; 40: 467–473.

[16]   Agid Y, Javoy-Agid F, Ruberg M. Biochemistry of neurotransmitter in Parkinson's disease. In: Marsden CD, Fahn S, eds. *Movement Disorder,* London: Butterworths 1987; 2: 166-230.

[17] Kish SJ, Shannak K, Hornykiewicz O. Uneven pattern of dopamine loss in the striatum of patients with idiopathic Parkinson's disease: pathophysiologic and clinical implications. *N. Engl. J. Med.* 1988; 318: 876–880.

[18] Damier P, Hirsch EC, Agid Y et al. The substantia nigra of the human brain. II. Patterns of loss of dopamine-containing neurons in Parkinson's disease. *Brain.* 1999; 122: 1437–1448.

[19] Alexi T, Borlongan CV, Faull RL, Williams CE, Clark RG, Gluckman PD, Hughes PE, Neuroprotective strategies for basal ganglia degeneration:Parkinson's and Huntington's diseases. *Prog. Neurobiol.* 2000; 60: 409- 470

[20] Cotzias CG, Van Woert MH, Schiffer LM Aromatic amino acids and modification of parkinsonism. *N. Engl. J. Med.* 1967; 276: 374–379.

[21] Olanow CW, Tatton WG. Etiology and pathogenesis of Parkinson's disease. *Annu. Rev. Neurosci.* 1999; 22: 123–144.

[22] Backlund EO, Granberg PO, Hamberger B et al. Transplantation of adrenal medullary tissue to striatum in parkinsonism. First clinical trials. *J. Neurosurg.* 1985; 62: 169–173.

[23] Madrazo I, León V, Torres C et al. Transplantation of fetal substantia nigra and adrenal medulla to the caudate nucleus in two patients with Parkinson's disease. *N. Engl. J. Med.* 1988; 318: 51.

[24] Lindvall O. Transplantation into the human brain: present status and future possibilities. *J. Neurol. Neurosurg. Psychiatry.* (suppl), 1989; 39–54.

[25] Date I, Imaoka T, Miyoshi Y et al. Chromaffin cell survival and host dopaminergic fiber recovery in a patient with Parkinson's disease treated by cografts of adrenal medulla and pretransected peripheral nerve. Case report. *J. Neurosurg.* 1996; 84: 685–689.

[26] Deacon T, Schumacher J, Dinsmore J et al. Histological evidence of fetal pig neural cell survival after transplantation into a patient with Parkinson's disease. *Nat. Med.* 1997; 3: 350–353.

[27] Mahowald MB, Areen J, Hoffer BJ et al. Transplantation of neural tissue from fetuses. *Science.* 1987; 235: 1307–1308.

[28] Spencer DD, Robbins RJ, Naftolin F et al. Unilateral transplantation of human fetal mesencephalic tissue into the caudate nucleus of patients with Parkinson's disease. *N. Engl. J. Med.* 1992; 327: 1541–1548.

[29] Freed CR, Breeze RE, Rosenberg NL et al. Survival of implanted fetal dopamine cells and neurologic improvement 12 to 46 months after transplantation for Parkinson's disease. *N. Engl. J. Med.* 1992; 327: 549–1555.

[30] Kordower JH, Freeman TB, Snow BJ et al. Neuropathological evidence of graft survival and striatal reinnervation after the transplantation of fetal mesencephalic tissue in a patient with Parkinson's disease. *N. Engl. J. Med.* 1995; 332: 1118–1124.

[31] Olanow CW, Kordower JH, Freeman TB Fetal nigral transplantation as a therapy for Parkinson's disease. *Trends Neurosci.* 1996; 19: 102–109.

[32] Kordower JH, Freeman TB, Chen EY et al. Fetal nigral grafts survive and mediate clinical benefit in a patient with Parkinson's disease. *Mov. Disord.* 1998; 13: 383–393.

[33] Hauser RA, Freeman TB, Snow BJ et al. Long-term evaluation of bilateral fetal nigral transplantation in Parkinson disease. *Arch. Neurol.* 1999; 56: 179–187.

[34] Lindvall O. Cerebral implantation in movement disorders: state of the art. *Mov. Disord.* 1999; 14: 201–205.

[35] Piccini P, Brooks DJ, Björklund A et al. Dopamine release from nigral transplants visualized in vivo in a Parkinson's patient. *Nat. Neurosci.* 1999; 2: 1137–1140.

[36] Freed CR, Greene PE, Breeze RE et al. Transplantation of embryonic dopamine neurons for severe Parkinson's disease. *N. Engl. J. Med.* 2001; 344: 710–719.

[37] Clarkson ED Fetal tissue transplantation for patients with Parkinson's disease: a database of published clinical results. *Drugs Aging.* 2001; 18: 773–785.

[38] Mendez I, Dagher A, Hong M et al. Simultaneous intrastriatal and intranigral fetal dopaminergic grafts in patients with Parkinson disease: a pilot study. Report of three cases. *J. Neurosurg.* 2002; 96: 589–596.

[39] Ben-Hur T, Idelson M, Khaner H et al., Transplantation of Human Embryonic Stem Cell-Derived Neural Progenitors Improves Behavioral Deficit in Parkinsonian Rats. *Stem Cells;* 2004; 22: 1246-1255;

[40] Greely HT, Hamm T, Johnson R et al. The ethical use of human fetal tissue in medicine. *N. Engl. J. Med.* 1989; 320: 1093–1096.

[41] Hendrickson AE, Van Brederode JF, Mulligan KA, Celio MR, Development of the calcium-binding protein parvalbumin and calbindin in monkey striate cortex. *J. Comp. Neurol.* 307: 626-646; 1991.

[42] Kathy EM, Mark LW, Brianna MM, Phillip M, Duane D, Lois M, Bryan H, Mark B, Khalil AE, Tammi H, Deryl T, Matrix Cells from Wharton's Jelly Form Neurons and Glia. *Stem cells.* 21: 50-60; 2003.

[43] Arsenijevic Y, Weiss S, Insulin-like growth factor-I is a differentiation factor for postmitotic CNS stem cell-derived neuronal precursors: distinct actions from those of brain-derived neurotrophic factor. *J. Neurosci.* 18: 2118-2128; 1998.

[44] Fraichard A, Chassande O, Bilbaut G, Dehay C, Savatier P, Samarut J, In vitro differentiation of embryonic stem cells into glial cells and functional neurons. *J. Cell Sci.* 108: 3181-3188; 1995.

[45] Mitchell KE. Weiss ML. Mitchell BM Matrix cells from Wharton's jelly form neurons and glia. *Stem Cells.* 2003; 21(1): 50 – 60.

[46] Strubing C, Ahnert-Hilger G, Shan J, Wiedenmann B, Hescheler J, Wobus AM, Differentiation of pluripotent embryonic stem cells into the neuronal lineage in vitro gives rise to mature inhibitory and excitatory neurons. *Mech. of Dev.* 53: 275-287; 1995.

[47] Stull ND, Jung JW, Iacovitti L, Induction of a dopaminergic phenotype in cultured striatal neurons by bone morphogenetic proteins. *Dev. Brain Res.* 130: 91-98; 2001.

[48] Nguyen L, Rigo J M, Rocher V, Belachew S, Malgrange B, Rogister B, Leprince P, Moonen G, Neurotransmitters as early signals for central nervous system development. *Cell and Tissue Res.* 305: 187-202; 2001.

[49] Woodbury D, Schwarz EJ, Prockop DJ, Black IB, (2000) Adult rat and human bone marrow stromal cells differentiate into neurons. *J. Neurosci. Res.* 61, 364-370

[50] White K, Bruckner JV, Guess WL, (1973) Toxicological studies of 2-mercaptoethanol. *J. Pharm. Sci.* 62: 237-241.

[51] Ni L, Wen Y, Peng X, Jonakait GM, (2001) Antioxidants N-acetylcysteine (NAC) and 2-mercaptoethanol (2-ME) affect the survival and differentiative potential of cholinergic precursors from the embryonic septal nuclei and basal forebrain: involvement of ras signaling. *Dev. Brain Res.* 130: 207-216.

[52] Sanchez-Ramos J, Song S, Cardozo-Pelaez F et al. Adult bone marrow stromal cells differentiate into neural cells in vitro. *Exp. Neurol.* 164: 247–256; 2000.

[53] Sarnat HB, Nochlin D, Born DE, Neuronal nuclear antigen (NeuN): a marker of neuronal maturation in early human fetal nervous system. *Brain and Dev.* 20, 88-94; 1998.

[54] Solbach S, Celio MR, Ontogeny of the calcium binding protein parvalbumin in the rat nervous system. *Anat. Embryol.* 184: 103-124; 1991.

[55] Gerhardt GA, Cass WA, Huettl PO, Brock S, Zhang Z, Gash DM, GDNF improves dopamine function in the substantia nigra but not the putamen of unilateral MPTP-lesioned rhesus monkeys. *Brain Res.* 817: 163-171; 1999.

[56] Beattie EC, Stellwagen D, Morishita W, Bresnahan JC, Ha B K, Von Zastrow M, Beattie MS, Malenka RC, Control of synaptic strength by glial TNFα. *Science.* 295: 2282-2285; 2002.

[57] Lee SH, Lumelsky N, Studer L et al. Efficient generation of midbrain and hindbrain neurons from mouse embryonic stem cells. *Nat. Biotechnol.* 2000; 218: 675–679.

[58] Zhang SC, Wernig M, Duncan ID et al., In vitro differentiation of transplantable neural precursors from human embryonic stem cells. *Nature Bio.* 2001; 19: 1129 – 1133.

[59] Kobayashi K, Kiuchi K, Ishii A et al. Expression of four types of human tyrosine hydroxylase in COS cells. *FEBS Letters.* 1988; 238(2):431-434.

[60] Haycock JW. Multiple forms of tyrosine hydroxylase in human neuroblastoma cells: Quantitation with isoform-specific antibodies. *J. Neurochem.* 1993; 60: 493–502.

[61] Gahn LG, Roskoski RJr. Tyrosine hydroxylase purification from rat PC 12 cells. *Protein expression and Purification.* 1991; 2(1): 10-14.

[62] Wang HS, Hung SC, Pong ST et al. Mesenchymal Stem Cells in Wharton Jelly of the Human Umbilical Cord. *Stem Cells.* 2004; 22: 1330-1337.

[63] Fu YS, Shih YT, Cheng YC et al. Transformation of Human Umbilical Mesenchymal Cells into Neurons in Vitro. *Journal of Biomedical Science.* 2004; 11: 652-660.

[64] Kim TE, Lee HS, Lee YB et al. Sonic hedgehog and FGF8 collaborate to induce dopaminergic phenotypes in the Nurr1-overexpressing neuronal stem cell. *Biochem. Biophys. Res. Commun.* 2003; 305: 1040-1048.

[65] Perrier AL, Tabar V, Barberi T et al. Derivation of midbrain dopamine neurons from human embryonic stem cells. *Proc. Natl. Acad. Sci. USA.* 2004; 101: 12543- 12548.

[66] Buytaert-Hoefen KA, Alvarez E, Freed CR. Generation of Tyrosine Hydroxylase Positive Neurons from Human Embryonic Stem Cells after Coculture with Cellular Substrates and Exposure to GDNF. *Stem Cells.* 2004; 22: 669-674.

[67] Rolletschek A, Chang H, Guan K et al. Differentiation of embryonic stem cell-derived dopaminergic neurons is enhanced by survival-promoting factors. *Mechanisms of Development.* 2001; 105(1-2): 93-104.

[68] Stull ND, Jung JW, Iacovitti L Induction of a dopaminergic phenotype in cultured striatal neurons by bone morphogenetic proteins. *Brain Research Developmental Brain Research.* 2001; 130: 91-98.

[69] Okabe S, Forsberg-Nilsson K, Spiro AC et al. Development of neuronal precursor cells and functional postmitotic neurons from embryonic stem cells in vitro. *Mech. Dev.* 1996; 59: 89–102

[70] Nikkhah G, Duan WM, Knappe U et al. Restoration of complex sensorimotor behavior and skilled forelimb use by a modified nigral cell suspension transplantation approach in the rat Parkinson model. *Neuroscience.* 1993; 56(1): 33-43.

[71] Olsson M, Nikkhah G, Bentlage C et al. Forelimb akinesia in the rat Parkinson model: differential effects of dopamine agonists and nigral transplants as assessed by a new stepping test. *Journal of Neuroscience.* 1995; 15(5 Pt 2): 3863-75

[72] Paxinos G, Watson C The rat brain in stereotaxic coordinates, 2nd edn. San Diego, CA: Academic Press. 1986

[73] Arbuthnott G, Fuxe K, Ungerstedt U. Central catecholamine turnover and self-stimulation behaviour. *Brain Research.* 1971; 27(2): 406-13.

[74] Ungerstedt U. Arbuthnott GW. Quantitative recording of rotational behavior in rats after 6-hydroxy-dopamine lesions of the nigrostriatal dopamine system. *Brain Research.* 1970; 24(3):485-93

[75] Ungerstedt U. Striatal dopamine release after amphetamine or nerve degeneration revealed by rotational behaviour. *Acta Physiologica Scandinavica.* Supplementum. 1971; 367: 49-68

[76] Kim JY, Koh HC, Lee JY et al. Dopaminergic neuronal differentiation from rat embryonic neural precursors by Nurr1 overexpression. *Journal of Neurochemistry.* 2003; 85(6): 1443-54.

[77] Nishimura F, Yoshikawa M, Kanda S et al. Potential Use of Embryonic Stem Cells for the Treatment of Mouse Parkinsonian Models: Improved Behavior by Transplantation of In Vitro Differentiated Dopaminergic Neurons from Embryonic Stem Cells. *Stem Cells.* 2003; 21: 171-180.

[78] Brundin P, Nilsson OG, Gage FH et al. Cyclosporin A increases survival of cross-species intrastriatal grafts of embryonic dopamine-containing neurons. *Experimental Brain Res.* 1985; 60(1): 204-8.

[79] Galpern WR, Burns LH, Deacon TW et al. Xenotransplantation of porcine fetal ventral mesencephalon in a rat model of Parkinson's disease: functional recovery and graft morphology. *Experimental Neurology.* 1996; 140(1): 1-13.

[80] Clarke DJ, Brundin P, Strecker RE et al. Human fetal dopamine neurons grafted in a rat model of Parkinson's disease: ultrastructural evidence for synapse formation using tyrosine hydroxylase immunocytochemistry. *Experimental Brain Research.* 1988; 73(1): 115-26.

[81] Bjorklund A. Neurobiology. Better cells for brain repair. *Nature.* 1993; 362(6419): 414-5.

In: Stem Cell Research Developments
Editor: Calvin A. Fong, pp. 229-272

ISBN: 978-1-60021-601-5
© 2007 Nova Science Publishers, Inc.

Chapter VIII

Human Oogenesis and Follicular Renewal from Ovarian Somatic Stem Cells

Antonin Bukovsky

Laboratory of Development, Differentiation and Cancer, Department of Obstetrics and Gynecology, The University of Tennessee Graduate School of Medicine, 1924 Alcoa Highway, Knoxville, Tennessee 37920, USA. buko@utk.edu

ABSTRACT

At present, it is widely believed that all primary follicles in adult human ovaries originate from the fetal period of life, since their numbers decline in aging females and fetal genetic abnormalities increase with advancement of maternal age. However, during 20 years of prime reproductive period (PRP; women between 18-38 years of age) the numbers of primary follicles do not show significant decline and fetal genetic abnormalities are rare, but their incidence begins to increase gradually thereafter. Our observations clearly demonstrate that during the PRP, but not thereafter, newly emerging germ and granulosa cells form new primary follicles, which replace aging follicles undergoing atresia (follicular renewal). The bipotent source of new germ and granulosa cells are ovarian surface epithelium (OSE) stem cells differentiating during adulthood by mesenchymal-epithelial transition from tunica albuginea mesenchymal cells. During follicular renewal, the OSE-derived germ cells enter peripheral blood circulation and assemble with granulosa cell nests associated with ovarian vessels. The follicular renewal during the PRP ensures that there are always fresh eggs available for the development of healthy progeny. *In vitro*, the OSE stem cells differentiate into distinct cell types (fibroblasts, epithelial, granulosa, and neural type cells) and oocytes. This suggests that OSE cells represent a new type of totipotent adult stem cells, which could be considered for autologous IVF treatment of premature or natural ovarian failure, and possibly for the local or systemic applications in distinct approaches of autologous regenerative medicine.

INTRODUCTION

It is still widely believed that oocytes in adult ovaries of higher vertebrates (birds, monotremes, and with few exceptions all eutherian mammals) persist from the early stage of ovarian development, i.e. from fetal period in humans and perinatal period in mice and rats [1-3].

However, this fifty year old storage doctrine was generally accepted after a one hundred year period of discussion on whether or not adult mammalian females exhibit formation of new eggs. From the evolutionary point of view the essential question is what the advantage of the egg storage from the early period of life for up to several decades in large mammals, including humans, might be as compared to the continued formation of new eggs in less evolved animal species. Our opinion is that the egg renewal exists during the prime reproductive period (PRP) throughout the animal kingdom (PRP theory, submitted), and it ceases after PRP termination, when the remaining eggs are stored until exhausted by a continuing ovarian function, i.e., cyclic follicular selection and ovulation.

Among invertebrates (flies and worms) and lower vertebrates (fishes and frogs) the germ cells develop in the same manner in both sexes. Large numbers of eggs and sperm are developed and ripened at the same rate and all are "discharged" either at once or within a very brief interval. In the males of higher vertebrates there is no great difference from such condition. In females of higher vertebrates, including mammals, however, a different state exists. Only several from numerous resting primary follicles present in ovaries are induced to grow during each cycle, and by the process of follicular selection only one or few are selected to ovulate. In addition, the ovarian ovulatory function in long living species, e.g. humans, is terminated at a certain age.

By why do such differences exist between lower and higher vertebrates? The difference between frogs and birds or humans is in the presence and absence of the maturation and discharge of all available oocytes. While frog progeny develops outside of the female body and independently of parental care, birds produce a certain (limited) number of eggs with respect to the need to take care for the development of limited progeny after hatching, and mammalian females ovulate a limited number of eggs, due to the limited capacity of the uterus to develop a certain number of fetuses. Also, with respect to age, the ovulation ceases earlier in mammals when compared to birds of similar size [4], probably because the hatching of the eggs is outside of the body but mammalian females appear to be naturally prevented from becoming pregnant during advanced age.

Terminology

In this article, the term primordial germ cells is utilized for the extragonadal cells migrating into gonads during the early embryonic period . The secondary or just germ cells means cells originating from the ovarian stem cells. The term primordial oocytes is utilized for the cells derived from primordial germ cells and primary for the oocytes derived from the ovarian stem cells. The ovarian stem cells are considered to be epithelial in nature, but could originate by mesenchymal-epithelial transition from the mesenchymal precursors in adult individuals of some species, e.g., humans [5]. In adult ovaries, it is virtually impossible to determine whether the resting follicles contain primordial or primary oocytes. Therefore, to make the issue more simple, we utilize the term primary follicles for the structures consisting of the oocyte and a single layer of granulosa cells, and growing follicles for the structures consisting of the oocyte and two or more layers of granulosa cells.

ORIGIN AND FATE OF PRIMORDIAL GERM CELLS

Female and male gametes represent a unique type of cells, since they are capable to undergo a meiotic division, which is not apparent in somatic cells. Hence, a question has initially been raised on whether the gametes can originate from somatic cell precursors or from a germline type of cells set apart during the earliest stage of embryonic development.

In 1849, Sir Richard Owen [6] studied development of invertebrates ("apterous larva" of Aphis), and indicated that there is a recognizable distinction between the general body mass and a cluster of cells, which he designated the germ mass. From this germ mass, the creative cells were suggested to come for the next generation. Owen wrote that "... the essential condition of the development of another embryo in this larva is the retention of part of the progeny of the primary impregnated germ-cell"(reviewed in [7]). Hence, no epigenetic mutations in the somatic cells were expected to be transmitted to the next generations of derived individuals. This indicates an extragonadal origin of germ cells but contrasts the definition of life and evolution of species indicating that living individuals are those who reproduce themselves, mutate, and are capable to transmit these mutations into the next generations. Owen's observations were elaborated further by Goette [8] and Nussbaum [9], and resulted in the "continuity of germ plasm" theory (see beneath).

The "Origin of Germ Cells from the Somatic Cells" Theory

Contrary to the Owen's view, Wilhelm von Waldeyer-Hartz in his book *Eierstock und Ei* presented evidence from mammalian females of successive stages of differentiation of germ cells from the somatic coelomic epithelium of the developing gonad [10], i.e. from the cells of the ovarian surface epithelium (OSE). He also expressed an opinion that such differentiation of germ cells is reserved for the period of early ovarian development and does not occur thereafter.

The "Continuity of Germ Plasm" Theory

In 1875, Goette [8] indicated that he had evidence supporting an extragonadal origin of germ cells in the toad, which exhibit a large size and for the first time, he indicated that they migrate into the developing gonads. Nussbaum in 1980 [9] discussed Waldeyer's opinion regarding the origin of germ cells from somatic cells [10] and maintained that the germ cells have a different character as compared to the somatic cells, since the somatic cells serve as nurse cells for the germ cells and can not be considered as progenitors of the germ cells.

In 1883, a series of papers from Weismann began dealing with the theory on the continuity of germ plasm [11]. Weismann's theory of germinal continuity, however, paid very little attention to the former cytological observations of Goette and Nussbaum (reviewed in [7]). Nevertheless, Weismann's view was a stimulating point for the series of investigations showing the physical continuity of the primordial germ cells in invertebrates and an extragonadal origin of primordial germ cells in vertebrates.

Extragonadal Origin of Primordial Germ Cells

Studies of Eigenmann [12], Nussbaum [9], and others showed that there is an extragonadal origin of the primordial germ cells, which migrate into the developing gonads. It was assumed that in the gonads, these primordial germ cells divide and produce definitive gametes for the following progeny.

Two Kinds of Germ Cells

Until the work of Dustin [13], there were no questions regarding the fate of primordial germ cells within developing ovaries. He recognized two kinds of cells in the germ-line history of amphibians: (1) primordial germ cells, which populated the developing gonad, differentiated into gonocytes, and degenerated, and (2) secondary germ cells originating from the OSE, which differentiated into definitive oocytes.

The Germ Cell Route

At the same time, Fedorov [14] and Rubaschkin [15] described the first appearance of primordial germ cells in the endoderm of the posterior part of the intestine (hind gut). Subsequently, based on studies of embryos from several mammalian species, Rubaschkin [16] suggested division of the history of the germ cell route (Keimbahn) into three periods. The first period begins with the differentiation of primordial germ cells, which, however, do not have a perspective to become definitive gametes (Urgeschlechtszellen). The gonadal development is associated with the establishment of the so called germinal epithelium (Keimepithel). The second period is associated with the appearance of female or male sex specific cells (Ureier or Ursamenzellen). The third period deals with the development of the sex-specific glands.

The germ cell route of Rubaschkin again raised a question of the fate of primordial germ cells [17]. Winiwarter and Sainmont [18] suggested that these cells degenerate after reaching the sex gland, and that definitive germ cells arise from the OSE. An alternative possibility considered, was that the primitive germ cells are destined from the time of cleavage to become definitive female or male germ cells [19].

In Firket's opinion [20], the primordial germ cells originate from the blastomeres, before the development of the genital ridge. They have an ability to migrate into sexual gland anlages, where they differentiate into sex cells, and then degenerate. The secondary germ cells do not descend from the primordial germ cells, but from the OSE. Swift reported that the primordial germ cells are found among the cells of the OSE from its very commencement. They are easily recognized, for they are quite different from the surrounding cylindrical cells. They are large, oval or round, have a large excentric nucleus, which appears vesicular and does not have much chromatin. The cytoplasm also stains faintly, and the germ cells of certain stages in the development of the chick scattered over the entire embryo, even in the blood vessels [21,22].

Although the extragonadal primordial germ cells may degenerate after entering the gonad, they nevertheless play an important role in the gonadal development. In the chick, the germ cells are first recognizable in the crescentic area of the germ-wall endoderm, as early as twenty four hours of incubation [21]. Reagan [23] cut out this crescentic area, in which the primordial germ cells were supposed to be located. The operated chicks were then further incubated and were killed for examination after varying lengths of time. In no instance where the removal of this sex cell area was complete did germ cells arise from somatic cells of the gonads, even after establishement of the OSE. In the normal chick, the OSE is well formed on the fourth day of incubation, and the primitive ova are clearly recognizable in it [24]. But in Reagan's operated chicks, even after five days of incubation, no germ cells at all were recognized [23].

The "Continuity of Germ Plasm" Theory Does Not Fit for the Mammals

Application of the "continuity of germ plasm" theory across the animal kingdom became dominant and persisted until the late 1970s [3,25]. However, following studies of mouse embryos, in which genetically marked cells were introduced at the 4- and 8-cell stage blastomere, have shown that such cells can either become germ cells or somatic cells [26]. This suggests that no specific germ cell commitment exists prior to implantation.

In non-mammalian species, removing either pole of the undivided egg prevents normal development: embryos may arrest early, lack organs, or the adults may be sterile. Such experiments have shown that spatial patterning of the egg is of utmost importance for subsequent development. However, when a substantial amount of material either from the animal (polar body-associated) or the vegetal (opposite) pole of the fertilized mouse egg was removed, the development of blastocysts was not affected, and after their transfer to the uteri of pseudo-pregnant foster mothers they can produce viable offspring. Furthermore, these develop into fertile adult mice. Hence, the mouse eggs have no essential components that are localized uniquely to the animal or the vegetal pole and, therefore, do not rely for their axial development on maternal determinants that are so localized in the fertilized egg. Thus the mammalian egg appears to be very unusual in the animal kingdom in that it establishes the embryonic axes after the zygote has begun development [27].

During the postimplantation period, mouse germ cells are not identifiable before ~7 days after fertilization [28]. The germ cells differentiate from somatic lineage [29]. It has also been shown that cellular differentiation of grafted embryonic cells does not depend on where the grafts were taken, but where they have been placed [30].

Additional studies suggest an important role in the development of germ cells for Bone Morphogenetic Protein 4 (BMP4), a member of TGFβ superfamily, as null BMP4 mouse embryos failed to develop primordial germ cells [31]. Utilization of newer techniques has shown that Weissmann's theory may fit invertebrates (*C. Elegans* and *Drosophila*) and some lower vertebrates (zebrafish and frogs) [32] and birds [33], but not mice, and possibly mammals in general [34,35].

An alternative opinion raised is, in present terms, that the migrating extragonadal primordial germ cells are, in reality, totipotent stem cells, which become tissue specific stem cells after settlement in the gonads [7]. Hence, the totipotent stem cells of any origin, if available during adulthood, might develop into germ cells and oocytes within the gonads. Indeed, oogenesis has recently been demonstrated in cultured mouse embryonic stem cells. Such oogonia entered meiosis, recruited adjacent cells to form follicle-like structures, and later developed into blastocysts [36,37]. Cultured mouse embryonic stem cells have also been reported to differentiate into haploid male gametes capable of fertilizing eggs and developing into blastocysts [38]. Human embryonic stem cells expressing *STELLAR* and *DAZL* genes originate from inner cell mass cells of the blastocyst expressing *STELLAR* only, and may differentiate either into germ cells expressing *VASA* gene or somatic cells [39].

In vivo, mouse primordial germ cells are induced to form around the proximal part of the epiblast adjacent to the extra-embryonic region. They are induced through cellular interactions during gastrulation, and then move through the primitive streak and invade the definitive endoderm, parietal endoderm and alantois. Next they are incorporated into the hintgut pocket, either by passive or active process. Finally, primordial germ cells emerge from the dorsal side of the hintgut and migrate towards and colonize the developing genital ridges. The primordial germ cells not reaching the genital ridge till certain stage of embryonic development are subjected to apoptosis and die. [35,40]. Human primordial germ cells expressing *VASA* and *c-kit* markers of germ cells were found to migrate into the region of the gonadal ridge between the 6 and 7th week of embryonic gestational age [41,42].

After the primordial germ cells enter the developing embryonic gonad, they commit to a developmental pathway that will lead them to become either eggs or sperm, depending not on their own sex chromosome constitution but on whether the gonad has begun to develop into an ovary or a testis, respectively. The sex chromosomes in the gonadal somatic cells determine which type of gonad will develop. A single *Sry* gene on the Y chromosome can redirect a female embryo to become a male (reviewed in [43]). These observations indicate that mammalian primordial germ cells originate from uncommitted (totipotent) stem cells, and their sex commitment is determined by local gonadal environment - signals produced by neighboring somatic cells.

During adulthood, the ovarian environment appears to be essential, since the germ cells have to assemble with granulosa cells to form primary follicles needed for oocyte survival, development, and maturation. Although the germ cells can utilize vascular transportation for distant destinations [44], the granulosa cells are not available elsewhere, except in the ovary. If the granulosa cell precursors are eliminated, for instance by radiation, the germ cells may not have a chance to establish primary follicles and rejuvenate the ovaries.

Summary on the Origin and Fate of Primordial Germ Cells in Mammalian Females

Altogether, two opinions regarding the origin of definitive eggs in ovaries of higher vertebrates emerged:

The first opinion argued that the somatic cells are never involved in gametogenesis, but that the extragonadal primordial germ cells are set apart at an early stage of ontogenesis in the endoderm of the hind gut. They migrate into a developing germ gland, where, after multiplication, they are directly transformed into the definitive oocytes, which persist in the gonads until and during sexual maturity. This opinion is consistent with the prevailing current view.

The second opinion contended that extragonadal primordial germ cells migrate into developing gonads, where they pass through the typical phases of the sex cells and degenerate. By so doing, the primordial germ cells somehow stimulate the production of definitive germ cells from the somatic cells of the OSE. This opinion is consistent with the author's view.

ORIGIN OF OOCYTES IN ADULT GONADS

During formation of views on the origin of definitive oocytes from extragonadal primordial germ cells or from the OSE somatic stem cells, some attention has also been made regarding the origin of oocytes in adult ovaries of higher vertebrates, including mammals.

Definitive Oocytes May Emerge Prior to or During Sexual Maturity

In 1917, based on the studies of the white mouse, Kingery [45] found that the definitive oocytes were derived from the OSE in the white mouse prior to sexual maturity. This observation was extended by Edgar Allen and Herbert M. Evans, who concluded their studies in adult ovaries of mice and other species as follows: "A cyclical proliferation of the germinal epithelium (OSE) gives rise to a new addition of young ova to the cortex of the adult ovary at each normal oestrous period" and defined the "continued formation" of oocytes theory [46] that states "New oocytes are formed throughout life, and in phase with the reproductive cycle, from germinal epithelium of the adult mammal, at the same time as vast numbers of already-formed oocytes become eliminated through atresia" [47].

Definitive Oocytes May Originate from Primordial Germ Cells in Developing Gonads

The current belief that in mammals there is never any increase in the number of oocytes beyond those differentiating during fetal or perinatal ovarian development ("storage" theory) was declared in 1921 [1]. During the 1950-1960s the dogma that all primary follicles in adult mammalian females were formed during the period of ovarian development [25,48] prevailed, primarily because of the overall diminution of primary follicle numbers with age reported by Block in the early 1950s [49]. However, Erik Block wrote: "In the age range eighteen to thirty-eight, the relation between the patient's age and the number of primordial follicles cannot be established statistically" [49]. This suggests that during the 20 years of the human female prime reproductive period, there is no significant change in the number of primary follicles. Nonetheless, this important part of Block's conclusions has not been appreciated by interpreters [25,48].

Meiotic Prophase Arrest

There are, however, several other issues contradicting the currently prevailing storage doctrine. During embryonic and fetal development, the female primordial germ cells multiply, and some of them pass into meiotic prophase, consisting of leptotene, zygotene, pachytene, and diplotene stages, with characteristic arrangement of chromosomes [25]. The principal milestone of the current dogma is the belief that all oocytes in developing ovaries pass meiotic prophase and persist in the diplotene stage with preserved chromosomes during resting stage till adulthood, and thereafter [3]. However, in mouse and rat females meiotically arrested oocytes disappear after postnatal day 3, and in the male gonads no fetal meiotic prophase is apparent, but meiosis is initiated at puberty (primary spermatocytes) and progresses without resting phase [25].

In addition, human fetuses show a peak of the oocyte numbers during the sixth month of intrauterine life (7×10^6 cells), and 5×10^6 oogonia undergo degeneration until birth. The degeneration affects a majority of oocytes at pachytene, but also at the diplotene stage, especially oocytes in primary follicles [25]. The chromosomes seen in the nuclei of human fetal oocytes are also not apparent in the adult human ovaries, until oocytes enter the initiation of meiosis in the Graafian follicles [25].

These observations indicate that entering meiotic prophase during fetal development is characteristic for the female but not for the male mammalian primordial gametes. An important aspect for unique meiotic activity of female germ cells appears to be a prevention of mesonephric cell migration and testis cord formation in developing ovaries [50]. Hence, arrest of some oocytes of developing ovaries in meiotic prophase appears to serve for the determination of the ovarian structure, just preventing the apparent tendency toward development of testicular morphology. Most of the fetal primordial/primary oocytes are not preserved till adulthood, but subjected to the process of perinatal demise. Nevertheless, it can not be excluded that fetal differentiation of oocytes and primordial/primary follicles, which are not functionally required until at least puberty and during sexual maturity, may play an important role in the programming of the time span for existence of periodical follicular renewal (FR) during the prime reproductive period (PRP) in adulthood [51].

Follicular Pool

Moreover, the evaluation of the follicular pool in adult mammalian ovaries revealed that 90% are primary follicles and 10% are follicles in certain stages of development [2]; the 50-70% of primary follicles are, however, undergoing atresia [52]. It is well known that primary follicles may persist for a long time, but growing follicles should either develop into Graafian follicles and ovulate, or degenerate. Therefore, assuming that at least 50% of the total follicular pool persists unaffected, and 10% enter growth phase during each cycle and ovulate or degenerate later, and that follicular development from the primary follicle toward ovulation is about three cycles [53], it is justified to say that the follicular pool will be exhausted within ~7 cycles. Yet, during the PRP, i.e., before the beginning of significant diminution of primary follicle numbers in the mouse [54] and human ovaries [49], there are about 35 and 300 ovarian ovulatory cycles, respectively.

Clinical Evidence for Follicular Renewal During Prime Reproductive Period

Finally, it is widely believed at present that all primary follicles in adult human ovaries originate from the fetal period of life, since their numbers decline in aging ovaries and fetal genetic abnormalities increase with the advancement of maternal age. However, during more than 20 years of the PRP, from 18 to 38 ±2 years of age, the numbers of human primary follicles did not show significant decline [49] and genetic abnormalities of the progeny are rare (0.5%). However, an incidence of fetal trisomy and other genetic alterations begin to increase exponentially within a few years thereafter, i.e., 6% in 40- 44-year-old mothers and 25% in the 45- 49-year-old age group (figure 1; reviewed in [44]).

Summary on the Origin of Oocytes in Adult Gonads

The advantage of the "storage" theory is that it is simple and easy to understand: The extragonadal primordial germ cells migrate into developing ovaries, achieve sex-specific properties, multiply, and complete meiotic prophase of oocytes, which form primordial follicles serving for reproductive function up to the menopause in human females. The essential disadvantage, however, is a requirement for the storage of female gametes in higher vertebrates for up to several decades prior to their utilization for the development of new progeny. Under such conditions, there is a high probability of accumulation of genetic alterations in stored oocytes due to the long lasting influence of environmental hazards. On the other hand, the "storage" doctrine supports evidence that in invertebrates and lower vertebrates the oogenesis continues throughout reproductive life. The most problematic issue here is what the advantage of the oocyte storage in higher vertebrates might be from the Darwinian evolutionary theory point of view on the development of animal species toward higher and more adaptive forms of life and reproduction, e.g. frogs vs. mammals.

The "continued formation" theory indicates that primordial germ cells degenerate and new oocytes originate during adulthood from cyclical proliferation of the ovarian surface epithelium (OSE) stem cells [45,46], and that new oocytes are formed throughout life, and in phase with the reproductive cycle, from germinal epithelium (OSE) of the adult mammal, at the same time as vast numbers of already-formed oocytes become eliminated through atresia [47]. The advantage of the "continued formation" theory is that it determines that there is a uniform ability of the oocyte and follicular renewal in all adult females throughout the animal kingdom species, making this doctrine acceptable from the evolutionary insight. The disadvantage is that it is not easy to follow a distinct pattern of this process between the species, e.g., apparent formation of new oogonia in adult prosimian primates [55-57], v.s. a more cryptic process in adult human females [44,58].

The "Prime Reproductive Period" Theory

Recently we attempted to establish a harmony between these two possibilities by proposing the "prime reproductive period" theory (submitted). According to the "PRP" theory, the "storage" doctrine fits to two periods of life in humans, that between the termination of fetal follicular development and the late puberty or premenarcheal period (about 10-12 years), and that following the end of PRP until menopause. On the other hand, the "continued formation" doctrine accounts for the follicular renewal during PRP, which ensures an availability of fresh oocytes for healthy progeny. During PRP, the number of primary follicles does not show a significant change in human [49] and mouse females [54] due to the replacement of aging primary follicles by follicular renewal [44,58,59]. Atresia of primary follicles declines during the premenopausal period [60], allowing a significantly reduced number of persisting primary follicles to remain functional in humans for another 10-12 years after termination of follicular renewal during PRP. While, however, there are no consequences of oocyte aging for the progeny during childhood, since ovulation is absent, the oocytes persisting after termination of PRP accumulate genetic alterations resulting in the exponentially growing incidence of fetal trisomies and other genetic abnormalities with advanced maternal age after PRP (figure 1).

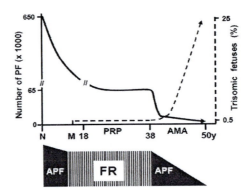

Figure 1. The incidence of trisomic fetuses exponentially increases with age after termination of follicular renewal through the prime reproductive period (PRP). PF, primary follicles; N, neonate; CH, childhood; M, menarche; AMA, advanced maternal age; APF, aging primary follicles; FR, follicular renewal. For data see Ref. [44].

HUMAN ADULT OVARIES

Structures in Adult Human Ovaries Contributing to Oogenesis and Follicular Renewal

The oogenesis and follicular renewal in adult human ovaries is still a controversial issue. In order to give the readers relevant information on prior observations, we are providing additional information on the structures in the human ovarian cortex that appear to play a role in this process and their behavior.

Tunica Albuginea, Surface Epithelium, and Derived Epithelial Structures in Human Ovarian Cortex

The human ovarian tunica albuginea (TA) is a thick fibrous subepithelial layer of loose connective-tissue cells. It does not begin to form until the end of intrauterine life [61] or several months after birth [62]. Even then it is not a true membrane, but merely a collection of loose connective-tissue cells [62]. In contrast to the OSE, supposedly the source of a variety of ovarian tumors [63], the TA has not been well studied.

In many animal species the ovarian cortex is covered by a layer of irregularly shaped special epithelial-like mesothelial cells [64], commonly referred to as the ovarian "germinal", superficial, or surface epithelium. This layer is attached to the basal lamina continuous with the subjacent TA by means of collagenous fibrils. Except in the ovaries of newborn animals, mitoses are essentially absent in the OSE [65]. In functional human ovaries the OSE is found in certain areas only, but in women with anovulatory cycles, or patients with polycystic or sclerotic ovaries, the ovarian surface is completely covered with OSE [66]. This is despite similar handling during surgical retrieval, suggested by Gillett [67] to cause ovarian denudation.

In scanning electron microscopy and submicroscopic studies of the OSE during ovulatory cycles, it has been reported that the ovarian surface is frequently evaginated into a series of villous-like projections or papillae, which may vary widely in the number, size, and distribution (reviewed in [64]). The OSE also invaginates into the ovarian cortex throughout the entire organ. This is true in all mammalian species, including humans. Cortical invaginations appear as small elongated clefts, subsurface channel-like crypts, and solid cords of epithelial cells. Crypts are hollow, tubular invaginations lined by cells possessing the same general features as OSE cells. However, the cord cells are very similar to some of the granulosa cells. In some areas of the ovary, cords fragment and appear as small 'nests' of epithelial cells. Typically, these epithelial nests (fragmented cords) lie in proximity to primary follicles [64,65]. In adult ovaries, the OSE retains a relatively embryonic structure [68]. The OSE-derived cords are in contact or penetrated by nerve terminals, and fragmented cords (nests) are suggested to contribute epithelial elements to ovarian follicles [65].

These data indicate that OSE exhibits a high degree of variability, by forming evaginations extending from the ovarian surface and invaginations into the stroma. Also, the crypt-like subsurface channels exist, which are lined by epithelial cells and retain the relatively embryonic structure of OSE cells. On the other hand, epithelial nests derived from epithelial cords appear to contribute epithelial cells to ovarian follicles.

Epithelio-Mesenchymal Transition In Vitro

In culture, the OSE cells undergo an epithelio-mesenchymal transition. The resulting mesenchymal type cells can be stimulated to differentiate back into the epithelial phenotype [69,70]. The OSE cells undergoing this epithelio-mesenchymal conversion are initially cytokeratin (CK) positive, but lose CK expression with time and passages in cultures [63]. Therefore, the diminution of CK expression appears to indicate a resting stage for OSE-derived mesenchymal cells.

Expression of Mitogen-Activated Protein Kinases

Normal OSE cells express mitogen-activated protein kinases (MAPK) [71], a group of serine/threonine kinases. MAPK are used throughout evolution to control the cellular responses to external signals such as growth factors, nutrient status, stress or inductive signals. Transcription factors are substrates for MAPK [72]. In adult human ovaries, we have reported prominent cytoplasmic MAPK expression in oocytes of heathy primary follicles, a diminution of oocyte MAPK expression during follicular atresia, and cytoplasmic and nuclear MAPK expression in growing secondary follicles [73]. Hence, cytoplasmic MAPK expression appears to be characteristic for resting healthy oocytes. Nuclear translocation signals oocyte growth and diminution of MAPK expression indicates oocyte degeneration.

Identification of Germ Cells in the OSE

Scanning and transmission electron microscopy have revealed numerous germ cells (10 μm in diameter) within the OSE of human fetuses from 7 to 24 weeks of intrauterine life. Germ cells are easily distinguished from smaller coelomic epithelial cells by their rounded contour, smooth surface and, in some instances, large amoeboid evaginations [61]. Using differential interference contrast (DIC) and immunohistochemistry, we previously reported the occurrence of similar putative germ cells within the OSE and cortex of adult human ovaries [58]. These data indicate that germ cells are present in the OSE. They may either invade OSE from adjacent structures and be extruded from the ovary [61], or originate in OSE and invade the ovarian cortex, or both [58].

Besides their characteristic morphology as outlined above, the germ cells can also be identified by alkaline phosphatase activity [30]. However, nonspecific alkaline phosphatase activity has been described in various tissues [74-77]. Zona pellucida (ZP) proteins are specific markers for oocytes. In postnatal rat ovaries, zona pellucidae first appear in primary follicles adjacent to keratin-positive granulosa cells [78]. Some ZP proteins, such as PS1, are also detected in the OSE of rabbit, cat, monkey, baboon and human, and in human ovarian cancers [79-82]. Hence, expression of ZP proteins in OSE cells suggests a relationship to the oocytes.

Intravascular Transport of Germ Cells

Germ cells are capable of migration by amoeboid movements, but in embryos of birds and large mammals they also utilize intravascular transport to reach distant destinations [25,33,83]. Why the cell leaves the circulating blood at certain sites remains unclear. It has been suggested that there is a trapdoor mechanism that prevents the germ cell from continuing to circulate, although adhesion of primordial germ cells ("cauliflower-like structures ") in the aortas of bovine embryos have been observed [83]. Hence, in certain species, germ cells may migrate to reach adjacent blood vessels, and then utilize vascular transport to reach distant destinations.

Balbiani Body

Oocytes in primary (resting) follicles show a single Balbiani body (named for the nineteenth century Dutch microscopist) in the cytoplasmic region near the nucleus where the majority of oocyte organelles are concentrated (reviewed in [84]). The Balbiani body contains aggregated mitochondria and can be observed in primary follicles in both fetal and adult ovaries [85-87]. In a study of turkey hens, no Balbiani body was detected in stage I oocytes, appeared in stage II oocytes, and diminished in the oocytes of growing follicles, coinciding with the dispersion of mitochondria throughout the ooplasm [85]. Similar observations were reported in human oocytes [86]. Balbiani bodies show immunostaining for CK 8, 18, and 19 [58,88]. In primary follicles of fetal and adult human ovaries, follicular (granulosa) cell extensions penetrate deep into the ooplasm, much like a sword in its sheath. There may be as many as 3-5 "intraooplasmic processes", even in one scanning microscopy plane. These intraoocytic invaginations are closely associated with a variety of organelles. They are close to the nuclear zone, and may help activate growth of the oocyte [89].

In mouse fetal ovaries, germ cells are arranged in special clusters (germline cysts) and dividing germ cells remain connected by intercellular bridges called "ring canals." The cysts may allow certain germ cells to specialize as nurse cells [90]. One possibility is that such nurse cells in germline cysts help provide oocytes with mitochondria [91]. It has been proposed that mitochondria with functional and defective genomes would be actively transported into different germ cells, and the quality of each cell's mitochondria might then determine whether it survived or entered apoptosis [46]. A recent study by Cox and Spralding indicates that during Drosophila oogenesis, follicular cells are a source of mitochondria, which enter the oocyte cytoplasm via the "ring canal" to form the Balbiani body, thereby supplying virtually all of the mitochondria of the oocyte [87].

It appears that the Balbiani body contributes to the resting state of the oocyte, since oocyte mitochondria are not released until the initiation of follicular growth. In addition, the contribution of granulosa cells to the formation of the Balbiani body in the oocyte cytoplasm is an indicator of the use of these cells in ongoing oocyte assembly.

Numbers of Ovarian Primary Follicles

In adult mammalian ovaries, 70-95% of oocytes are in various stages of degeneration [52,92]. Block's quantitative morphological investigations of follicles in women [49] showed wide individual variation, but the numbers in the right and left ovaries are similar, with a tendency to decline with age. However, in the eighteen to thirty eight year age range, a relationship between age and the number of primary follicles could not be statistically proven [49]. The number of primary follicles in both ovaries varied between 8100 and 290000. This lack of significant numerical change during the reproductive period also has been reported in cattle [92]. Gougeon used the data of Block and his own observations and concluded that the depletion of the primary follicle pool is caused mainly by atresia in younger women and by a decrease in the growing pool in older women, with the changing point at 38 ± 2.4 years of age [60]. These observations suggest that in human females new cohorts of primary follicles may replace follicles undergoing atresia until about 38 years of age, and a lack of follicular replacement after that period may cause a significant decrease in the pool of primary follicles.

We used the immunohistochemical detection of the CK marker of epithelial cells and DIC to study the mesenchymal-epithelial transition of TA mesenchymal cells in adult human ovaries and the development and distribution of epithelial aggregates in the cortex. We also investigated the association of oocytes with CK positive epithelial nests in ovarian cortex by double color immunohistochemistry, and the expression of OSE/oocyte shared ZP proteins and mitogen activated protein kinases in putative germ cells. In addition, triple color immunohistochemistry was employed on serial sections to study vascular involvement in oocyte transportation. This study expanded our earlier and recent observations and views on the formation of germ cells in adult human ovaries [58,73,93,94]. Our data supported further the concept of the formation of new ovarian primary follicles during the human reproductive period.

Human Tunica Albuginea Stem Cells Produce Somatic (Granulosa) Cells and Germ Cells

The long-held belief that the total number of oocytes present in the mammalian ovary is generated during fetal ovarian development with no additional oocyte formation during reproductive life [1,2] has been recently challenged (reviewed in [95]). At present, there are two proposed mechanisms for the generation of new oocytes in postnatal mammals [96]:

1. New oocytes are produced via germline stem cells that reside in an extraovarian location, the bone marrow [97]. Germline progenitors are released to the peripheral circulation, and these progenitor cells home to the ovary, where they may engraft as

new oocytes within new follicles. The question of developmental potential of labeled oocytes after bone marrow transplantation remains unclear [98].

2. New oocytes and granulosa cells are produced by a transformative mechanism. Bipotential progenitor mesenchymal cells exist near the surface of the adult human ovary in the tunica albuginea, and produce both somatic (granulosa) cells of the ovary and new oocytes [44,58,99].

It has been indicated [95] that the studies of adult stem cells in TA of adult human ovaries [44,58,99] deserve the merit of being the first report to challenge the above mentioned consensus that the total number of oocytes present in human ovaries is generated during fetal ovarian development with no additional oocyte formation during reproductive life. In addition, it has been also indicated that time will tell whether a modern proposal for a transformative mechanism of oocyte and granulosa cell development from the TA/OSE stem cells in the human ovary is to be regarded as a start of "unequivocal" evidence for a human neo-oogenesis that has been lacking for more than 100 years [96].

Relationship of Tunica Albuginea, Surface Epithelium and Ovarian Cortex

The TA shows a variable thickness, ranging from almost undetectable to more than 50 μm [44]. Cytokeratin expression of various density is detected in mesenchymal cells of some TA segments, particularly in segments showing an appearance of OSE cells; in contrast, no CK expression is detected in mesenchymal cells of the ovarian cortex [44]. The development of OSE-derived cortical nests of primitive granulosa cells [64,65] coincides with the appearance of OSE cells directly connected to the ovarian cortex (without interference of TA), and with appearance of TA flaps extending over the OSE [44].

Origin of Nests of Primitive Granulosa Cells

The TA mesenchymal cells, which show CK immunoexpression, differentiate into OSE cells by a process of mesenchymal-epithelial transition (see figure 2A). However, depending on additional unknown factors, this process may result in either the formation of primitive granulosa cell nests, or the differentiation of OSE cells covering the TA surface (precursors of germ cells). The nests of primitive granulosa cells descend into the deeper ovarian cortex, where they eventually associate with oocytes to form primary follicles [44]. Figure 3, a panoramic view of the ovarian surface and adjacent cortex (ovc), shows a thick segment of TA (ta) and CK expression in TA fibroblasts associated with the differentiation of OSE (left white arrow). No OSE is apparent above TA lacking CK+ fibroblasts (right white arrow). The upper ovarian cortex contains a row of longitudinally (arrows) or perpendicularly viewed solid epithelial cords (arrowheads; as evidenced from serial sections), precursor structures of nests of primitive granulosa cells.

Figure 4 shows formation of epithelial channels (arrowhead), longitudinally (dashed arrowhead) and perpendicularly viewed solid epithelial cords (white arrowheads and right inset), and follicle like structures containing stromal elements (solid box, see left top inset for detail) in the upper cortex (uc). These structures were arranged in a surprisingly straight row (see also figure 3). In some ovaries a similar orientation of primary follicles was observed in the lower ovarian cortex (lc).

Hence, the formation of new primary follicles in adult human ovaries is more complex as compared to more primitive association of oocytes with clusters of granulosa cells available in human fetal or adult rat ovaries [100].

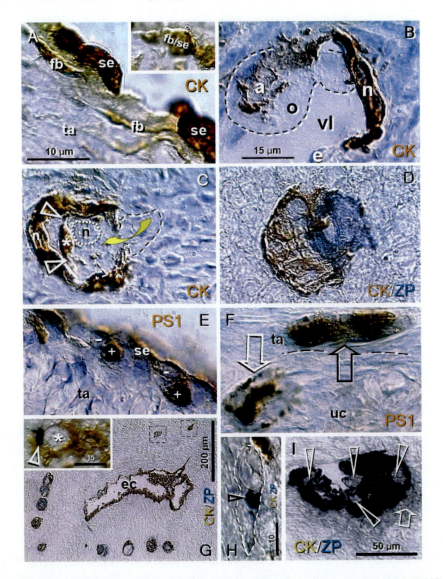

Figure 2. Follicular renewal in adult human ovaries. A) Some fibroblasts (fb) in TA (ta) show CK18 expression and transition into OSE (se) cells. Inset shows a cell in mesenchymal-epithelial transition (fb/se). B) The CK+ epithelial nest (n) wall inside the vascular lumen (vl) pocket, which is lined with endothelial cells (e), extends an arm (a) to catch the oocyte (o, dashed line). C) The nest body (n) with closing "gate" and a portion of the oocyte (dashed line) still outside of the nest-oocyte complex (arched arrow). The oocyte contains intraooplasmic CK+ (brown color) extensions from the nest wall (arrowheads), which contribute to the formation of CK+ paranuclear (Balbiani) body (asterisk); the nucleus is indicated by a dotted line. D)

Occupied "bird's" nest indicates a halfway oocyte-nest assembly. CK (brown)/ ZP (blue). E) Segments of OSE show cytoplasmic PS1 (brown) expression (-nuclei) and give rise to cells exhibiting nuclear PS1 (+ nuclei, asymmetric division), which descend into TA. F) In TA, the putative germ cells show symmetric division (black arrow) and exhibit also development of cytoplasmic PS1 when entering (white arrow) the upper cortex (uc). G) Primary follicles develop around the OSE cortical epithelial crypt (ec); dashed boxes indicate unassembled epithelial nests. Inset shows the emergence of CK- germ cell (asterisk) with ZP+ intermediate segment (arrowhead) among crypt CK+ epithelial cells. H) Migrating tadpole-like germ cell shows no CK staining but ZP+ intermediate segment (arrowhead). I) Accumulation of multiple ZP+ oocytes with unstained nuclei (arrowheads) in a medullary vessel. A-C and E, hematoxylin counterstain. Reprinted from Ref. [99], Antonin Bukovsky copyright.

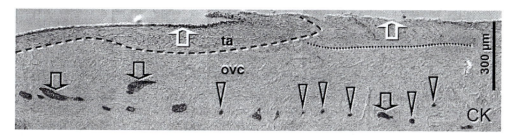

Figure 3. Ovarian surface and adjacent TA and cortex in adult human ovary. Parallel (black arrows) and perpendicular (arrowheads) view of epithelial cords in the upper ovarian cortex (ovc). Dashed line indicates a segment of CK+ TA with flap and differentiating OSE cover (left white arrow). Dotted line indicates CK- segment lacking OSE cover (right white arrow). Reprinted from Ref. [99], Antonin Bukovsky copyright.

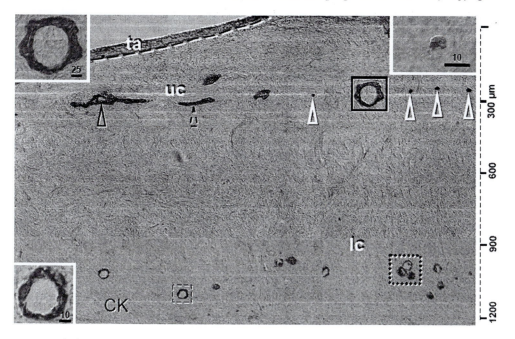

Figure 4. Distribution of epithelial cords and primary follicles in the ovarian cortex. Panoramic view composed of nine images shows ovarian TA filled with CK18+ mesenchymal cells, upper cortex (uc) with epithelial channels (black arrowhead), cords (dashed and white arrowheads - see right inset) and follicle-like structure lacking oocyte (solid box, see upper left inset for detail). Lower cortex (lc) shows isolated (dashed box - see lower left inset) and grouped primary follicles (dotted box). Bars in insets indicate μm. Cytokeratin 18 immunostaining, hematoxylin counterstain. Reprinted from Ref. [99], Antonin Bukovsky copyright.

Development of Balbiani Body During Follicular Renewal

Studies of Motta and collaborators [64,65] have shown that in some areas of the ovary, epithelial cords fragment and appear as small nests of epithelial cells which lie in proximity to primary follicles. We observed that in the lower ovarian cortex, some epithelial nests associated with the lumen of ovarian venules, and these nests exhibited a stretch of intravascular oocytes (figure 2B). During oocyte-nest assembly the Balbiani body was formed by granulosa cell extensions penetrating deep into the ooplasm (figure 2C).

Origin of New Oocytes and Their Assembly with Epithelial Nests

We also visualized the assembly of oocytes with epithelial nests using double color immunohistochemistry for CK in epithelial nests and ZP glycoproteins expressed in oocytes, and showed an association of the oocytes with epithelial nests resembling occupied bird's nests [44] (figure 2D).

Most of the OSE cells showed CK immunostaining, but immunoexpression of ZP proteins was restricted to certain OSE segments. While most ZP proteins were also detected in the zona pellucida of oocytes during and after assembly within epithelial nests (including primary, secondary, preantral and antral follicles), the meiotically expressed porcine ZP oocyte carbohydrate antigen named PS1 [80] was detected in OSE segments but not in zona pellucida of oocytes in human ovarian follicles [44].

The immunoexpression of PS1 in human OSE cells was cytoplasmic. However, cells descending from the OSE into TA also showed nuclear PS1 staining (figure 2E). The dividing OSE cells showed an asymmetric distribution of meiotically expressed nuclear PS1, suggesting meiotic activity. Double color immunostaining for PS1 and CK revealed an asymmetric distribution of PS1 in putative germ cells descending from the OSE, resulting in two distinct (CK+ or PS1+) daughter cells [44]. Larger putative germ cells with nuclear PS1 staining were detected in the TA. Such cells divided symmetrically (both daughter cells expressed PS1; figure 2F) and entered the adjacent ovarian cortex. In the cortex, the putative germ cells showed a translocation of nuclear PS1 immunoexpression to cytoplasmic staining, and an association with cortical vasculature showing minute amounts of PS1 immunoexpression in adjacent endothelial cells. In addition, PS1 immunoexpression was detected in germ cells migrating from CK+ epithelial crypts into the adjacent cortex - an alternative pathway for germ cell origin [44].

These observations indicate that in adult human females, there are no persisting oogonia or germline stem cells, but new germ cells originate from asymmetrically dividing OSE cells. Such germ cells symmetrically divide in the TA (crossing over), enter ovarian vasculature or migrate from OSE cortical crypts to reach nests of primitive granulosa cells and form new primary follicles. Such follicular renewal replaces earlier primary follicles undergoing atresia.

Follicular Atresia

Follicular atresia and luteal regression are essential mechanisms required for the elimination of unnecessary and aged structures, as well as for normal ovarian function. Elimination of antral follicles undergoing atresia and of degenerating corpora lutea during reproductive years in human females is a fast process, associated with infiltration by activated macrophages [101,102], and there is no reason to expect that the similar process accompanying regression of primary and secondary follicles [44] will last longer than several days. If at least 50% of oocytes in adult ovaries are in various stages of degeneration [52], one may conclude that without follicular renewal the ovarian function will cease in human females within a few months. However, in aging ovaries, the elimination of degenerating ovarian structures appears to be affected [103], possibly due to the age-induced alterations of the immune system function [103]. Alternatively, the atresia of aged primary follicles may be initiated during follicular renewal, and if such renewal is absent, aging primary follicles may persist. Hence, atresia may not affect primary follicles in aging ovaries [60], and such follicles may persist in spite of an accumulation of spontaneously arising or environmentally induced genetic alterations of oocytes.

During the prime reproductive period, the degeneration may affect groups of primary and secondary follicles. Immunohistochemically, the follicles undergoing atresia release ZP proteins into the neighboring stroma. This is associated with an altered oocyte morphology and disorganization of the follicular CK+ granulosa layer. In addition, there is a considerable influx of large macrophages into the area from accompanying vessels [44]. Some investigators have claimed that characteristic morphological features of primary follicle atresia are often difficult to determine (reviewed in [25]), while others are more confident [60].

In our immunohistochemical study, the assembly of oocytes with epithelial nests was also associated with some release of ZP proteins. Formation of new follicles was characterized by a well-defined oocyte nucleus, intraooplasmic CK+ extensions from the nest cell wall, and formation of the Balbiani body, i.e., structures and processes not apparent during follicular regression. Resting primary follicles and growing secondary/preantral follicles show a regular morphology, with no leakage of ZP proteins, and only occasional small tissue macrophages associated with the developing theca [44].

Enhanced follicular atresia was accompanied by the appearance of epithelial nests (fragmented epithelial cords) in adjacent segments of the ovarian cortex. We have shown that these nests are small CK+ spheroidal cell clusters of 20-30 μm in diameter. There were also epithelial crypts, likely originating from deep OSE invaginations. These do not communicate with the ovarian surface, as evidenced from serial sections. The movements of epithelial nests and crypts appear to be caused by a rearrangement of stromal bundles, and their migration is probably guided by HLA-DR+ (activated) tissue macrophages.

Origin of Oocytes from OSE Crypts

We have also described an alternative germ cell origin from epithelial crypts in the lower ovarian cortex (inset, figure 2G), accompanied by migration of tadpole like germ cells with ZP+ intermediate segment (arrowhead figure 2H), presence of epithelial cell nests without oocytes (dashed boxes, figure 2G), and accumulation of primary follicles in the neighborhood of epithelial crypts [44] (figure 2G).

These observations indicate that adult human ovaries exhibiting atresia of primary and secondary follicles initiate formation of new epithelial nests with granulosa cell features [65]. This is one of the prerequisites for formation of new primary follicles. Cortical crypts, consisting of epithelial cells retaining a relatively embryonic structure of OSE cells [65,68], appear to be an alternate source of germ cells. Germ cells entering the vasculature may reach epithelial nests at distant destinations, although vascular proximity is not a requirement for follicular development from nests approaching the cortical epithelial crypts producing germ cells.

Adult Oogenesis Exceeds Follicular Renewal

An important question is whether the number of newly formed follicles in adult human ovaries is determined by the number of available epithelial nests or the number of generated germ cells. In the first instance, the isolated nests will either persist or degenerate. In the second, degenerating oocytes not utilized in new follicle formation might be detected. To answer this question we utilized double color immunohistochemistry to search for ZP+ oocytes not assembled with CK+ structures.

We observed [44] an accumulation of degenerating ZP+ oocytes in medullary vessels (figure 2I). Accumulation of oocytes in occasional ovarian medullary vessels was observed in four of twelve cases studied (33%). This suggests that the differentiation of oocytes during the reproductive period is a relatively frequent event. These ovarian samples showed either preparation for, or the ongoing formation of new primary follicles. The accumulation of oocytes in some medullary vessels was present in the samples from both ovaries. Yet, there were eight cases showing no such activity. These ovaries rarely showed primary follicles in the ovarian cortex [44]. This agrees with the observations of Block [49], who observed a similarity between oocyte numbers in the right and left ovaries but wide variation between cases during the prime reproductive period.

Our observations support the idea that the formation of new primary follicles in adult human ovaries is a periodical process, which may occur during a certain phase of the ovarian cycle. This idea was first proposed by Evans and Swezy [47]. Although we did not study a large number of patients, our observations indicate that new primary follicles are likely to be formed during the late luteal phase, as evidenced from the patient's history, ovarian corpus luteum immunohistochemistry, and endometrium morphology [44]. However, the preparation for follicular renewal consists of two sequential steps: formation of primitive granulosa nests, followed later by differentiation of new germ cells, which may be initiated earlier during the ovarian cycle. For example follicular atresia is most prominent during the late follicular phase (follicular selection), when the formation of epithelial nests may be initiated, followed by an appearance of germ cells during midcycle (estradiol and LH peaks), and formation of primary follicles thereafter.

An "Ovary-within-the Ovary" Pattern and Thy-1 Differentiation Protein (Thy- Dp)

The Thy-1 dp consists of a single variable Ig domain and belongs to a group of glycosylphosphatidylinositol-anchored molecules involved in primitive recognition at the cell surface, with the consequences of recognition being due to the differentiated state of the cells [104,105]. Our observations indicate that the Thy-1 dp produced by vascular pericytes accompanies early stages of cellular differentiation [106].

Why do primary follicles form in the lower ovarian cortex, not just near the origin of their components, primitive granulosa and germ cells? We have reported previously that groups of follicles lie in isolated areas of the cortex, exhibiting an oval arrangement of stromal elements [58]. In a recent study, staining for Thy-1 dp revealed that groups of primary follicles reside in the center of rounded areas, extending ~400-1200 μm from the ovarian surface, exhibiting low stromal Thy-1 dp immunoexpression, and showing an ovary-within-the ovary pattern (ov-in-ov, figure 5A). In addition, growth of some follicles in a given cohort is associated with Thy-1 dp+ vasculature (arrows, figure 5A and detail 5B vs. arrowhead figure 5A and detail 5C). Hence, a lack of Thy-1 dp may be required to maintain primary follicles in the resting state, and the presence of Thy-1 dp may stimulate follicular growth. Note strong Thy-1 dp immunostaining of the TA fibroblasts (ta, figure 5A).

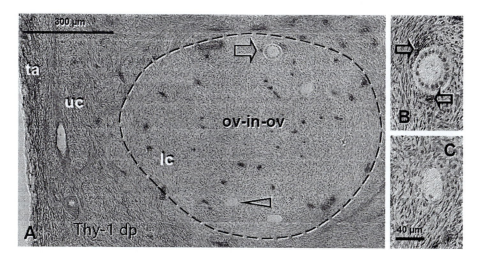

Figure 5. Distribution of Thy-1 dp in the ovarian cortex - an "ovary within the ovary" pattern. A) Thy-1 dp is strongly expressed by TA fibroblasts (ta), and moderately in the upper (uc) and lower ovarian cortex (lc) except for areas showing an "ovary within the ovary" pattern (ov-in-ov) with virtually no Thy-1 dp immunoexpression except for vascular pericytes and smooth muscle cells. These areas characteristically contained primary follicles (arrowhead and C), some of which showed an increase in size accompanied by Thy-1 dp+ pericytes (arrows in A and B). Hematoxylin counterstain, details in text. Reprinted from Ref. [99], Antonin Bukovsky copyright.

Cessation of Adult Oogenesis

Our observations [44] indicate that epithelial nests of primitive granulosa cells derived from the OSE cells contribute to the follicular renewal in adult ovaries. We also studied ovaries of premenopausal and postmenopausal women for CK expression in order to determine whether formation of these nests is associated exclusively with follicular renewal, or if it persists after cessation of this process [94]. During optimal reproductive period (< 38 ± 2 years of age), both epithelial nests and primary follicles have been detected in deeper ovarian cortex. In older (premenopausal) females, only primary follicles were detected. During the premenopausal period, most ovaries (92%) did not show the formation or presence of epithelial nests. Only a single case, from 12 patients investigated (8%), showed formation of epithelial nests in the proximity of the OSE, as well as occurrence of epithelial nests in the deeper cortex, but these nests showed degenerative changes and no adjacent primary follicles were detected [94].

Therefore, it appears that the formation of epithelial nests and their migration into the deeper cortex during the premenopausal period usually does not occur. Premenopausal women show OSE segments with more or less pronounced hyperplasia, and such OSE behavior persists in postmenopausal women. One may speculate that hyperplasia of the OSE in aging women reflects an attempt of a homeostatic mechanism (TCS, see below) to initiate formation of new primary follicles in the ovaries. In other words, a failure of the TCS to stimulate formation of new primordial follicles in adult ovaries may result in the stimulation of OSE proliferation and development of ovarian cancer.

Another important question is whether the premenopausal and postmenopausal ovaries are capable to produce new germ cells and oocytes from persisting OSE stem cells *in vivo*. They are certainly able to do so under *in vitro* conditions, even when derived from ovaries of over 60 year old females [107], and we have occasionally observed degenerating oocytes in the medullary vessels in perimenopausal ovaries lacking epithelial cell nests (unpublished observations).

Altogether, it appears that pre- and postmenopausal ovaries may have a capacity to produce new oocytes, and rarely epithelial nests, but events required for their association and follicle formation are missing, either because the oocytes and germ cell do not have a chance to assemble with epithelial nests, or *vice versa*.

HUMAN FETAL OVARIES

The surface of the human fetal ovary is covered by a serous membrane made of OSE which is continuous with the peritoneal mesothelium. During the early stages of ovarian development there is a rapid proliferation of OSE cells, resulting in cellular stratification, nuclear pleomorphism and nuclear irregularities [108].

The fetal OSE has been implicated in the formation of oocytes [10,109], and it has been suggested that the OSE is a source of granulosa cells in adult ovaries [65,110]. Some immunohistochemical observations, reported and interpreted previously (see [100] and [5] for details), are provided beneath.

Origin of Primitive Granulosa and Germ Cells in Midpregnancy Human Fetal Ovaries

Primitive granulosa cells (pgc, figure 6A) show a decrease of CK expression when compared to the OSE cells. They originate from sprouts of OSE cells extending into the ovary between mesenchymal cell cords (mcc) of rete ovarii. The mesenchymal cell cords are rich in expression of Thy-1 dp, which plays an important role in the stimulation of early cellular differentiation (see above). The primitive granulosa cells associate with oocytes in the deeper ovarian cortex to form primary follicles (asterisks, panel E).

Germ cells originate by asymmetric division of OSE cells (white arrowhead) and show a diminution of major histocompatibility complex class 1 antigen (MHC-1; black vs. white asterisks, figure 6B). Subsequently, the germ cells undergo symmetric division (black arrowhead and s-s') required for crossing over of chromosomes. Next, their size substantially increases under the OSE layer, where they exhibit a tadpole-like shape (dashed line) and enter the ovarian cortex. Note a lack of TA layer.

Association of Immune System Related Cells with Fetal Oogenesis

An essential question is why only some OSE cells are transformed into germ cells. It has been suggested that to become a germ cell, the OSE stem cell should receive an impulse from the ovary-committed monocyte derived cells (MDC) and T lymphocytes, i.e. ovary-committed monocytes and T cells (OCMT), assuming a milieu of favorable systemic (hormonal) conditions ([100] and table 1). During ovarian development the immune system related cells migrate through the rete ovarii and interact with resident MDC (figure 6C and G), and this may result in their ovarian commitment. Apparently, the MDC accompany origination of germ cells from the OSE (figure 6D), as well as T cells (figure 6H) and Thy-1 dp (figure 6I). The OSE also shows a high binding of immunoglobulins (figure 6J), which may prevent them from a spontaneous transformation into germ cells, and activated MDC accompany growing primary follicles (figure 6F). Altogether, the origination of the germ cells from the OSE appears not to be an accidental but OCMT driven process. In other words, the number of OCMT interacting with the OSE cells appears to determine the number of germ cells originating in the ovaries as well as the number of growing primary follicles.

Cessation of Oogenesis in Prenatal Human Ovaries

The origination of new human oocytes and primary follicles ceases after the second trimester of fetal intrauterine life, possibly due to the diminution of circulating human chorionic gonadotropin (hCG) in the fetal blood due to the development of the placental "hCG barrier" [100]. Thereafter (perinatally), the layer of loose mesenchymal cells forming ovarian TA develops, exhibiting some features of the OSE cells (CK expression), and hence possibly originating from epithelial-mesenchymal transition of the OSE cells [5,44], as described in OSE cultures [63]. Under certain conditions [100] these TA mesenchymal cells could be transformed back into the OSE cells by mesenchymal-epithelial transition, i.e., into bipotent stem cells capable to differentiate into germ and granulosa cells in adult human ovaries. This, however, may not happen prior to puberty or around menarche [100].

Table 1. Working model on age-associated changes of ovary-committed MDC & T cells (OCMT) and hormonal signals (LH/hCG & E2) required for the initiation & resumption of oogenesis in human ovaries

Period of life	OCMT[c]	LH/hCG[d]	E_2[e]	Oogenesis
First trimester - midpregnancy	yes	yes	yes	yes[f]
Last trimester - newborn	yes	no	yes	no[f]
Postnatal - menarche	yes	no	no	no[g]
Reproductive period[a]	yes	yes	yes	yes[f]
Premenopause[b]	no	yes	yes	no[g]
Postmenopause	no	yes	no	no[f]

[a] From menarche till 38 ± 2 years of age

[b] From 38 ± 2 years till menopause

[c] OCMT with commitment for stimulation of OSE to germ cell transformation

[d] Levels corresponding to the mid cycle LH peak, or more [hCG levels should be 10x more, since it has a 10% affinity to the LH receptor compared to that of LH (see Ref. [147])

[e] Levels corresponding to the preovulatory E_2 peak, or more

[f] Confirmed

[g] Predicted; Reprinted from Ref. [100], with permission of Humana Press, Inc.

IMMUNE CELLS INFLUENCE COMMITMENT OF ADULT OSE STEM CELLS

Like in fetal ovaries, the OCMT show association with oogenesis in adult human ovaries. The primitive MDC and CD8+ T cells accompany origination of germ cells from OSE stem cells during adulthood (figure 7A and B). The MDC are also associated with symmetric division of germ cells in tunica albuginea and germ cells entering the upper cortex (figure 7C). These observations also show that primitive MDC may initiate asymmetric division of OSE cells and symmetric division of germ cells, since they associate with both daughter cells (arrowheads, figure 7A and C). On the other hand, the CD8 T cells appear to be required for the commitment of emerging germ cells toward the oocyte lineage, as evidenced from the association with one of the daughter cells only (arrowheads, figure 7B), which descends into the TA and exhibits marked increase in size (black asterisk, figure 7B; see also figure 6H).

Activated MDC are associated with migrating germ cells (figure 7D), and such cells associate with the cortical vasculature (figure 7E) and utilize vascular transportation to reach distant destinations (figure 7F; see also figure 2B).

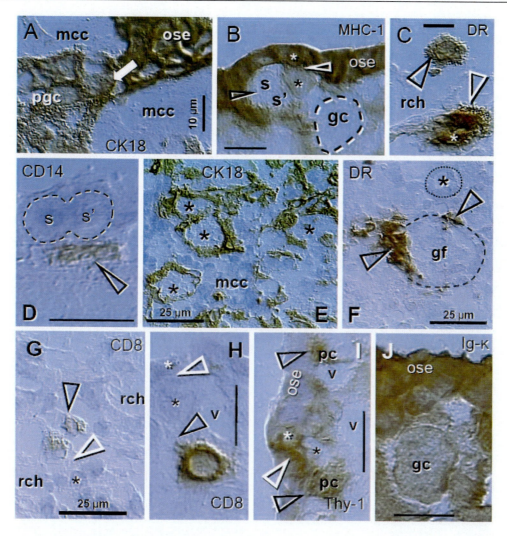

Figure 6. Oocytes and granulosa cells originate from OSE stem cells (ose) in midpregnancy human fetuses. A) Cytokeratin (CK) staining of a cluster of primitive granulosa cells (pgc) descending from the OSE (arrow) between mesenchymal cell cords (mcc). B) Major histocompatibility complex class one (MHC-1) immunostaining, no hematoxylin counterstain. Asymmetric division (white arrowhead) gives rise to MHC-I positive OSE (white asterisk) and MHC-I negative germ (black asterisk) daughter cells. Symmetric division (black arrowhead) produces two MHC negative (s and s') germ cells (crossing over). Larger (tadpole-like) germ cell (dashed line) enters the ovarian cortex. C) HLA-DR+ (activated) monocyte type cells (black arrowhead) migrate through the rete channels (rch) and interact (white arrowhead) with resident monocyte derived cells (MDC; asterisk). D) CD14 primitive monocyte-derived cells (MDC) associate (arrowhead) with symmetric division of germ cells (dashed line; hematoxylin counterstain). E) Small (primordial) follicles (asterisks) with CK+ granulosa cells in the lower cortex. F) HLA-DR cells intimately associate with growing primary follicles (gf), but not non-growing ones (asterisk). G) CD8 T cells (black arrowhead) in rete channels interacting with resident cells (white arrowhead), and beneath the OSE (H) associating (arrowhead) with emerging germ cell (black asterisk; v, vessel). I) Thy-1 differentiation protein (Thy-1) is secreted (arrowheads) from vascular pericytes (pc) among OSE cells with emerging germ cells (asterisks). J) Immunoglobulins (Ig-κ) have a low affinity to germ like cells (gc) but bind heavily to the OSE cells. Bars in A-D, and H-J = 10 μm. Adapted from Ref. [100], with permission of Humana Press Inc.

The rete ovarii is absent in adult ovaries and OCMT during adulthood could originate from bone marrow and lymphoid tissues. It has been suggested that during the fetal immune adaptation an "ovarian" memory is built within the developing immune system for support of follicular renewal by OCMT during adulthood [5]. With its utilization, such memory could be exhausted between 35-40 years of age, and follicular renewal terminated. It appears that termination of follicular renewal occurs at about 38 years of age (figure 1), resulting in a significant decline of oocyte numbers in human ovaries [49] and an abrupt change in the exponential rate of primary follicle loss [111].

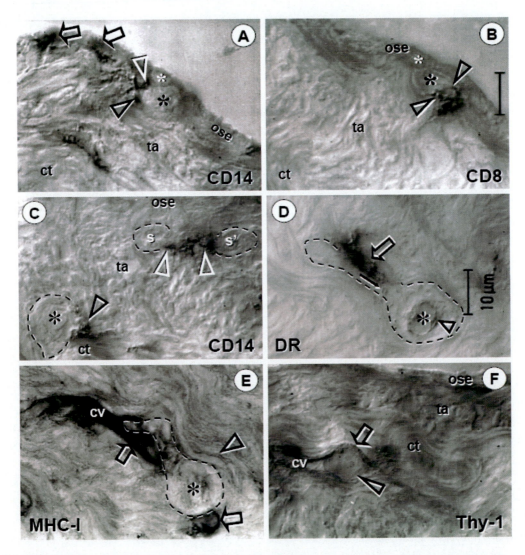

Figure 7. Immune cells influence commitment of OSE stem cells. Staining of the adult human OSE (ose), tunica albuginea (ta), and adjacent cortex (ct) for CD14 of primitive MDC and HLA-DR of activated MDC, CD8 of cytotoxic/suppressor T cells, MHC class I heavy chain, and Thy-1 glycoprotein of pericytes, as indicated in panels. Large asterisks and dashed lines indicate putative germ cells. A) Primitive MDC associate with OSE (arrows) and accompany (arrowheads) origination of germ cells by asymmetric division of OSE stem cells (asterisks). B) Asymmetric division is also accompanied by extensions from T cells (arrowheads). C) Primitive MDC accompany (white arrowheads) symmetric division (s-s') of germ cells in

tunica albuginea and their migration into the adjacent cortex (ct). D) Migrating tadpole-like germ cells are accompanied by activated MDC (open arrow), and HLA-DR material is apparent in the cytoplasm (solid arrow) and in the nuclear envelope (arrowhead). E) The germ cells associate with cortical vasculature (cv) strongly expressing MHC-I (arrows vs. arrowhead), enter and are transported by the bloodstream (F). Adapted from Ref. [58], with permission of Blackwell Publishing, Oxford, UK.

Immune Adaptation and Determination of Ovarian Functional Lifespan

It is possible that ovarian development is influenced by mesenchymal-epithelial interactions, which accompany differentiation of epithelial cells in adult tissues [106]. This may depend on the ability of OCMT, first to recognize and memorize the character of primordial germ cells, which populate the gonadal anlage from the extragonadal source during embryonal development, and then to induce replication of this process within fetal ovaries. Ovarian surface epithelium, due to its rapid proliferation and pleomorphism, as well as its capacity to differentiate into various cell types (ovarian cancers), might be a target of OCMT in this process.

In normal individuals, the first organ affected by aging is the thymus [112] and next is the ovary [113,114]. There is a striking correlation between the period at which an organ is present during early ontogeny and that organ's functional longevity. For instance the heart, which differentiates very early, can in human beings function over one hundred years. However, the ovary, which differentiates later, does not function for more than half of that period. We have suggested that the later the differentiation of certain type of tissue occurs during early ontogeny, the earlier its function expires during adulthood [115].

During immune adaptation (through the end of the second trimester of intrauterine life in humans [116]), the differentiating tissues are recognized by the developing lymphoid (immune) system as self. However, depending on the time at which a certain tissue arises during immune adaptation, a memory could be built for how long such tissue would be supported by tissue-specific mesenchymal cells to function thereafter. Immune system related cells (MDC and T cells) are present in peripheral tissues, and influence the differentiation of tissue cells [106], including formation of germ and granulosa cells and differentiation of primary follicles [58,100].

Monocyte-derived cells play an important role in the regulation of the immune system. These cells control function of tissue lymphocytes associated with differentiation of tissue specific cells [106]. Lymphoid tissues not only produce cells promoting differentiation of tissue-specific epithelial and parenchymal cells, but also receive information from peripheral tissues via afferent lymph. This information is transmitted by veiled MDC, a subpopulation of tissue macrophages. They are low phagocytic, HLA-DR positive, and are highly immunogenic, since they present antigens to T cells in the draining lymph nodes [117-120].

In the fetal ovary, presumptive memory cells reside in the rete ovarii, and immature MDC and T cells migrate through rete channels toward the ovarian surface and participate in the development of germ cells from the OSE [100]. Similar interaction of immune cells with OSE was described in the ovaries of adult women [58]. During adulthood, however, no rete is present in ovaries, so the memory cells may reside in the lymphoid tissues, sources of circulating immune cells. The immune system shows significant functional decrease between

35 and 40 years of age [121] and concomitantly the ovarian follicular renewal appears to cease [44].

Thymus and Reproduction

The thymus plays an important role in the immune system, and it has been suggested that thymic peptides play a role in determining reproductive lifespan in females [122,123]. Relationship of age-associated thymic involution with diminution of ovarian function is supported by the alteration of ovarian function in neonatally thymectomized mice [124]. In addition, in congenitally athymic (nude) mice, follicular loss is first evident at 2 months of age and this is specifically due to a reduction in the numbers of primary follicles. The first ovulation is delayed until two and a half months of age, compared to the first ovulation in the one and a half month old normal mouse females. By four months, an overall reduction in all fractions of the follicle population occurs in nude mice, and ovulation ceases [125]. Interestingly, the absence of the thymus might also be responsible for the lack of hair in nude mice, due to the lack of thymus-derived T cells, which might be required for hair development. Similarly, baldness may develop in aging men, but less likely in women, since the immune system in females works more efficiently and effectively longer than in males [126].

WORKING HYPOTHESIS

Our working hypothesis on the role of the gonadal environment in the regulation of human oogenesis is presented in figure 8. After the indifferent gonad is populated by primordial germ cells (figure 8A), the rete ovarii develops and stimulates differentiation of oocytes from primordial germ cells (panel B). During immune adaptation (IA), the rete is populated by uncommitted MDC and T cells (uMT), from which the MDC may differentiate into the veiled cells. The veiled cells transmit information on oocytes from the rete into the developing lymphoid tissues (curved arrowhead, B). The MDC in rete ovarii then become ovarian memory cells able to convert u-MT passing through the rete channels into committed OCMT. These OCMT, along with appropriate hormonal signaling, induce the development of germ cells from the OSE (panel C). The number of veiled cells populating lymphoid tissues increases further.

When the IA is terminated, the rete ovarii degenerates and oogenesis ceases due to the diminution of hormonal signaling (fetal hCG barrier [100]). The ovarian TA develops from OSE cells (epithelial-mesenchymal transformation), and the number of ovarian memory cells (om; the transformed veiled cells) in lymphoid tissues is set (panel D). Around menarche, and during the prime reproductive period, the hormonal signaling and OCMT resume cyclic oogenesis to replace aging primary follicles undergoing atresia (panel E). The cyclic follicular renewal during adulthood requires a cyclic supply of OCMT, and their generation in lymphoid tissues causes depletion of the pool of memory cells. Hence, from this point of view, the pool of ovarian memory cells in lymphoid tissues, but not the pool of primary fetal follicles, is what is set during mammalian fetal development. Once the available pool of ovarian memory cells is consumed, the oogenesis and follicular renewal cease, in spite of the presence of hormonal signaling (panel F). Remaining primary follicles persist and are utilized until gone. However, the aging oocytes accumulate genetic alterations and may become unsuitable for ovulation and fertilization. The postmenopausal ovaries were reported to carry occasional follicles with degenerated oocytes (reviewed in [113]).

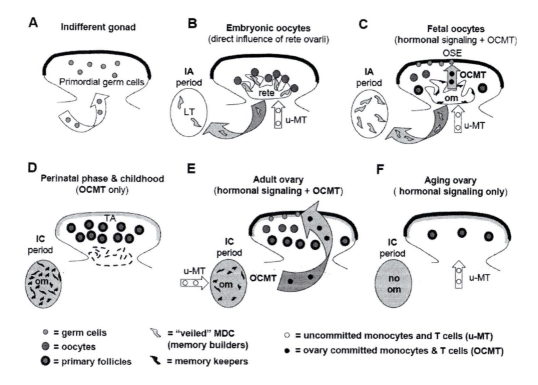

Figure 8. Development of ovaries during immune adaptation (IA) and immune competence (IC). LT, lymphoid tissues; om, ovarian memory. Details in text. Adapted from Ref. [51], with permission of Bentham Science Publishers Ltd.

The initial pool of ovarian memory cells in lymphoid tissues may occasionally be reduced, due to the retardation of normal ovarian development during embryonal and fetal immune system adaptation. If the period for which the primary follicles differentiate during immune adaptation is shorter (delayed or terminated earlier), the period of follicular renewal after menarche ceases earlier compared to normal ovaries, and premature ovarian failure (POF) with secondary amenorrhea results. Advanced restriction of primary follicle development during adaptation may result in the lack of follicular renewal after menarche and primary amenorrhea (early POF). Primary follicles and ovarian memory in the lymphoid system can also be depleted by cytostatic chemotherapy. Interestingly, the incidence of POF after such chemotherapy increases with age. In women <20 years old the incidence is 13%, in 20-30 years is 50%, and >30 years is 100% [127]. This indicates a diminution of the ovarian memory in lymphoid system with age and its increasing sensitivity to chemotherapy.

Altogether, we speculate that a lack of follicular renewal may be caused by age associated exhaustion of specific memory cells in the lymphoid system, which are required to generate effector cells migrating to ovaries and stimulating transformation of OSE cells into primitive granulosa and germ cells. Premature ovarian failure may be caused by a delayed ovarian development during immune adaptation, by earlier termination of immune adaptation, or by cytostatic chemotherapy affecting both the existing pool of primary follicles and OCMT required for follicular renewal. Patients with POF have been found to have abnormalities in function of circulating monocytes, activated lymphocytes, NK cells, and exhibited other immune abnormalities [128-130], suggesting a relationship of the immune system alteration to POF development.

POF Ovaries with Primary Follicles and Animal Models

Premature ovarian failure, as described above, is a result of the lack of primary follicles within the ovaries of women under 40 years of age. However, POF is also often associated with follicular resistance to gonadotropins, called "hypergonadotropic amenorrhea", where ovaries contain normal primary or even antral follicles not responding to gonadotropins by production of estrogens. None of the women with primary amenorrhea have been reported to ever ovulate or conceive with their own oocytes, but over one third of the women with secondary amenorrhea were pregnant at least once before developing hypergonadotropic POF. A quarter of them had evidence of ovulation after the diagnosis was established, and 8% of those with secondary amenorrhea later conceived [130].

Laboratory animal models (rats and mice) indicate that there are two types of POF with primary and antral follicles within the ovaries. The first one, persistent ovarian immaturity, can be induced by inhibition of ovarian development (inhibition of androgen receptor expression with estrogens) during immune adaptation, while the second one, premature ovarian aging, can be induced by acceleration of ovarian development (premature expression of androgen receptor) with androgens [131,132].

The Tissue Control System Theory and a "Stop-Effect" of MDC

The tissue control system (TCS) theory [73,102,106,132-134] deals with the role of vascular pericytes, MDC, and T and B cells in the regulation of tissue function. It proposes that MDC participate in the stimulation of early differentiation of tissue specific (epithelial, parenchymal, neural, and muscle) cells. The MDC also regulate expression of epitopes of specific tissue cells, and in that way control their recognition by circulating tissue-committed T cells and antibodies. Such T cells and antibodies are suggested to participate in the stimulation of advanced differentiation of tissue cells, which may ultimately result in the aging and degeneration of these cells [106].

By the end of the immune adaptation in early ontogeny, the MDC are supposed to encounter the most differentiated tissue cells in a tissue specific manner, and then prevent them from differentiating beyond the encoded state by the so called "stop effect." The nature of the "stop effect" may reside in the inability of monocyte-derived cells to stimulate differentiation of tissue cells beyond the encoded stage. Retardation or acceleration of certain tissue differentiation during immune adaptation is suggested to cause a rigid and persisting alteration of this tissue function. The ability of monocytes to preserve tissue cells in the functional state declines with age, and this is accompanied by functional decline of various tissues within the body, including the ovary, resulting in increased incidence of degenerative diseases and menopause in human beings.

In large mammals, including primates, immune adaptation is terminated during intrauterine life, while in small laboratory rodents (rats and mice) immune adaptation continues for several postnatal days, ending about one week after birth [116]. Estrogens given to neonatal rats or mice inhibit ovarian development, and during adulthood such rat females exhibit persisting ovarian immaturity characterized by retardation of follicular development [73] in spite of normal serum levels of gonadotropins [135,136]. This indicates that suppression of early ovarian development results in persisting ovarian immaturity, which resembles POF associated with gonadotropin resistence of ovarian follicles. Injection of estrogens to neonatal mice (days 0-3) caused permanent anovulation, but mice injected later (days 3-6; closer to the end of immune adaptation) showed resumption of ovulatory cycles after initial anovulation [137]. Hence, persisting ovarian immaturity can result in a delay of normal ovarian function. Since incidence of degenerative diseases increases with age, one may expect that there is a tendency of the "stop-effect" to shift with age (arrowheads, figure 9). This may explain how persisting ovarian immaturity may switch to the functioning ovary.

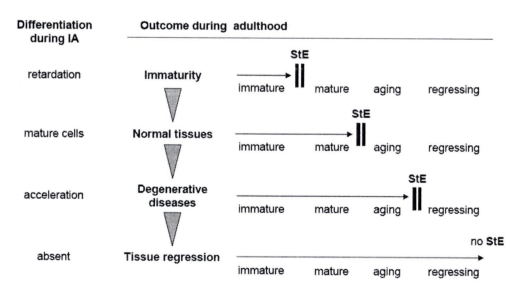

Figure 9. Stage of cell differentiation during immune adaptation (IA) sets TCS "stop effect" (StE) for tissue physiology and pathology during adulthood. Arrowheads indicate a tendency to StE "shifts" with age. Adapted from Refs. [73,131,134,146].

On the other hand, injection of androgens causes premature ovarian aging persisting during adulthood. However, androgen induced anovulation can be prevented by neonatal injection of thymic cell suspension from immunocompetent prepubertal normal female donors, but not if given from animals prior to completion of immune adaptation [138,139]. This suggests that certain thymic cells (thymocytes, or thymic MDC) of normal immunocompetent females carry information on appropriate differentiation of ovarian structures, and this information can be transferred to immunologically immature neonatal rats.

However, when a low dose of androgens is injected during immune adaptation, the rats exhibit so called delayed anovulatory syndrome. Ovaries exhibit onset of normal function after puberty (~40 days of age), but premature aging of the ovary occurs between 60-100 days [140]. This delayed manifestation of ovarian dysfunction resembles human POF with secondary amenorrhea, as well as some human degenerative diseases with autoimmune character, which also occur after a shorter (juvenile diabetes mellitus) or longer (Alzheimer's disease) period of normal tissue function.

A simplified application of the TCS theory on the regulation of tissue function via "stop effect" (StE) is depicted in figure 9 - see also Ref. [106,131,132]. In normal tissues, the mature cells are present during immune adaptation and the tissue-specific cells are "parked" in the mature state during adulthood. However, a retardation of cell differentiation during adaptation results in persisting immaturity (POF with primary amenorrhea) and acceleration in premature aging (POF with secondary amenorrhea, degenerative diseases). If the tissues were absent during adaptation (corpus luteum), they are handled as a "graft."

The Immune System vs. Brain Memory and Aging of the Body

The "ovarian memory" built within the lymphoid system can be viewed as a charged battery, which is drained by periodical follicular renewal. The higher the charge during the immune adaptation, the longer it will last, and vice versa. The possible involvement of immune adaptation in the programming of ovarian function and various types of POF can be extrapolated toward other tissues in the body as well. From this point of view, the degenerative changes of the immune system with advancing age can be responsible for the aging of other tissues and the whole body in general. In contrast, however, the "brain memory" can be viewed as a computer's hard drive, which is initially empty, and gradually filled during life. Hence, while the "ovarian memory" within the lymphoid system is diminishing and eventually lost, the capacity of the "brain memory" may suffer from a shortage of unused neuronal cells, unless there is a persistence of neuronal cell renewal with age advancement.

HUMAN OOGENESIS *IN VITRO* AND POSSIBLE UTILIZATION IN POF TREATMENT

After studies of oogenesis in fetal and adult human ovaries, we wondered if a similar potential for OSE cells could be demonstrated *in vitro*. Our recent observations indicate that OSE cultures consist of undifferentiated cells on day 3 (figure 10A). Thereafter, they may differentiate into distinct cell types, including neural, epithelial and mesenchymal cells, and oocytes [99]. Presence of oocytes was not observed prior to day four of culture, indicating that they do not originate from follicular oocytes. Oocyte type cells show distinct sizes (arrows, figure 10B and C), and are often accompanied by fibroblasts (arrowheads). Cells resembling secondary oocytes figure 10D) were found to develop in OSE cultures from premenopausal and postmenopausal ovaries, and we also observed a development of oocytes into parthenogenetic morulae [99,107], a phenomenon occasionally occurring during cultivation of human follicular oocytes [141].

These observations indicate that even OSE cultures from postmenopausal ovaries lacking any follicles can produce new oocytes with parthenogenetic potential similar to that observed in follicular oocyte cultures. However, it remains to be investigated whether OSE-derived oocytes can be utilized for IVF treatment in order to provide genetically related children to women with POF, or with ovarian sterility due to the alteration of oocytes in aging ovaries.

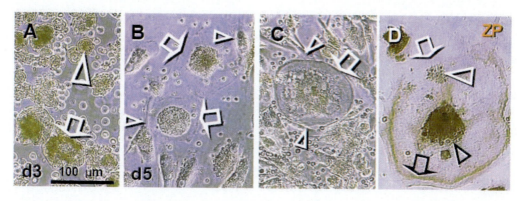

Figure 10. OSE cultures. A) Undifferentiated cells in day 3 (d3) OSE culture. B and C) Day 5 cultures contain oocyte type cells of distinct sizes (arrows) and associated fibroblasts (arrowheads). D) Secondary oocyte in 5 day culture stained for ZP; note poorly defined nuclear envelope (black arrowhead) expulsion of polar body (white arrowhead) toward surface with lack of expression of ZP (white arrow). Reproduced from Ref. [99], Antonin Bukovsky copyright.

ARE THERE ALTERNATIVE SOURCES OF GERM CELLS FOR POF TREATMENT?

In 2004, follicular renewal was also described in the ovaries of juvenile mice, and large (40 μm) germline stem cells persisting among OSE cells were suggested to be a source of oocytes [59]. This view has been subjected to immediate critique [44,142], since such large cells among OSE cells resemble oocytes known to leave perinatal and adult mammalian ovaries [58,143]. The persistence of germline stem cells in OSE has recently been found by the same research team untenable, and replaced by the proposal that the sources of oocytes in adult mice and humans are stem cells in bone marrow [97].

Following publication, the authors widely extrapolated their observations to the formation of allogeneic oocytes after bone marrow (or blood) transplant in ovaries of adult mice treated with cytostatics. They proposed in the public media such clinical implications as using these transplants in the treatment of human ovarian infertility. Yet, the proposal on the origin of oocytes from bone marrow has been found even more controversial, and interpretation of the data presented questionable [144,145].

For instance, the molecular markers studied are not specific for germ cells, but also expressed in other cell types and organs, including brain and bone, so they cannot be considered as germ cell markers, but rather stem cell markers [145]. Evidence that germ cell formation in bone marrow disappears in ovariectomized mice [97] raises by itself solid doubts on the bone marrow origin of oocytes [144]. Since germ cells developing from the OSE cells of adult human ovaries during follicular renewal enter blood vessels (see Ref. [44,58] and figure (1) panels D and F), they also contaminate peripheral blood and hence bone marrow. Therefore, the collection of peripheral blood, with its periodic autologous germ cells and circulating OCMT, which are capable of initiating oogenesis, could be used in women prior to cytostatic chemotherapy [144]. The blood can be returned thereafter in hope of resuming the wave(s) of periodical follicular renewal. However, the majority of women already exhibiting POF do not belong to this clinical category.

In contrast to the utilization of autologous blood transfusion in infertile women for follicular renewal [97], with its questionable effectiveness [145], *in vitro* production of new autologous eggs from the OSE cells of human ovaries, which is age independent [99,100,107], and their *in vitro* fertilization and subsequent utilization of embryos for intrauterine implantation, may represent a more suitable variant for providing genetically related children to women with ovarian infertility, and is worthy of consideration and further exploration [144].

CONCLUSION

Primordial mammalian germ cells originate from somatic stem cell precursors, and primordial oocytes differentiate under the influence of neighboring ovarian somatic cells. In midpregnancy human fetuses the oocytes and granulosa cells begin to differentiate from bipotent OSE stem cells covering fetal gonads, and associate to contribute to the pool of fetal primary follicles. In adult women, however, OSE cells differentiate from ovarian TA mesenchymal cells, which may represent an environmentally and morphologically more stable cell type as compared to the OSE cells and oocytes. Periodical oogenesis in adult ovaries and differentiation of granulosa cell nests from OSE stem cells contribute to the replacement of older primary follicles (follicular renewal) until the end of the prime reproductive period. A survey of human oogenesis is given in figure 11.

Differentiation of tissue specific cells from stem cells *in vivo* depends on tissue committed immune cells. If tissue-specific cells and structures differentiate later during immune adaptation in early ontogeny (oocytes, granulosa cells, and primary follicles), their regeneration and survival during adulthood ceases earlier as compared to the earlier differentiating tissues (heart). Furthermore, tissues which were absent during immune adaptation, such as ovarian corpus luteum, do not regenerate. Fetal and adult oocytes differentiate by asymmetric division of OSE cells in the presence of the OSE-committed monocytes (tissue macrophages) and T cells, and oogenesis may also require increased levels of luteinizing hormone/chorionic gonadotropin and estrogens.

Embryo

Totipotent stem cells are influenced by neighboring cells to become primordial germ cells migrating into developing gonads. Sex commitment of primordial germ cells is determined by somatic cells of the gonads.

Midpregnancy Fetuses

Secondary female germ cells differentiate from OSE under the influence of OCMT (Fig. 8). Pegs of OSE cells descending into the cortex become primitive granulosa cells. Association of oocytes with primitive granulosa cells results in the formation of fetal primary follicles. The later primary follicles begin to develop, the earlier follicular renewal during adulthood is terminated (POF).

Perinatal period

Formation of new primary follicles ceases and TA (OSE precursors) develops by epithelial-mesenchymal transition of OSE cells.

Childhood

Formation of new primary follicles may not occur until menarche, when persisting fetal primary follicles are expected to degenerate.

Prime reproductive period

The TA is a source of OSE cells (mesenchymal-epithelial transition). Under the influence of OCMT, the OSE cells sequentially differentiate into nests of primitive granulosa cells and germ cells. Germ cells differentiate into oocytes, which associate with granulosa cell nests to form new primary follicles replacing older follicles undergoing atresia. This follicular renewal ensures that fresh eggs are always available for ovulation and healthy progeny.

Premenopausal period

Follicular renewal ceases physiologically between 35 and 40 years of age, or earlier in POF. Persisting primary follicles may accumulate genetic alteration in oocytes. Genetic mutations in fetus increase with advancement of maternal age.

Postmenopausal period

Onset of postmenopause (or POF) is a result of the exhaustion of the pool of functional primary follicles remaining after diminution of follicular renewal. New oocytes may still differentiate in OSE cultures from ovaries lacking functional follicles and serve for autologous IVF purposes.

Figure 11. Survey of human oogenesis. OSE, ovarian surface epithelium; OCMT, ovary-committed MDC and T cells; TA, tunica albuginea; POF, premature ovarian failure; IVF, in vitro fertilization. Adapted from Ref. [51], with permission of Bentham Science Publishers Ltd.

Fetal oogenesis ceases after the second trimester of intrauterine life, and it may not resume again until menarche, due to the low hormonal levels during childhood. Adult oogenesis ceases between 35-40 years of age, possibly due to the lack of generation of committed ovary-specific mesenchymal cells. Earlier deficit of these cells (idiopathic or induced by cytostatic chemotherapy) may cause premature ovarian failure. Factors responsible for the diminution of follicular renewal may be responsible for the aging of other tissues and the whole body in general. Premenopausal primary follicles persist until gone, but persisting oocytes accumulate genetic alterations with age. However, *in vitro* cultured OSE stem cells from premenopausal and postmenopausal ovaries differentiate into various cell types, including neural, epithelial and mesenchymal cells, and oocytes. Some of these oocytes develop into parthenogenetic morulae, indicating their functional potential. Therefore, fresh oocytes from ovarian cultures may be suitable for autologous treatment of POF or age associated alteration of oocytes.

ACKNOWLEDGMENTS

Supported by the Physicians' Medical Education and Research Foundation, Knoxville, TN. The technical skills and assistance of Marta Svetlikova, M.S. and Rachel S. White, B.S. are highly appreciated and acknowledged, as well as proof reading of the manuscript by Rachel S. White.

REFERENCES

[1]   Pearl, R., and Schoppe, W. F. (1921). Studies on the physiology of reproduction in the domestic fowl. XVIII. Further observations on the anatomical basis of fecundity. *J. Exp. Zool.,* 34, 101-1189.

[2]   Zuckerman, S. (1951). The number of oocytes in the mature ovary. *Recent Prog. Horm. Res,* 6, 63-109.

[3]   Zuckerman, S., and Baker, T. G. (1977). The development of the ovary and the process of oogenesis. In: S. Zuckerman and B. J. Weir (Eds.), *The Ovary,* Volume I. (pp. 41-67). New York: Academic Press,

[4]   Holmes, D. J., Thomson, S. L., Wu, J., and Ottinger, M. A. (2003). Reproductive aging in female birds. *Exp. Gerontol.,* 38, 751-756.

[5]   Bukovsky, A., Copas, P., and Virant-Klun, I. (2006). Potential new strategies for the treatment of ovarian infertility and degenerative diseases with autologous ovarian stem cells. Expert Opin Biol Ther, 6, 341-365.

[6]   Owen, R. (1843). Lectures on the comparative anatomy and physiology of the invertebrate animals, delivered at the Royal College of Surgeons. From notes by William White Cooper. London: Longman, Brown, Green, and Longmans.

[7]   Simkins, C. S. (1923). On the origin and migration of the so-called primordial germ cells in the mouse and the rat. *Acta zool. Stockh.,* 4, 241-278.

[8]   Goette, A. W. (1875). Die Entwicklungsgeschichte der Unke (Bombinator igneus) als Grundlage einer vergleichenden Morphologie der Wirbeltiere. Leipzig: Voss.

[9]   Nussbaum, M. (1880). Zur Differenzierung des Geschlechts im Terreich. *Arch. mikrosk. Anat. EntwMech.,* 18, 121-1.

[10]   Waldeyer, W. (1870). *Eierstock und Ei.* Leipzig: Engelmann.

[11]   Weismann, A. (1885). Die Continuitat des Keimplasmas als Grundlage einer Theorie der Vererbung. Jena: Fischer-Verlag.

[12]   Eigenmann, C. H. (1891). On the precocious segregation of the sex-cells in Micrometrus. aggregatus, Gibbons. *J. Morphol.,* 5, 481-492.

[13] Dustin, A. P. (1907). Recherches sur l'Oringine des Gonocytes chez les Amphibiens. *Arch. de Biol.,* 23, 411-522.

[14] Federow, V. (1907). Uber die Wanderung der Genitalzellenbei Salmo fario. *Anat Anz.,* 30, 219-223.

[15] Rubaschkin, W. (1907). Uber das erste Auftreten und Migration der Keimzellen bei Vogelembryonen. *Anat. Hefte, Abt.* 1, 35, 241-261.

[16] Rubaschkin, W. (1909). Uber die Urgeschlechtszellen bei Saugetieren. *Anat. Hefte, Abt.* 1, 39, 603-652.

[17] Dustin, A. P. (1910). L'origine et l'evolution des Gonocytes chez les Reptiles (Chrysemis marginata). *Arch. de Biol.,* 25, 495-534.

[18] von Winiwarter, H., and Sainmont, G. (1908). Uber die ausschliesslich post fetale Bildung der definitiven Eier bei der Katze. *Anat. Anz.,* 32, 613-616.

[19] Spuler, A. (1910). Uber die normale Entwicklung des weiblichen Genitalapparats. In: J. F. Bergmann (Ed.), *Handbucher Gynakologie von Veit,* Vol. 5.:

[20] Firket, J. (1914). Recherches sur l'organogenese des glandes sexuelles chez les oiseaux. *Arch. Biol.,* 29, 201-351.

[21] Swift, C. H. (1914). Origin and early history of the primordial germ-cells of the chick. *Am. J. Anat.,* 15, 483-516.

[22] Swift, C. H. (1916). Origin of the sex-cords and definitive spermatogonia in the male chick. *Am. J. Anat.,* 20, 375-410.

[23] Reagan, F. P. (1916). Some results and possibilities of early embryonic castration. *Anat. Rec.,* 11, 251-267.

[24] Lillie, F. R. (1908). The development of the chick. New York: Henry Holt and Co.

[25] Baker, T. G. (1972). Oogenesis and ovarian development. In: H. Balin and S. Glasser (Eds.), *Reproductive Biology.* (pp. 398-437). Amsterdam: Excerpta Medica,

[26] Kelly, S. J. (1977). Studies of the developmental potential of 4- and 8-cell stage mouse blastomeres. *J. Exp. Zool.,* 200, 365-376.

[27] Zernicka-Goetz, M. (1998). Fertile offspring derived from mammalian eggs lacking either animal or vegetal poles. *Development,* 125, 4803-4808.

[28] Ginsburg, M., Snow, M. H., and McLaren, A. (1990). Primordial germ cells in the mouse embryo during gastrulation. *Development,* 110, 521-528.

[29] Lawson, K. A., and Hage, W. J. (1994). Clonal analysis of the origin of primordial germ cells in the mouse. *Ciba Found. Symp.,* 182, 68-84.

[30] Tam, P. P., and Zhou, S. X. (1996). The allocation of epiblast cells to ectodermal and germ-line lineages is influenced by the position of the cells in the gastrulating mouse embryo. *Dev. Biol.,* 178, 124-132.

[31] Lawson, K. A., Dunn, N. R., Roelen, B. A., Zeinstra, L. M., Davis, A. M., Wright, C. V., Korving, J. P., and Hogan, B. L. (1999). Bmp4 is required for the generation of primordial germ cells in the mouse embryo. *Genes Dev.,* 13, 424-436.

[32] Wylie, C. (2000). *Germ cells. Curr. Opin. Genet. Dev.,* 10, 410-413.

[33] Tsunekawa, N., Naito, M., Sakai, Y., Nishida, T., and Noce, T. (2000). Isolation of chicken vasa homolog gene and tracing the origin of primordial germ cells. *Development,* 127, 2741-2750.

[34] McLaren, A. (1999). Signaling for germ cells. *Genes Dev.,* 13, 373-376.

[35] Raz, E. (2000). The function and regulation of vasa-like genes in germ-cell development. *Genome Biol.,* 1, REVIEWS1017.

[36] Hubner, K., Fuhrmann, G., Christenson, L. K., Kehler, J., Reinbold, R., De La, F. R., Wood, J., Strauss, J. F., III, Boiani, M., and Scholer, H. R. (2003). Derivation of oocytes from mouse embryonic stem cells. *Science,* 300, 1251-1256.

[37] Toyooka, Y., Tsunekawa, N., Akasu, R., and Noce, T. (2003). Embryonic stem cells can form germ cells in vitro. *Proc. Natl. Acad. Sci. U. S. A,* 100, 11457-11462.

[38] Geijsen, N., Horoschak, M., Kim, K., Gribnau, J., Eggan, K., and Daley, G. Q. (2004). Derivation of embryonic germ cells and male gametes from embryonic stem cells. *Nature,* 427, 148-154.

[39] Clark, A. T., Bodnar, M. S., Fox, M., Rodriquez, R. T., Abeyta, M. J., Firpo, M. T., and Pera, R. A. (2004). Spontaneous differentiation of germ cells from human embryonic stem cells in vitro. *Hum. Mol. Genet.,* 13, 727-739.

[40] Molyneaux, K., and Wylie, C. (2004). Primordial germ cell migration 1. *Int. J. Dev. Biol,* 48, 537-544.

[41] Castrillon, D. H., Quade, B. J., Wang, T. Y., Quigley, C., and Crum, C. P. (2000). The human VASA gene is specifically expressed in the germ cell lineage. *Proc. Natl. Acad. Sci. U. S. A,* 97, 9585-9590.

[42] Hoyer, P. E., Byskov, A. G., and Mollgard, K. (2005). Stem cell factor and c-Kit in human primordial germ cells and fetal ovaries 1. *Mol. Cell Endocrinol,* 234, 1-10.

[43] Alberts, B., Johnson, A., Lewis, J., Raff, M., Roberts, K., and Walter, P. (2002). *Molecular Biology of the Cell.* New York: Garland Science.

[44] Bukovsky, A., Caudle, M. R., Svetlikova, M., and Upadhyaya, N. B. (2004). Origin of germ cells and formation of new primary follicles in adult human ovaries. *Reprod. Biol. Endocrinol.,* 2, 20-http://www.rbej.com/content/2/1/20.

[45] Kingery, H. M. (1917). Oogenesis in the white mouse. *J. Morphol.,* 30, 261-315.

[46] Allen, E. (1923). Ovogenesis during sexual maturity. *Am. J. Anat.,* 31, 439-481.

[47] Evans, H. M., and Swezy, O. (1931). Ovogenesis and the normal follicular cycle in adult mammalia. *Mem. Univ. Calif.,* 9, 119-224.

[48] Franchi, L. L., Mandl, A. M., and Zuckerman, S. (1962). The development of the ovary and the process of oogenesis. In: S. Zuckerman (Ed.), *The Ovary.* (pp. 1-88). London: Academic Press,

[49] Block, E. (1952). Quantitative morphological investigations of the follicular system in women. Variations at different ages. *Acta Anat.* (Basel), 14, 108-123.

[50] Yao, H. H., DiNapoli, L., and Capel, B. (2003). Meiotic germ cells antagonize mesonephric cell migration and testis cord formation in mouse gonads. Development, 130, 5895-5902.

[51] Bukovsky, A. (2006). Oogenesis from human somatic stem cells and a role of immune adaptation in premature ovarian failure. *Curr. Stem Cell Res. Ther.,* 1, 289-303.

[52] Ingram, D. L. (1962). Atresia. In: S. Zuckerman (Ed.), *The Ovary.* (pp. 247-273). London: Academic Press,

[53] Gougeon, A. (1996). Regulation of ovarian follicular development in primates: facts and hypotheses. *Endocr. Rev.,* 17, 121-155.

[54] Kerr, J. B., Duckett, R., Myers, M., Britt, K. L., Mladenovska, T., and Findlay, J. K. (2006). Quantification of healthy follicles in the neonatal and adult mouse ovary: evidence for maintenance of primordial follicle supply. *Reproduction.,* 132, 95-109.

[55] Gerard, P. (1920). Contribution a l'etude de l'ovarie des mammiferes. L'ovaire de *Galago mossambicus* (Young). *Arch. Biol.,* 43, 357-391.

[56] Rao, C. R. N. (1928). On the structure of the ovary and the ovarian ovum of Loris lydekkerianus Cabr. *Qaurt. J. Micr. Sci.,* 71, 57-73.

[57] Zuckerman, S., and.Weir, B. J. (1977). The Ovary. Second Edition, Volume I. New York: Academic Press.

[58] Bukovsky, A., Keenan, J. A., Caudle, M. R., Wimalasena, J., Upadhyaya, N. B., and Van Meter, S. E. (1995). Immunohistochemical studies of the adult human ovary: possible contribution of immune and epithelial factors to folliculogenesis. *Am. J. Reprod. Immunol.,* 33, 323-340.

[59] Johnson, J., Canning, J., Kaneko, T., Pru, J. K., and Tilly, J. L. (2004). Germline stem cells and follicular renewal in the postnatal mammalian ovary. *Nature,* 428, 145-150.

[60] Gougeon, A., Echochard, R., and Thalabard, J. C. (1994). Age-related changes of the population of human ovarian follicles: increase in the disappearance rate of non-growing and early- growing follicles in aging women. *Biol. Reprod.,* 50, 653-663.

[61] Motta, P. M., and Makabe, S. (1986). Germ cells in the ovarian surface during fetal development in humans. A three-dimensional microanatomical study by scanning and transmission electron microscopy. *J. Submicrosc. Cytol.,* 18, 271-290.

[62] Simkins, C. S. (1932). Development of the human ovary from birth to sexual maturity. *J. Anat.,* 51, 465-505.

[63] Auersperg, N., Wong, A. S., Choi, K. C., Kang, S. K., and Leung, P. C. (2001). Ovarian surface epithelium: biology, endocrinology, and pathology. *Endocr. Rev.,* 22, 255-288.

[64] Van Blerkom, J., and.Motta, P. M. (1979). The Cellular Basis of Mammalian Reproduction. Baltimore-Munich: Urban and Schwarzenberg.

[65] Motta, P. M., Van Blerkom, J., and Makabe, S. (1980). Changes in the surface morphology of ovarian 'germinal' epithelium during the reproductive cycle and in some pathological conditions. *J. Submicrosc. Cytol.,* 12, 407-425.

[66] Makabe, S., Iwaki, A., Hafez, E. S. E., and Motta, P. M. (1980). Physiomorphology of fertile and infertile human ovaries. In: P. M. Motta and E. S. E. Hafez (Eds.), *Biology of the Ovary.* (pp. 279-290). The Hague: Martinus Nijhoff Publishers,

[67] Gillett, W. R. (1991). Artefactual loss of human ovarian surface epithelium: potential clinical significance. *Reprod. Fertil. Dev.,* 3, 93-98.

[68] Mossman, H. W., and Duke, K. L. (1973). Some comparative aspects of the mammalian ovary. In: R. O. Greep (Ed.), Handbook of Physiology, Sect. 7: *Endocrinology.* (pp. 389-402). Washington: Am. Physiol. Soc.,

[69] Dyck, H. G., Hamilton, T. C., Godwin, A. K., Lynch, H. T., Maines-Bandiera, S., and Auersperg, N. (1996). Autonomy of the epithelial phenotype in human ovarian surface epithelium: changes with neoplastic progression and with a family history of ovarian cancer. *Int. J. Cancer,* 69, 429-436.

[70] Auersperg, N., Pan, J., Grove, B. D., Peterson, T., Fisher, J., Maines-Bandiera, S., Somasiri, A., and Roskelley, C. D. (1999). E-cadherin induces mesenchymal-to-epithelial transition in human ovarian surface epithelium. *Proc. Natl. Acad. Sci. U. S. A,* 96, 6249-6254.

[71] Choi, K. C., Auersperg, N., and Leung, P. C. (2003). Mitogen-activated protein kinases in normal and (pre)neoplastic ovarian surface epithelium. *Reprod. Biol. Endocrinol.,* 1, 71.

[72] Treisman, R. (1996). Regulation of transcription by MAP kinase cascades. *Curr. Opin. Cell Biol.,* 8, 205-215.

[73] Bukovsky, A., Caudle, M. R., and Keenan, J. A. (1997). Regulation of ovarian function by immune system components: the tissue control system (TCS). In: P. M. Motta (Ed.), *Microscopy of Reproduction and Development: A Dynamic Approach.* (pp. 79-89). Roma: Antonio Delfino Editore,

[74] Picher, M., Burch, L. H., Hirsh, A. J., Spychala, J., and Boucher, R. C. (2003). Ecto 5'-nucleotidase and nonspecific alkaline phosphatase. Two AMP-hydrolyzing ectoenzymes with distinct roles in human airways. *J. Biol. Chem.,* 278, 13468-13479.

[75] Ziomek, C. A., Lepire, M. L., and Torres, I. (1990). A highly fluorescent simultaneous azo dye technique for demonstration of nonspecific alkaline phosphatase activity. *J. Histochem. Cytochem.,* 38, 437-442.

[76] Quinones, J. A., and van Bogaert, L. J. (1979). Nonspecific alkaline phosphatase activity in normal and diseased human breast. *Acta Histochem.,* 64, 106-112.

[77] Page-Roberts, B. A. (1972). Changes in nonspecific alkaline phosphatase activity in the rat urinary bladder wall in response to experimental filling. *Invest. Urol.,* 9, 385-389.

[78] Pan, J., and Auersperg, N. (1998). Spatiotemporal changes in cytokeratin expression in the neonatal rat ovary. *Biochem. Cell Biol.,* 76, 27-35.

[79] Skinner, S. M., and Dunbar, B. S. (1992). Localization of a carbohydrate antigen associated with growing oocytes and ovarian surface epithelium. *J. Histochem. Cytochem.,* 40, 1031-1036.

[80] Skinner, S. M., Lee, V. H., Kieback, D. G., Jones, L. A., Kaplan, A. L., and Dunbar, B. S. (1997). Identification of a meiotically expressed carbohydrate antigen in ovarian carcinoma: I. Immunohistochemical localization. *Anticancer Res.,* 17, 901-906.

[81] Skinner, S. M., Kieback, D. G., Chunn, J., Jones, L. A., Metzger, D. A., Malinak, L. R., and Dunbar, B. S. (1997). Identification of a meiotically expressed carbohydrate antigen in ovarian carcinoma: II. Association with proteins in tumors and peritoneal fluid. *Anticancer Res.,* 17, 907-911.

[82] Dunbar, B. S., Timmons, T. M., Skinner, S. M., and Prasad, S. V. (2001). Molecular analysis of a carbohydrate antigen involved in the structure and function of zona pellucida glycoproteins. *Biol. Reprod,* 65, 951-960.

[83] Wartenberg, H. (1983). Germ cell migration induced and guided by somatic cell interaction. *Bibl. Anat.,* 24, 67-76.

[84] Zamboni, L. (1970). Ultrastructure of mammalian oocytes and ova. *Biol. Reprod. Suppl,* 2, 44-63.

[85] Carlson, J. L., Bakst, M. R., and Ottinger, M. A. (1996). Developmental stages of primary oocytes in turkeys. *Poult. Sci.,* 75, 1569-1578.

[86] Motta, P. M., Nottola, S. A., Makabe, S., and Heyn, R. (2000). Mitochondrial morphology in human fetal and adult female germ cells. *Hum. Reprod,* 15 Suppl 2, 129-147.

[87] Cox, R. T., and Spradling, A. C. (2003). A Balbiani body and the fusome mediate mitochondrial inheritance during Drosophila oogenesis. *Development,* 130, 1579-1590.

[88] Santini, D., Ceccarelli, C., Mazzoleni, G., Pasquinelli, G., Jasonni, V. M., and Martinelli, G. N. (1993). Demonstration of cytokeratin intermediate filaments in oocytes of the developing and adult human ovary. *Histochemistry,* 99, 311-319.

[89] Motta, P. M., Makabe, S., Naguro, T., and Correr, S. (1994). Oocyte follicle cells association during development of human ovarian follicle. A study by high resolution scanning and transmission electron microscopy. *Arch. Histol. Cytol.,* 57, 369-394.

[90] Pepling, M. E., and Spradling, A. C. (2001). Mouse ovarian germ cell cysts undergo programmed breakdown to form primordial follicles. *Dev. Biol.,* 234, 339-351.

[91] Pepling, M. E., and Spradling, A. C. (1998). Female mouse germ cells form synchronously dividing cysts. *Development,* 125, 3323-3328.

[92] Erickson, B. H. (1966). Development and senescence of the postnatal bovine ovary. *J. Anim. Sci.,* 25, 800-805.

[93] Bukovsky, A., and Presl, J. (1977). Origin of "definitive" oocytes in the mammal ovary. *Cesk. Gynekol.,* 42, 285-294.

[94] Bukovsky, A. (2006). Immune system involvement in the regulation of ovarian function and augmentation of cancer. *Microsc. Res. Tech.,* 69, 482-500.

[95] Romeu, M., Simon, C., and Pellicer, A. (2006). Adult stem cells in the human ovary: hope or fiction? In: C. Simon and A. Pellicer (Eds.), *Stem Cells in Reproductive Medicine: Basic Science and Therapeutic Potential.* (pp. 45-52). London: Informa Healthcare,

[96] Johnson, J. (2006). Stem cell support of ovary function and fertility. In: C. Simon and A. Pellicer (Eds.), *Stem Cells in Reproductive Medicine: Basic Science and Therapeutic Potential.* (pp. 31-44). London: Informa Healthcare,

[97] Johnson, J., Bagley, J., Skaznik-Wikiel, M., Lee, H. J., Adams, G. B., Niikura, Y., Tschudy, K. S., Tilly, J. C., Cortes, M. L., Forkert, R., Spitzer, T., Iacomini, J., Scadden, D. T., and Tilly, J. L. (2005). Oocyte generation in adult mammalian ovaries by putative germ cells in bone marrow and peripheral blood. *Cell,* 122, 303-315.

[98] Eggan, K., Jurga, S., Gosden, R., Min, I. M., and Wagers, A. J. (2006). Ovulated oocytes in adult mice derive from non-circulating germ cells. *Nature,* 441, 1109-1114.

[99] Bukovsky, A., Svetlikova, M., and Caudle, M. R. (2005). Oogenesis in cultures derived from adult human ovaries. *Reprod. Biol. Endocrinol.,* 3, 17- http://www.rbej.com/content/3/1/17.

[100] Bukovsky, A., Caudle, M. R., Svetlikova, M., Wimalasena, J., Ayala, M. E., and Dominguez, R. (2005). Oogenesis in adult mammals, including humans: a review. *Endocrine,* 26, 301-316.

[101] Bukovsky, A., Caudle, M. R., Keenan, J. A., Wimalasena, J., Foster, J. S., and Van Meter, S. E. (1995). Quantitative evaluation of the cell cycle-related retinoblastoma protein and localization of Thy-1 differentiation protein and macrophages during

follicular development and atresia, and in human corpora lutea. *Biol. Reprod.*, 52, 776-792.

[102] Bukovsky, A., Caudle, M. R., Keenan, J. A., Wimalasena, J., Upadhyaya, N. B., and Van Meter, S. E. (1995). Is corpus luteum regression an immune-mediated event? Localization of immune system components, and luteinizing hormone receptor in human corpora lutea. *Biol. Reprod.*, 53, 1373-1384.

[103] Bukovsky, A., Caudle, M. R., Keenan, J. A., Wimalasena, J., Upadhyaya, N. B., and Van Meter, S. E. (1996). Is irregular regression of corpora lutea in climacteric women caused by age-induced alterations in the "tissue control system"? *Am. J. Reprod. Immunol.*, 36, 327-341.

[104] Williams, A. F., and Barclay, A. N. (1988). The immunoglobulin superfamily--domains for cell surface recognition. *Annu. Rev. Immunol.*, 6, 381-405.

[105] Cohen, F. E., Novotny, J., Sternberg, M. J. E., Campbell, D. G., and Williams, A. F. (1981). Analysis of structural similarities between brain Thy-1 antigen and immunoglobulin domains. *Biochem. J.*, 195, 31-40.

[106] Bukovsky, A., Caudle, M. R., Keenan, J. A., Upadhyaya, N. B., Van Meter, S., Wimalasena, J., and Elder, R. F. (2001). Association of mesenchymal cells and immunoglobulins with differentiating epithelial cells. *BMC Dev. Biol.*, 1, 11.-http://www.biomedcentral.com/1471-213X/1/11.

[107] Bukovsky, A. (2005). Origin of germ cells and follicular renewal in adult human ovaries. Presented at Microscopy and Microanalysis Conference 2005 - July 31 - August 4, Honolulu, Hawaii (Invited).

[108] Peters, H., and.McNatty, K. P. (1980). The Ovary. A Correlation of Structure and Function in Mammals. Berkeley and Los Angeles, California: University of California Press.

[109] Simkins, C. S. (1928). Origin of the sex cells in man. *Am. J. Anat.*, 41, 249-253.

[110] Brambell, F. W. R. (1927). The development and morphology of the gonads of the mouse. Part 1. The morphogenesis of the indifferent gonad and of the ovary. *Proc. Roy. Soc.*, 101, 391-409.

[111] Faddy, M. J. (2000). Follicle dynamics during ovarian ageing. *Mol. Cell Endocrinol*, 163, 43-48.

[112] Kay, M. M. (1979). An overview of immune aging. *Mech. Ageing Dev.*, 9, 39-59.

[113] Talbert, G. B. (1968). Effect of maternal age on reproductive capacity. *Am. J. Obstet. Gynecol.*, 102, 451-477.

[114] Kirkwood, T. B. (1998). Ovarian ageing and the general biology of senescence. *Maturitas*, 30, 105-111.

[115] Bukovsky, A., and Caudle, M. R. (2002). Immunology: animal models. In: D. J. Ekerdt (Ed.), *Encyclopedia of Aging.* (pp. 691-695). New York: Macmillan Reference USA,

[116] Klein, J. (1982). Immunology: The Science of Self-Nonself Discrimination. New York: John Wiley and Sons, Inc.

[117] Balfour, B. M., Drexhage, H. A., Kamperdijk, E. W., and Hoefsmit, E. C. (1981). Antigen-presenting cells, including Langerhans cells, veiled cells and interdigitating cells. *Ciba. Found. Symp.*, 84, 281-301.

[118] Hoefsmit, E. C., Duijvestijn, A. M., and Kamperdijk, E. W. (1982). Relation between Langerhans cells, veiled cells, and interdigitating cells. *Immunobiology,* 161, 255-265.

[119] Knight, S. C., Farrant, J., Bryant, A., Edwards, A. J., Burman, S., Lever, A., Clarke, J., and Webster, A. D. (1986). Non-adherent, low-density cells from human peripheral blood contain dendritic cells and monocytes, both with veiled morphology. *Immunology,* 57, 595-603.

[120] Howard, C. J., and Hope, J. C. (2000). Dendritic cells, implications on function from studies of the afferent lymph veiled cell. *Vet. Immunol. Immunopathol.,* 77, 1-13.

[121] Mathe, G. (1997). Immunity aging. I. The chronic perduration of the thymus acute involution at puberty? Or the participation of the lymphoid organs and cells in fatal physiologic decline? *Biomed. Pharmacother.,* 51, 49-57.

[122] Rebar, R. W. (1982). The thymus gland and reproduction: do thymic peptides influence the reproductive lifespan in females? J. Am. Geriatr. Soc., 30, 603-606.

[123] Suh, B. Y., Naylor, P. H., Goldstein, A. L., and Rebar, R. W. (1985). Modulation of thymosin beta 4 by estrogen. *Am. J. Obstet. Gynecol.,* 151, 544-549.

[124] Nishizuka, Y., and Sakakura, T. (1969). Thymus and reproduction: sex-linked dysgenesis of the gonad after neonatal thymectomy in mice. *Science,* 166, 753-755.

[125] Lintern Moore, S., and Pantelouris, E. M. (1975). Ovarian development in athymic nude mice. The size and composition of the follicle population. *Mech. Ageing Dev.,* 4, 385-390.

[126] Aspinall, R. (2000). Longevity and the immune response. *Biogerontology.,* 1, 273-278.

[127] Lo, P. A., Ruvolo, G., Gancitano, R. A., and Cittadini, E. (2004). Ovarian function following radiation and chemotherapy for cancer. *Eur. J. Obstet. Gynecol. Reprod. Biol.,* 113 Suppl 1, S33-S40.

[128] Hoek, A., van Kasteren, Y., de Haan-Meulman, M., Schoemaker, J., and Drexhage, H. A. (1993). Dysfunction of monocytes and dendritic cells in patients with premature ovarian failure. *Am. J. Reprod. Immunol.,* 30, 207-217.

[129] Hoek, A., van Kasteren, Y., de Haan-Meulman, M., Hooijkaas, H., Schoemaker, J., and Drexhage, H. A. (1995). Analysis of peripheral blood lymphocyte subsets, NK cells, and delayed type hypersensitivity skin test in patients with premature ovarian failure. *Am. J. Reprod. Immunol.,* 33, 495-502.

[130] Rebar, R. W. (2000). Premature ovarian failure. In: R. A. Lobo, J. Kesley, and R. Marcus (Eds.), *Menopause Biology and Pathobiology.* (pp. 135-146). San Diego: Academic Press,

[131] Bukovsky, A., Ayala, M. E., Dominguez, R., Keenan, J. A., Wimalasena, J., McKenzie, P. P., and Caudle, M. R. (2000). Postnatal androgenization induces premature aging of rat ovaries. *Steroids,* 65, 190-205.

[132] Bukovsky, A., Ayala, M. E., Dominguez, R., Keenan, J. A., Wimalasena, J., Elder, R. F., and Caudle, M. R. (2002). Changes of ovarian interstitial cell hormone receptors and behavior of resident mesenchymal cells in developing and adult rats with steroid-induced sterility. *Steroids,* 67, 277-289.

[133] Bukovsky, A., Michael, S. D., and Presl, J. (1991). Cell-mediated and neural control of morphostasis. *Med. Hypotheses,* 36, 261-268.

[134] Bukovsky, A., Caudle, M. R., and Keenan, J. A. (2000). Dominant role of monocytes in control of tissue function and aging. *Med. Hypotheses,* 55, 337-347.

[135] Nagasawa, H., Yanai, R., Kikuyama, S., and Mori, J. (1973). Pituitary secretion of prolactin, luteinizing hormone and follicle-stimulating hormone in adult female rats treated neonatally with oestrogen. *J. Endocrinol.,* 59, 599-604.

[136] Matsumoto, A., Asai, T., and Wakabayashi, K. (1975). Effects of x-ray irradiation on the subsequent gonadotropin secretion in normal and neonatally estrogenized female rats. Endocrinol. *Jpn.,* 22, 233-241.

[137] Deshpande, R. R., Chapman, J. C., and Michael, S. D. (1997). The anovulation in female mice resulting from postnatal injections of estrogen is correlated with altered levels of CD8+ lymphocytes. *Am. J. Reprod. Immunol.,* 38, 114-120.

[138] Kincl, F. A. (1965). Permanent Atrophy of Gonadal Glands Induced by Steroid Hormones (Ph.D. Thesis). Prague.: Charles University.

[139] Kincl, F. A., Oriol, A., Folch Pi, A., and Maqueo, M. (1965). Prevention of steroid-induced sterility in neonatal rats with thymic cell suspension. *Proc. Soc. Exp. Biol. Med.,* 120, 252-255.

[140] Swanson, H. E., and van der Werff ten Bosch, J. J. (1964). The "early-androgen" syndrome; differences in response to prenatal and postnatal administration of various doses of testosterone propionate in female and male rats. *Acta Endocrinol.* (Copenh), 47, 37-50.

[141] Santos, T. A., Dias, C., Henriques, P., Brito, R., Barbosa, A., Regateiro, F., and Santos, A. A. (2003). Cytogenetic analysis of spontaneously activated noninseminated oocytes and parthenogenetically activated failed fertilized human oocytes--implications for the use of primate parthenotes for stem cell production. *J. Assist. Reprod. Genet.,* 20, 122-130.

[142] Gosden, R. G. (2004). Germline stem cells in the postnatal ovary: is the ovary more like a testis? Hum. Reprod. Update, 10, 193-195.

[143] Motta, P. M., and Makabe, S. (1986). Elimination of germ cells during differentiation of the human ovary: an electron microscopic study. *Eur. J. Obstet. Gynecol. Reprod. Biol.,* 22, 271-286.

[144] Bukovsky, A. (2005). Can ovarian infertility be treated with bone marrow- or ovary-derived germ cells? *Reprod. Biol. Endocrinol.,* 3, 36-http://www.rbej.com/content/3/1/36.

[145] Telfer, E. E., Gosden, R. G., Byskov, A. G., Spears, N., Albertini, D., Andersen, C. Y., Anderson, R., Braw-Tal, R., Clarke, H., Gougeon, A., McLaughlin, E., McLaren, A., McNatty, K., Schatten, G., Silber, S., and Tsafriri, A. (2005). On regenerating the ovary and generating controversy. *Cell,* 122, 821-822.

[146] Bukovsky, A. (2000). Mesenchymal cells in tissue homeostasis and cancer. *Mod. Asp. Immunobiol.,* 1, 43-47.

[147] Bousfield, G. R., Butnev, V. Y., Gotschall, R. R., Baker, V. L., and Moore, W. T. (1996). Structural features of mammalian gonadotropins. *Mol. Cell Endocrinol,* 125, 3-19.

In: Stem Cell Research Developments
Editor: Calvin A. Fong, pp. 273-293

ISBN: 978-1-60021-601-5
© 2007 Nova Science Publishers, Inc.

Chapter IX

Gastric Stem Cells

Yoshikiyo Akasaka[*1] *and Toshiharu Ishii*[2]

[1] Department of Pathology, School of Medicine,
Toho University, 5-21-16 Omori-Nishi, Ohta-City, Tokyo 143-8540, Japan
[2] Department of Pathology, School of Medicine, Toho University,
5-21-16 Omori-Nishi, Ohta-City, Tokyo 143-8540, Japan

ABSTRACT

Cells of the gastric mucosa undergo constant renewal. This process is thought to be regulated by multipotent stem cells, which give rise to all gastric epithelial cell lineages and can regenerate whole gastric glands by production of committed precursor cells. Molecular studies are beginning to reveal the pathways that regulate the proliferation and differentiation of gastrointestinal stem cells. The Wnt/β-catenin signaling pathway and downstream molecules such as APC, Tcf-4, fkh-6, Cdx-1, and Cdx-2 play an important role in the differentiation and proliferation of gastrointestinal epithelial cells. Recent evidence indicates that gastric stem cells occupy a niche in the isthmus of gastric glands, which might regulate the function of gastric stem cells through mesenchymal-epithelial interactions. Due to the lack of reliable stem cell markers at the single-cell level, the precise nature of gastric stem cells is difficult to define and characterize precisely, and data about numbers and positions of gastric stem cells remain unclear. Identification of the stem cell marker, Musashi-1, in both the intestine and stomach will provide a clear insight into the properties of gastric stem cells in humans.

---

[*] Correspondence: Yoshikiyo Akasaka, M.D., Department of Pathology, School of Medicine, Toho University, 5-21-16 Omori-Nishi, Ohta City, Tokyo, Japan. Telephone: int. +81-3-3762-4151 (ext.) 2383; Fax: int. +81-3-5493-5414; E-mail: akasakay@med.toho-u.ac.jp.

INTRODUCTION

The cells of gastric glands undergo constant renewal. Although stem cells are the most important cell type in the gastric gland, they have not yet been identified. It is thought that a single stem cell gives rise to a clone of differentiated epithelial cells in every gastric gland [1,2]. These cells undergo division to produce the specialized epithelial lineages, which will form the foveolar, isthmus, neck, and basal regions of the gastric gland. Accumulated evidence has shown that multipotent stem cells are present in specific zones, or niches, within gastric glands [3,4,5,6,7]. It is probable that extracellular matrix (ECM) factors regulate the differentiation and self-renewal of stem cells through mesenchymal-epithelial interactions [8]. Although studies are beginning to identify the molecular mechanisms that regulate the development of the gastrointestinal tract, the Wnt/β-catenin signaling pathway and downstream molecules such as APC, Tcf-4, fkh-6, Cdx-1, and Cdx-2 are important for function of the gastrointestinal epithelial cell lineage [9,10,11,12,13,14,15,16,17,18]. The molecular pathways that determine the differentiation of committed progenitor cells into specific epithelial cell lineages are beginning to be investigated; the Notch-Delta signaling pathways involving the transcription factors Hes1 and Math1 regulate the differentiation of normal gastrointestinal epithelial cells. Although much evidence for the presence of stem cells in gastric glands has been reported, the stem cells themselves remain unidentified at the single-cell level, mainly because of a lack of reliable stem cell markers [19,20]. Recently, a putative stem cell marker in the gastric gland, Musashi-1, has been identified in humans [21]. This review also describes the process that led to the discovery of Musashi-1, which is considered to be a significant contribution to studies of stem cell biology.

GASTRIC EPITHELIAL CELL LINEAGES

In the stomach, the epithelial lining forms long, tubular glands divided into foveolar, isthmus, neck, and basal regions. Gastric foveolar cells are located on the mucosal surface and in the foveola. The mucus neck cells are situated within the neck and isthmus of the gastric glands. The peptic-chief or zymogenic cells are located in the base of the glands in the fundic and body regions of the stomach. In the murine stomach, several lines of evidence indicate that multipotent stem cells and undifferentiated granular-free progenitor cells (committed precursor cells) reside in the isthmus [22]. It is thought that migration of cell progenitors to form gastric epithelial cells is bi-directional from the neck/isthmus region [23,24]. Thus, the pre-pit precursor differentiates into mucous cells of the foveola, or pit, as it moves up the isthmus, while the pre-neck cell precursor differentiates into parietal cells and then zymogenic cells as it migrates downwards. The precursor cell population including gastric epithelial progenitor cells and multipotent stem cells make up approximately 3% of the gastric epithelium in adult mice [6].

CLONAL POPULATIONS IN THE GASTRIC GLAND

Mouse embryo aggregation chimeras are readily made, wherein the two populations can be easily distinguished. The lectin *Dolichos biflorus* agglutinin (DBA) binds to sites on B6-derived, but not Swiss Webster (SWR)-derived, cells in C57BL/6J Lac (B6) ↔ SWR mouse embryo aggregation chimeras, and it can be used to distinguish the two parental strains in gut epithelial cells. Thompson and colleagues showed that epithelial cell lineages in the antral gastric mucosa of the mouse stomach, including the endocrine cells, are derived from a common stem cell, using XX/XY chimeric mice, which have easily identifiable male- and female-derived regions [25]. This finding was confirmed by Tatematsu and colleagues, who used CH3 ↔ BALB/c chimeric mice and found that each gastric gland was composed entirely of either CH3 or BALB/c cells and that there were no mixed glands. Although contradicting hypothesis had been reported previously [26], these findings support the contention that murine gastric glands are clonally derived [27].

Nomura and colleagues used X-inactivation mosaic mice expressing a *LacZ* receptor gene to study the clonality of gastric glands in the fundic and pyloric regions of the developing mouse stomach [28]. They indicated that most glands are initially polyclonal with three or four stem cells per gland, but become monoclonal during the first 6 weeks of life, possibly due to purification of the gland, where division of one stem cell eventually overrides all other stem cells, or by gland fission. A population of approximately 5-10% of mixed, polyclonal glands persists into adulthood. This population may have gone undetected in previous studies using aggregation chimeras, due to reduced survival rates of cells of different genotypes. The mixed glands may not undergo fission or may have reduced fission rates, or perhaps have an increased number of stem cells during development, thereby maintain a higher number of stem cells after gland fission.

The first study of glandular clonality in the human intestine was done using the human colorectal carcinoma cell line HRA19 [29]. This malignant epithelial cell line is multipotential and can produce every differentiated epithelial cell type in the human colorectal mucosa *in vitro* and *in vivo*. However, such results cannot be applied to normal human gastrointestinal epithelia, because of the difference in clonality between normal development and neoplasma.

With regard to glandular clonality in the human stomach, Nomura and colleagues have used X-chromosome-linked inactivation to study fundic and pyloric glands in the stomach of human females [30]. The X-chromosome-linked phosphoglycerate kinase (PGK) gene and polymorphism of the androgen receptor gene (HUMARA) allow distinction between the two X-chromosomes. These analyses have revealed that while pyloric glands appear homotypic for the PGK or HUMARA locus, and thus monoclonal, about half of the fundic glands are heterotypic for the PGK and HUMARA loci, and thus polyclonal. These findings indicate a more complex situation than studies of gastric clonality in chimeric mice, and suggest regional differences in clonality during the development of the human gastric glands.

STEM CELL NICHE IN THE GASTRIC GLAND

It is generally accepted that stem cells reside within a "niche" or group of cells and extracellular substrates, which provide a microenvironment in which the stem cells can give rise to their differentiated cells. In the small intestine, it has been suggested that stem cells reside in the base of the crypts of Lieberkuhn, just superior to the Paneth cells [31]. In the large intestine, they are presumed to be located in the mid-crypt of the ascending colon, and crypt base of the descending colon [31]. However, within the gastric glands, migration of cells is bidirectional from the neck/isthmus region to form simple mucous epithelial cells of the foveola, or pit, and cells that migrate downwards to form parietal cells and chief cells [23,24]. Therefore, the stem cells are believed to lie within the neck/isthmus region of the gastric gland [3,4,5,6,7]. The gastric stem cell niche is presumably formed and maintained by the underlying cells of the lamina propria and their secreted growth factors, which regulate stem cell behavior through the paracrine secretion of growth factors and cytokines, whose receptors are expressed on gastric epithelial cells. Intestinal subepithelial myofibroblasts are closely adherent to the intestinal epithelium. These cells secrete hepatocyto growth factor (HGF), transforming growth factor-β (TGF-β), and keratinocyte growth factor (KGF), but the receptors for these growth factors are located on the epithelial cells [32]. Platelet-derived growth factor-α (PDGF-α), which is expressed in intestinal epithelial cells, acts by paracrine signaling through its mesenchymal receptor, platelet-derived growth factor receptor-α (PDGFR-α), to regulate epithelial-mesenchymal interactions during development [33]. The subepithelial myofibroblasts surround the base of the neck-isthmus of the gastric gland, a commonly proposed location for the gastric stem cell niches. Thus, it has been proposed that subepithelial myofibroblasts influence gastric epithelial cell proliferation and differentiation through epithelial-mesenchymal interactions and that these cells play an important role in determination of epithelial cell fate [5,6].

MOLECULAR PATHWAYS IN THE GASTROINTESTINAL TRACT

Although the precise molecular mechanisms by which gastric stem cells differentiate into epithelial cell lineages remains unclear, recent molecular biology has identified a large number of genes and receptors that are involved in the regulatory molecular pathways of proliferation and differentiation of gastrointestinal stem cells [5,6]. This leads to an improved understanding of the molecular pathways that regulate proliferation and differentiation of cells in the gastrointestinal tract.

The Wnt/β-Catenin Signaling Pathway

The Wnt genes encode a large family of secreted molecules that play important roles in controlling tissue patterning, cell fate, and cell proliferation within a broad range of embryonic contexts, including the gastrointestinal tract [9]. Studies of knock-out mice have provided evidence that the Wnt pathway is important for maintaining a dividing small-intestinal stem cell population, and that Notch signaling is involved in specification of its descendant secretary cell lineages. To date, 19 members of the Wnt family have been identified in humans, along with 10 members of the frizzled (Fz) family, serpentine transmembrane cell surface receptors through which the Wnt signaling cascade is initiated. Under normal growth conditions, the multifunctional protein β-Catenin interacts with a glycogen synthase kinase 3-β (GSK3β), axin, and adenomatous polyposis coli (APC) tumor suppressor protein complex [34].

Wnt ligand binding to a Fz receptor activates the cytoplasmic phosphoprotein disheveled, which in turn initiates a signaling cascade that results in increased cytosolic levels of β-catenin due to negative regulation of GSK3β [35]. β-catenin then translocates to the cell nucleus, where it forms a transcriptional activator by combining with members of the T-cell factor/lymphocyte enhancer factor (Tcf/LEF) DNA-binding protein family, and by activating specific genes, ultimately results in the proliferation of target cells.

The interactions of Wnt ligands and Fz receptors are modulated by the secreted Wnt antagonisits (sWAs), which can be divided into two functional classes: the soluble frizzled related protein (sFRR) class and the dickkopf (Dkk) class. Members of the sFRR family include Wnt inhibitory factor-1 (Wif1), sFRP1, 2, 4, and 5, and frisbee (FrzB, sFRP3). These bind directly to Wnts, thus altering their ability to bind to Fz receptors. Four members of the Dkk family, Dkk1-4, bind to low-density lipoprotein receptor-related proteins (LRP5 and 6) contained within the Wnt receptor-related complex and influence Wnt signaling by preventing normal LRP-Fz-Wnt interactions [36]. The various secreted Wnt antagonists interact to effect Wnt signaling and influence a wide variety of biological processes, including developmental cell fate, differentiation, and tumorigenesis.

One of the main functions of the APC genes appears to be destabilization of β-catenin. Many genes, including c-myc, cyclin D1, c-Jun, CD44, Fra-1, and urokinase-type plasminogen receptor receptor, have been identified as targets of the β-catenin/Tcf/LEF nuclear complex, although the precise mechanisms that lead to carcinogenesis are not entirely understood [37,38,39].

The TCf/LEF DNA Binding Protein Family

The Tcf/LEF family of transcription factors has four members: Tcf-1, LEF-1, Tcf-3, and Tcf-4. Tcf-4 is expressed at high levels in the developing intestine and in the epithelial cells of adult small intestine, colon, and colon carcinomas [40]. Mice with targeted disruption of the Tcf-4 gene have no proliferating cells within their small-intestinal crypts and therefore lack a functional stem cell compartment [41]. This suggests that Tcf-4 is responsible for establishing stem cell populations within the crypts, most probably activated by a Wnt signal from the underlying mesenchymal cells in the stem cell niche.

Chimeric ROSA26 mice express a fusion protein containing the HMG box domain of Lef-1 linked to the trans-activation domain of β-catenin (Lef-1/β-cat), and thereby undergo increased β-catenin signaling without being retained in the cytoplasm by interaction with the GSKβ/axin/APC complex. These B6-ROSA26⇔129/Sv (Lef-1/β-cat) chimeras display increased intestinal epithelial apoptosis specifically in 129/Sv cells throughout crypt morphogenesis, unrelated to enhanced cell proliferation. On completion of crypt formation and in adult mice, there is complete loss of all 129/Sv cells. Stem cell selection is biased towards the unmanipulated ROSA26 cells in their chimeras, suggesting that an adequate threshold level of β-catenin during development permits sustained proliferation and selection of cells, thus establishing a stem cell hierarchy. Increased β-catenin expression appears to induce an apoptotic response. Thus the stem cell niche is unaffected by increased Lef-1/β-cat during intestinal crypt development [42].

Cdx-1 and Cdx-2 Homeobox Genes

Candidates for the control of intestinal development and differentiation include caudal genes. Caudal genes are necessary for determination of anteroposterior polarity during early *Drosophila* development, and caudal-type homeobox (Cdx) 1 and Cdx2 are mammalian members of the caudal-related homeobox gene family [43,44]. The Cdx1 and Cdx2 genes are intestinal transcription factors that regulate the proliferation and differentiation of intestinal epithelial cells. In both the adult mouse and human, expression is strictly confined to the gut, from the duodenum to the rectum [45,46].

The Cdx1 and Cdx2 proteins are expressed predominantly in the small intestine and colon, and not in the normal adult stomach. However, Silberg and colleagues have reported the presence of Cdx1 protein in intestinal metaplastic lesions of the human stomach [47]. Mizoshita and colleagues have also demonstrated the expression of Cdx1 and Cdx2 proteins in intestinal metaplastic lesions of the human stomach [48]. Recent studies have clearly shown that Cdx2 acts as master regulator of intestinal development and differentiation [49]. Loss of Cdx2 expression leads to focal gastric differentiation in the colon [46]. This indicates a possible homeotypic shift in stem cell phenotype. Tcf-4 knockout mice do not express Cdx-1 in the small-intestinal epithelium; thus, the Wnt/β-catenin complex directly confers Cdx-1 transcription in association with Tcf-4 during the development of intestinal crypts [50].

The Forkhead Family of Transcrition Factors

The winged helix/forkhead family of transcription factors is essential for proper development of the ectodermal and endodermal regions of the gut. There are nine murine forkhead family members, which give rise to the Fox (forkhead box) proteins [51]: three homologues of the rat hepatic nuclear factors 3 gene, HNF3α, -β, and -γ, and six novel genes referred to as fkh-1 to fkl-6 [52]. The forkhead homologue 6 (fkh-6) gene, expressed exclusively in gastrointestinal mesenchymal cells, encodes the Fox1 protein [53]. Fox1 knockout mice have dramatically altered gastrointestinal epithelial cells, with branched and elongated glands in the stomach, elongated villi, hyperproliferative crypts, and goblet cell hyperplasia due to increased epithelial cell proliferation [54]. These mice have markedly up-regulated levels of heparin sulfate proteoglycans, which increase the efficacy of Wnt binding to the frizzled receptors on gastrointestinal epithelial cells, thereby overactivating the Wnt/β-catenin pathway and increasing nuclear β-catenin. The resulting β–catenin/Tcf/LEF complex activates cyclin D1 and c-myc, which increase epithelial cell proliferation. Therefore, Fox1 regulates the Wnt/β-catenin pathway indirectly by increasing heparin sulphate proteoglycans.

The Math1 and Hes1 Signalling Pathway

Math1 is a basic loop-helix transcription factor and downstream component of the Notch signaling pathway. Deletion of Math1 causes depletion of the goblet, Paneth, and enteroendocrine cell lineages in the small intestine, suggesting that Math1 is essential for progenitor cell commitment to one of three epithelial cell types in the adult intestine. This experiment also indicates that Math1-negative progenitors become enterocytes [55]. High levels of Notch switch on the Hes1 transcription repressor, which blocks expression of Math1, causing cells to remain as progenitors and ultimately to become enterocytes. In contrast, low Notch expression increases the levels of its ligand, which induces Math1 expression by blocking Hes1, causing cells to become goblet cells, Paneth cells, or enteroendocrine cells [56]. Hes1 null mice have elevated Math1 expression, with increased enteroendocrine and goblet cells and fewer enterocytes. These findings indicate that Math1 can regulate the determination of cell fate through a Notch signaling pathway [57].

While gastric stem cells have not been isolated at the single cell level, genetic analysis of an enriched mouse gastric epithelial progenitor cell population has helped to clarify some of the molecular pathways that regulate this precursor cell proliferation and differentiation in the murine stomach. Transgenic mice with mutant diphtheria toxin A fragment-ablation of partial cells have an increased number of gastric epithelial cell progenitors. This is increased in transgenic embryonic animals [58]. Gene-chip analysis of epithelial progenitor cell populations has demonstrated that growth factor response pathways and regulators of protein turnover pathways are prominent in these cells [59]. Real-time quantitative RT-PCR analysis of laser capture microdissected cells retrieved from the niche have revealed that growth factor response pathways, such as the insulin-like growth factor (IGF) signaling pathway, regulating protein turnover (ubiquitin proteosomal, sumoylation, and neddylation) pathway, and controlling RNA processing and localization pathway are prominent in murine gastric epithelial lineage progenitor cells. This indicates the importance of growth factor signaling in the progenitor cells in mice, and their ability to communicate specifically with different epithelial cell types.

Stem Cell Markers of Gastric Glands

Due to the lack of specific molecular markers for human gastric stem cells, their exact location remains unclear and no technique exists for isolating human gastric stem cells or epithelial progenitor cells at the single cell level. Unlike the mouse, the molecular pathways that regulate the proliferation and differentiation of stem cells in the human stomach also remain unresolved. Thus, there is a need to identify putative stem cell markers in human gastric glands [6].

BMI-1

Polycomb genes are transcriptional repressors that control development by regulation of cell growth and differentiation genes [60]. Several polycomb genes, such as BMI-1, are involved in the preservation of a variety of stem cell types [61]. Indeed, BMI-1 is required for self renewal of hematopoietic cells and neural stem cells. BMI-1 deficiency leads to a strong reduction of hematopoietic stem cells and neural stem cells in postnatal BMI-1-/- mice [62,63]. This indicates that BMI-1 is indispensable for self renewal of hematopoietic stem cells and of stem cells in the central and peripheral nervous system. Therefore, Reinisch and colleagues examined whether BMI-1 expression may be indicative of stem cell properties in the human gastrointestinal tract [64]. They found weak expression in the isthmus region of the stomach and in the crypts of the intestines, indicating that stem cell compartments of the gastrointestinal tract are BMI-1-positive. In contrast, a number of highly differentiated cells such as parietal cells, neuroendocrine cells of the pylorus, Paneth cells and a subset of goblet cells were also BMI-1-positive. BMI-1 has been suggested to contribute to differentiation of a variety of cell types by stabilization of cell type-specific gene expression [65]. Therefore, Reinisch et al. indicate that BMI-1 is not only a stem cell marker but can also be regarded as a differentiation marker of a variety of cell types in the adult gastrointestinal tract. They also indicate that BMI-1 expression can hardly be used to demonstrate the precise distribution of stem cells and progenitor cells in the gastrointestinal tract [64].

Musashi-1

Musashi-1 is selectively expressed in neural progenitor cells, including neural stem cells. Musashi-1 is thought to be involved in the early asymmetric divisions that generate differentiated cells from neural stem cells [66,67,68]. Recent studies have demonstrated that Musashi-1 is a distinctive marker of epithelial stem cells in the crypts of the mouse small intestine and human colon [69,70,71]. These results provide a clear insight into the properties of gastrointestinal stem cells. In this review, we summarize the process that led to the discovery of this stem cell marker in the nervous system as well as in the gastrointestinal tract.

Function of Drosophila MUSASHI Gene

Musashi-1 is an RNA-binding protein family that is strongly expressed in the nervous system and whose primary structure and expression pattern have been conserved among species such as *C. elegans, Drosophila melanogaster, Ciona intestinalis,* and in vertebrates as a whole [66,72,73,74,75,76]. Based on loss-of-function phenotypes of the musashi gene in *Drosophila*, this gene was demonstrated to play an essential role in the asymmetrical division of sensory organ precursor cells, which are precursor cells of the ectodermal system that are common to both neural and non-neural cell lineages. Okano and colleagues were able to clarify the regulatory mechanism of the asymmetric cell division by the Musashi gene product of *Drosophila* [77]. The Musashi gene product was found to induce differentiation of neural precursor cells by selectively repressing translation of the mRNA of the neural differentiation inhibitory factor Tramtrack69 (TTK69). Later, the investigators succeeded in identifying the RNA base sequence that is the binding-target of Musashi protein. After cloning and sequencing of the cDNA for the RNA molecule that is the binding target of Musashi protein, it was concluded that Musashi protein binds specifically to a binding sequence that is present on ttk69 mRNA, and by repressing translation to TTK69 protein, which is a repressor of neural differentiation, maintains the potential of neural precursor cells for neural differentiation. The Musashi gene is also expressed in proliferating neural stem cells/progenitor cells (neuroblasts) in the larval brain of *Drosophila* [66,78]. Overexpression of Musashi in the neural stem/progenitor cells of *Drosophila* causes proliferation of undifferentiated cells. Unlike the asymmetrical division, the induction of proliferation of neural stem/progenitor cells in the larval brain of *Drosophila* by overexpression of Musashi is difficult to explain by repression of translation of ttk69 mRNA alone, and thus a different function of Musashi is postulated.

Musashi-1 as a Marker of Mammalian Neural Stem Cells

Okano and colleagues first cloned the mouse homologue of Musashi-1 and then analyzed its pattern of expression in detail [67,68,79]. Musashi-1 is strongly expressed in neural stem cells (NSCs) in the periventricular area or undifferentiated neural precursor cells of vertebrates as a whole. A detailed analysis in the mouse has revealed strong expression of Musashi-1 in the ventricular zone of the neural tube in the embryo stage, when NSC and progenitor-cell division is very active in the central nervous system (CNS) [67,68]. The Musashi-1 protein in postnatal CNS is expressed in periventricular ependymal cells and astrocytes, which have been reported to possess stem cell characteristics in the adult brain [80,81]. Goldman and colleagues succeeded in identifying NSCs and progenitor cells in the adult human brain [82]. Thus, Musashi-1 protein is continuously expressed in neural stem-cell-like cells. Strong expression is also demonstrated in neurogenic sites within the postnatal brain including the rostral migratory stream. The evidence indicates that Musashi-1 is not only a marker of neural stem cells, but is also involved in regulating the properties of NSCs [83].

Function of Musashi-1 Protein

Musashi-1 protein has been found to activate Notch signaling by repressing translation of the mRNA of the intracellular Notch signal repressor m-Numb, and to maintain the self-renewal ability of NSCs. Analysis of the RNA base sequence that is the binding-target of Musashi protein has also revealed that the Musashi-1 protein-binding sequence is present in the 3'-UTR of the m-Numb mRNA and that Musashi-1 protein binds to m-Numb mRNA *in vivo* as well as *in vitro* [84]. Because m-Numb is a modulator that exerts a repressive effect on the Notch signal [84], Musashi-1 protein was expected to positively regulate Notch signaling, but in fact was confirmed that Musashi-1 protein induces transactivation of the promoter of the Notch signal target Hes-1 gene [72,86]. It is clear that activation of the Notch signal positively regulates neural stem-cell self-renewal, and therefore Musashi-1 is thought to contribute to retention of the properties of NSCs [87,88,89].

Musashi-1 as an Intestinal Stem Cell Marker

Comparison of the Musashi-1 genes in humans and mice has revealed that the Tcf/Lef binding sequence (Wnt signal response sequence) and Sox binding sequence are present in the regions that have been conserved outside the protein-coding region. Wnt signaling and the Sox family transcription factors have each been found to play important roles in the induction and maintenance of intestinal stem cells, hematopoietic stem cells, certain types of neural stem/progenitor cells [41,90,91], and undifferentiated neural precursor cells [78,82].

Assuming that Musashi-1 plays a general role in crosstalk with the signal systems involved in maintaining stem cells, it may contribute to maintaining stem-cell systems other than NSCs. Northern blot analysis has revealed that the expression of Musashi-1 mRNA in various organs other than the CNS is high in the adult small intestine [67]. Potten and Clarke have provided evidence that Musashi-1 is a marker of intestinal epithelial stem cells and mammary stem cells [70]. It has been suggested that nuclear localization of β-catenin reaches its highest level as a result of activation of the canonical pathway of the Wnt signal in the 4th cells from the bottom of the crypts, which is the stem-cell position. In the small intestine, they observed the expression of Musashi-1 in cells up to the 4th-6th position (especially the 4th) from the bottom of the crypts of the small intestine, and in the cells in the deepest portion of the large intestine, where stem cells are presumed to be present [92]. These results indicate that Musashi-1 can be used as a stem cell marker, especially in the epithelial cells of the mucosa of the small intestine [70]. In the intestinal epithelial cell of mutants with functional deficiency of the APC molecule, Musashi-1 expression is increased. Considering that the APC molecule constitutively activates the Wnt signal, it is suggested that the Wnt signal pathway performs an important function in expression of Musashi-1 in intestinal epithelial stem cells. Musashi-1 is also expressed in mammary epithelial stem cells. Clevers and colleagues suggested that Tcf-4, a transcriptional factor that functions in the canonical pathways of the Wnt signal, plays an important role in stem cells of the mammary epithelium as well as the intestine [93]. The fact that the Musashi-1 gene contains many Tcf binding consensus sequences in its 5'-upstream region suggests transcription repression of the Musashi-1 gene.

Musashi-1 as a Gastric Stem Cell Marker

Musashi-1 is also expressed in the progenitor cells of amphibian stomach epithelium during metamorphosis before final differentiation [94]. Asai and colleagues examined Musashi-1 expression in the mouse stomach during embryonic, fetal and postnatal development [95]. They demonstrated that Musashi-1 expression diminished during the latter half of fetal development and that there was no expression during the postnatal period. In the glandular stomach, the epithelium forms simple glands and the cell proliferation zone develops at the neck of the glands. The localization of Musashi-1-positive cells overlapped partially with the area of proliferating cells, indicating that Musashi-1 may be expressed in stem cells. However, Musashi-1 expression was also found in the deeper regioins of the glands where differentiating cells, such as parietal cells and chief cells, reside. Nagata and colleagues examined the expression of Musashi-1 in the rat stomach and demonstrated that it was present in the luminal compartment of the corpus mucosa [96]. Most of the Musashi-1-positive cells were located in the isthmus, where the epithelial progenitor cells are thought to be present. Musashi-1 expression was not found in the antrum. The Musashi-1-positive cells seemed to be distinct from other epithelial cell lineages in the stomach, except for parietal cells. Ablation of mature parietal cells has been reported to be associated with a four to fivefold increase in the number of granular-free cell precursors in the isthmus and neck [58]. Therefore, they speculated that Musashi-1 synthesized in the parietal cells may be involved in proliferation and differentiation of isthmus-lineage precursors. The same investigators also demonstrated that Musashi-1 was coexpressed with Hes5. Hes5 and Hes1 play an important role in Notch activity in regulation of neural stem cell differentiation, and Musashi-1 activates Notch signaling by repressing translation of the Notch inhibitor m-Numb [97]. These findings support the hypothesis that Musashi-1 has a role in maintaining stem cells in the rat stomach.

By analogy, it would be expected that Musashi-1 is expressed in the predicted stem cell regions of the human stomach. Akasaka and colleagues examined whether Musashi-1 is expressed in the putative stem cell regions in human gastric glands, as in the murine intestine [21]. They demonstrated that Musashi-1 is expressed strongly in epithelial cells of the isthmus/neck region in the adult human antrum. In contrast, Musashi-1 expression was not found in any regions of the fundic glands. The surface epithelium in the upper part of the pit and the epithelium in the basal regions of the glands were also negative for Musashi-1 expression. During the development of the human stomach, Musashi-1 expression was limited to the basal regions of fetal pyloric glands. In the adult antrum, Musashi-1-positive cells were intermingled with proliferating cell nuclear antigen (PCNA)-positive cells in the isthmus/neck region, but did not coexpress PCNA. The specific expression of Musashi-1 within the proliferative regions in the isthmus/neck region indicates that Musashi-1 can be a marker for progenitor cells in the human stomach.

Musashi-1 Expression in Intestinal Metaplasia

Intestinal metaplasia (IM) is defined histologically by the presence of intestinal-type cells such as goblet cells, Paneth cells, and absorptive cells and is often encountered in chronic gastritis. IM in the human stomach has long been believed to be a premalignant condition and therefore extensively studied [98,99,100,101]. Several classifications of IM have been suggested. Kawachi and colleagues first proposed division into complete and incomplete types on the basis of morphology [102,103]. Inada and colleagues have proposed a new classification of IM based on the presence or absence of gastric-type cells in IM glands, which they have subdivided into two major types: a mixed gastric and intestinal type (GI-mixed-type) and a solely intestinal type (I-type) [104,105]. In GI mixed-type IM, gastric surface mucous cells, intestinal absorptive cells and goblet cells are found in the upper glandular portion from the proliferative zone, and pyloric gland cells and Paneth cells are found in the lower glandular portions from the proliferative zone [105]. Yuasa and colleagues clearly demonstrated a phenotypic shift from GI mixed-type to an I-type IM upon sequential observation of X-irradiated rat stomach [106]. Their findings suggest that GI mixed-type IM may be composed of a mixture of cells with various degrees of intestinal phenotypic shift rather just a random mixture of gastric and intestinal-type cells. This allowed them to introduce the notion that IM might be the consequence of abnormal differentiation of stem cells that can produce both gastric and intestinal-type cells, with the normal cell migration pattern preserved. Supportive evidence for this was obtained in the study by Akasaka and colleagues [21]. It is clear that Musashi-1 is expressed in the predicted stem cell regions of murine and human intestinal crypts [69,70] as well as in the isthmus/neck (proliferative) region of the adult human antrum [21]. However, Musashi-1 expression is markedly decreased in IM cells of the human stomach. The difference in the expression patterns of Musashi-1 between normal intestinal cells and intestinal metaplastic cells in the human stomach supports the assumption that IM is a consequence of abnormal differentiation, in which stem cells or progenitor cells may not differentiate into any of the normal intestinal epithelial phenotypes [21].

CONCLUSION

The molecular events that regulate the development of the gastrointestinal tract are beginning to be identified. It is clear that the Wnt/β-catenin signaling pathway and downstream molecules such as APC, Tcf-4, Fkh-6, Cdx-1, and Cdx-2 are important for normal gastrointestinal function. The identification of molecular pathways that determine further differentiation of progenitor cells into specific epithelial cell lineages is now underway: The Notch-Delta signaling pathways involving Hes1 and Math1 transcription factors regulate differentiation of goblet, Paneth, and enteroendocrine cells in the small intestine. Although it is believed that stem cells are present in the gastric glands, the stem cells remains unidentified at the single-cell level, mainly because of a lack of reliable stem cell markers. Musashi-1 has been revealed to be a distinctive marker of epithelial stem cells in the crypts of mouse small intestine and human colon. Recent studies have demonstrated that Musashi-1 is expressed especially in the putative position of stem cells (isthmus/neck region) in the adult antrum, indicating that Musashi-1 can be a marker of progenitor cells in the human stomach. The identification of Musashi-1 expression in putative progenitor cells in human gastric glands will provide a clear insight into the differentiation mechanisms of stem cells or progenitor cells in the human stomach.

REFERENCES

[1]   Cheng H, Leblond CP 1974 Origin, differentiation and renewal of the four main epithelial cell types in the mouse small intestine. III. Entero-endocrine cells. *Am. J. Anat.* 141:503–19.

[2]   Winton DJ, Ponder BA 1990 Stem-cell organization in mouse small intestine. *Proc. R. Soc. Lond. B. Biol. Sci.* 241:13–18.

[3]   Kirkland SC 1988 Clonal origin of columnar, mucous, and endocrine cell lineages in human colorectal epithelium. *Cancer.* 61: 1359–63.

[4]   Ponder BA, Schmidt GH, Wilkinson MM, Wood MJ, Monk M, Reid A 1985 Derivation of mouse intestinal crypts from single progenitor cells. *Nature.* 313: 689–91.

[5]   Brittan M, Wright NA 2002 Gastrointestinal stem cells. *J. Pathol.* 197: 492–509.

[6]   Modlin IM, Kidd M, Lye KD, Wright NA 2003 Gastric stem cells: an update. *Keio J. Med.* 52: 134–37.

[7]   Brittan M, Wright NA 2004 Stem cell in gastrointestinal structure and neoplastic development. *Gut.* 53: 899–910.

[8]   Lin H 2002 The stem-cell niche theory: lessons from flies. *Nat. Rev. Genet.* 3:931–40.

[9]   Cadigan KM, Nusse R 1997 Wnt signaling: a common theme in animal development. *Genes Dev.* 11:3286–305.

[10] Polakis P 1999 The oncogenic activation of beta-catenin. *Curr. Opin. Genet. Dev.* 9: 15–21.

[11] Barker N, Huls G, Korinek V, Clevers H 1999 Restricted high level expression of Tcf-4 protein in intestinal and mammary gland epithelium. *Am. J. Pathol.* 154: 29–35.

[12] Korinek V, Barker N, Moerer P, van Donselaar E, Huls G, Peters PJ, Clevers H 1998 Depletion of epithelial stem-cell compartments in the small intestine of mice lacking Tcf-4. *Nature Genet.* 19: 379–383.

[13] Kaestner KH, Bleckmann SC, Monaghan AP, Schlondorff J, Mincheva A, Lichter P, Schutz G 1996 Clustered arrangement of winged helix genes fkh-6 and MFH-1: possible implications for mesoderm development. *Development.* 122: 1751–58.

[14] Lickert H, Domon C, Huls G, Wehrle C, Duluc I, Clevers H, Meyer BI, Freund JN, Kemler R 2000 Wnt/(beta)-catenin signaling regulates the expression of the homeobox gene Cdx1 in embryonic intestine. *Development.* 127: 3805–13.

[15] Beck F, Chawengsaksophak K, Waring P, Playford RJ, Furness JB 1999 Reprogramming of intestinal differentiation and intercalary regeneration in Cdx2 mutant mice. *Proc. Natl. Acad. Sci. U S A.* 96: 7318–23.

[16] Yang Q, Bermingham NA, Finegold MJ, Zoghbi HY 2001 Requirement of Math1 for secretory cell lineage commitment in the mouse intestine. *Science.* 294: 2155–58.

[17] van Den Brink GR, de Santa Barbara P, Roberts DJ 2001 Development. Epithelial cell differentiation – a mather of choice. *Science.* 294: 2115–16.

[18] Jensen J, Pedersen EE, Galante P, Hald J, Heller RS, Ishibashi M, Kageyama R, Guillemot F, Serup P, Madsen OD 2000 Control of endodermal endocrine development by Hes-1. *Nature Genet.* 24: 36–44.

[19] Brittan M, Wright NA 2004 Stem cell in gastrointestinal structure and neoplastic development. *Gut.* 53:899-910.

[20] Karam SM, Straiton T, Hassan WM, Leblond CP 2003 Defining epithelial cell progenitors in the human oxyntic mucosa. *Stem Cells.* 21: 322–36.

[21] Akasaka Y, Saikawa Y, Fujita K, Kubota T, Ishikawa Y, Fujimoto A, Ishii T, Okano H, Kitajima M 2005 Expression of a candidate marker for progenitor cells, Musashi-1, in the proliferative regions of human antrum and its decreased expression in intestinal metaplasia. *Histopathology.* 47: 348-56.

[22] Karam SM, Leblond CP 1993 Dynamics of epithelial cells in the corpus of the mouse stomach. II. Outward migration of pit cells. *Anat. Rec.* 236; 280–96.

[23] Hattori T, Fujita S 1976 Tritiated thymidine autoradiographic study of cell migration and renewal in the pyloric mucosa of golden hamsters. *Cell Tissue Res.* 175: 49–57.

[24] Karam SM, Leblond CP 1993 Dynamics of epithelial cells in the corpus of the mouse stomach. I. Identification of proliferative cell types and pinpointing of the stem cell. *Anat. Rec.* 236: 259–79.

[25] Thompson M, Fleming KA, Evans DJ, Fundele R, Surani MA, Wright NA 1990 Gastric endocrine cells share a clonal origin with other gut cell lineages. *Development* 110: 477–81.

[26] Pearse AG. Endocrine Tumours. In: Polak JM, Bloom SL, editors Edinburgh: Churchill Livingstone; 1984; 82–94.

[27] Tatematsu M, Fukami H, Yamamoto M, Nakanishi H, Masui T, Kusakabe N, Sakakura T 1994 Clonal analysis of glandular stomach carcinogenesis in C3H/HeN<BALB/c chimeric mice treated with N-methyl-N-nitrosourea. *Cancer Lett.* 83: 37–42.

[28] Nomura S, Esumi H, Job C, Tan SS 1998 Lineage and clonal development of gastric glands. *Dev. Biol.* 204: 124–135.

[29] Kirkland S 1988 Polarity and differentiation of human rectal adenocarcinoma cells in suspension and collagen gel cultures. *Cancer.* 61: 1359–63.

[30] Nomura S, Kaminishi M, Sugiyama K, Oohara T, Esumi H 1996 Clonal analysis of isolated single fundic and pyloric gland of stomach using X-linked polymorphism. *Biochem. Biophys. Res. Commun.* 226: 385–90.

[31] Karam SM 1999 Lineage commitment and maturation of epithelial cells in the gut. *Frontiers Biosci.* 4: 286–98.

[32] Powell DW, Mifflin RC, Valentich JD, Crowe SE, Saada JI, West AB 1999 Myofibroblasts II. Intestinal subepithelial myofibroblasts. *Am. J. Physiol.* 277: C183–C201.

[33] Karlsson L, Lindahl P, Heath JK, Betsholtz C 2000 Abnormal gastrointestinal development in PDGF-A and PDGFR-(alpha) deficient mice implicates a novel mesenchymal structure with putative instructive properties in villus morphogenesis. *Development.* 127: 3457-66.

[34] Polakis P 1999 The oncogenic activation of beta-catenin. *Curr. Opin. Genet. Dev.* 9: 15–21.

[35] Kinzler KW, Vogelstein B 1996 Lessons from hereditary colorectal cancer. *Cell.* 87:159–70.

[36] Kawano Y, Kypta R 2003 Secreted antagonists of the Wnt signaling pathway. *J. Cell Sci.* 116:2627–34.

[37] He T-C, Sparks AB, Rago C, Hermeking H, Zawel L, da Costa LT, Morin PJ, Vogelstein B, Kinzler KW 1988 Identification of c-MYC as a target of the APC pathway. *Science.* 281:1509–11.

[38] Tetsu O, McCornick F 1999 Beta-catenin regulates expression of cyclin D1 in colon carcinoma cells. *Nature* 398:422–26.

[39] Mann B, Gelos M, Siedow A, Hanski ML, Gratchev A, Ilyas M, Bodmer WF, Moyer MP, Riecken EO, Buhr HJ, Hanski C 1999 Target genes of beta- catenin-T cell-factor/lymphoid-enhancer-factor signaling in human colorectal carcinomas. *Proc. Natl. Acad. Sci. U S A.* 96: 1603–8.

[40] Barker N, Huls G, Korinek V, Clevers H 1999 Restricted high level expression of Tcf-4 protein in intestinal and mammary gland epithelium. *Am. J. Pathol.* 154: 29–35.

[41] Korinek V, Barker N, Moerer P, van Donselaar E, Huls G, Peters PJ, Clevers H 1998 Depletion of epithelial stem-cell compartments in the small intestine of mice lacking Tcf-4. *Nature Genet.* 19: 379–83.

[42] Wong MH, Huelsken J, Birchmeier W, Gordon JI 2002 Selection of multipotent stem cells during morphogenesis of small intestinal crypts of Lieberkuhn is perturbed by stimulation of Lef-1/ β-catenin signalling. *J. Biol. Chem.* 277: 15843–50.

[43] Macdonald PM, Struhl G 1986 A molecular gradient in early Drosophila embryos and its role in specifying the body pattern. *Nature.* 324: 537–45.

[44] Mallo GV, Rechreche H, Frigerio JM, Rocha D, Zweibaum A, Lacasa M, Jordan BR, Dusetti NJ, Dagorn JC, Iovanna JL 1997 Molecular cloning, sequencing and expression of the mRNA encoding human Cdx1 and Cdx2 homeobox. Downregulation of Cdx1 and Cdx2 mRNA expression during colorectal carcinogenesis. *Int. J. Cancer.* 74: 35–44.

[45] James R, Kazenwadel J 1991 Homeobox gene expression in the intestinal epithelium of adult mice. *J. Biol. Chem.* 266: 3246–51.

[46] Freund JN, Domon-Dell C, Kedinger M, Duluc I 1998 The Cdx-1 and Cdx-2 homeobox genes in the intestine. *Biochem. Cell Biol.* 76: 957–69.

[47] Silberg DG, Furth EE, Taylor JK, Schuck T, Chiou T, Traber PG 1997 CDX1 protein expression in normal, metaplastic, and neoplastic human alimentary tract epithelium. *Gastroenterology.* 113:478–86.

[48] Mizoshita T, Inada K, Tsukamoto T, Kodera Y, Yamamura Y, Hirai T, Kato T, Joh T, Itoh M, Tatematsu M 2001 Expression of Cdx1 and Cdx2 mRNAs and relevance of this expression to differentiation in human gastrointestinal mucosa–with special emphasis on participation in intestinal metaplasia of the human stomach. *Gastric Cancer.* 4:185–91.

[49] Beck F, Chawengsaksophak K, Waring P, Playford RJ, Furness JB 1999 Reprogramming of intestinal differentiation and intercalary regeneration in Cdx2 mutant mice. *Proc. Natl. Acad. Sci. U S A.* 96: 7318–23

[50] Lickert H, Domon C, Huls G, Wehrle C, Duluc I, Clevers H, Meyer BI, Freund JN, Kemler R 2000 Wnt/(beta)-catenin signaling regulates the expression of the homeobox gene Cdx1 in embryonic intestine. *Development.* 127: 3805–3813.

[51] Kaestner KH, Knochel W, Martinez DE 2000 Unified nomenclature for the winged helix/forkhead transcription factors. *Genes Dev.* 14: 142–6.

[52] Kaestner KH, Lee KH, Schlondorff J, Hiemisch H, Monaghan AP, Schutz G 1993 Six members of the mouse forkhead gene family are developmentally regulated. *Proc. Natl. Acad. Sci. U S A.* 90: 7628–31.

[53] Kaestner KH, Bleckmann SC, Monaghan AP, Schlondorff J, Mincheva A, Lichter P, Schutz G 1996 Clustered arrangement of winged helix genes fkh-6 and MFH-1: possible implications for mesoderm development. *Development.* 122: 1751–58.

[54] Kaestner KH, Silberg DG, Traber PG, Schutz G 1997 The mesenchymal winged helix transcription factor Fkh6 is required for the control of gastrointestinal proliferation and differentiation. *Genes Dev.* 11: 1583–95.

[55] Yang Q, Bermingham NA, Finegold MJ, Zoghbi HY 2001 Requirement of Math1 for secretory cell lineage commitment in the mouse intestine. *Science.* 294: 2155–58.

[56] van Den Brink GR, de Santa Barbara P, Roberts DJ 2001 Development. Epithelial cell differentiation – a mather of choice. *Science.* 294: 2115–16.

[57] Jensen J, Pedersen EE, Galante P, Hald J, Heller RS, Ishibashi M, Kageyama R, Guillemot F, Serup P, Madsen OD 2000 Control of endodermal endocrine development by Hes-1. *Nature Genet.* 24: 36–44.

[58] Li Q, Karam SM, Gordon JI 1996 Diphtheria toxin-mediated ablation of parietal cells in the stomach of transgenic mice. *J. Biol. Chem.* 271: 3671–76.

[59] Mills JC, Andersson N, Hong CV, Stappenbeck TS, Gordon JI 2002 Molecular characterization of mouse gastric epithelial progenitor cells. *Proc. Natl. Acad. Sci. USA.* 99: 14819 – 24.

[60] Mahmoudi T, Verrijzer CP 2001 Chromatin silencing and activation by Polycomb and trithorax group proteins. *Oncogene.* 20:3055-66.

[61] Iwama A, Oguro H, Negishi M, Kato Y, Nakauchia H 2005 Epigenetic regulation of hematopoietic stem cell self-renewal by polycomb group genes. *Int. J. Hematol.* 81:294-300.

[62] Lessard J, Sauvageau G 2003 Bmi-1 determines the proliferative capacity of normal and leukaemic stem cells. *Nature.* 423:255-60.

[63] Park IK, Qian D, Kiel M, Becker MW, Pihalja M, Weissman IL, Morrison SJ, Clarke MF 2003 Bmi-1 is required for maintenance of adult self-renewing haematopoietic stem cells. *Nature.* 423: 302-5.

[64] Reinisch C, Kandutsch S, Uthman A, Pammer J 2006 BMI-1: a protein expressed in stem cells, specialized cells and tumors of the gastrointestinal tract. *Histol. Histopathol.* 21:1143-49.

[65] Raaphorst FM, Otte AP, van Kemenade FJ, Blokzijl T, Fieret E, Hamer KM, Satijn DP, Meijer CJ 2001 Distinct BMI-1 and EZH2 expression patterns in thymocytes and mature T cells suggest a role for Polycomb genes in human T cell differentiation. *J Immunol.* 15: 5925-34.

[66] Nakamura M, Okano H, Blendy JA, Montell C 1994 Musashi, a neural RNA-binding protein required for Drosophila adult external sensory organ development. *Neuron.* 13:67– 81.

[67] Sakakibara S, Imai T, Hamaguchi K, Okabe M, Aruga J, Nakajima K, Yasutomi D, Nagata T, Kurihara Y, Uesugi S, Miyata T, Ogawa M, Mikoshiba K, Okano H 1996 Mouse-Musashi-1, a neural RNA-binding protein highly enriched in the mammalian CNS stem cell. *Dev. Biol.* 176: 230 – 42.

[68] Sakakibara S, Okano H 1997 Expression of neural RNA-binding proteins in the postnatal CNS: implications of their roles in neuronal and glial cell development. *J. Neurosci.* 17: 8300 – 12

[69] Kayahara T, Sawada M, Takaishi S, Fukui H, Seno H, Fukuzawa H, Suzuki K, Hiai H, Kageyama R, Okano H, Chiba T 2003 Candidate markers for stem and early progenitor cells, Musashi-1 and Hes1, are expressed in crypt base columnar cells of mouse small intestine. *FEBS Lett.* 535: 131–5.

[70] Potten CS, Booth C, Tudor GL, Booth D, Brady G, Hurley P, Ashton G, Clarke R, Sakakibara S, Okano H 2003 Identification of a putative intestinal stem cell and early lineage marker; Musashi-1. *Differentiation.* 71: 28 – 41.

[71] Sakatani T, Kaneda A, Iacobuzio-Donahue CA, Carter MG, Witzel SB, Okano H, Ko MSH, Ohlsson R, Longo DL, Feinberg AP 2005 Loss of imprinting of Igf 2 alters intestinal maturation and tumorigenesis in mice. *Science.* 307: 1976 –78.

[72] Okano H, Imai T, Okabe M 2002 Musashi: a translational regulator of cell fates. *J. Cell Sci.* 115: 1355 – 59.

[73] Yoda A, Sawa H, Okano H 2000 MSI-1, a neural RNA-binding protein, is involved in the male mating behavior in Caenorhabditis elegans. *Genes Cells.* 5: 885 – 95.

[74] Hirota Y, Okabe M, Imai T, Kurusu M, Yamamoto A, Miyao S, Nakamura M, Sawamoto K, Okano H 1999 Musashi and Seven in absentia downregulate Tramtrack through distinct mechanisms in Drosophila eye development. *Mech. Dev.* 87: 93 – 101.

[75] Kawashima T, Murakami AR, Ogasawara M, Tanaka KJ, Isoda R, Sasakura Y, Nishikata T, Okano H, Makabe KW 2000 Expression patterns of musashi homologues of the ascidians, Halocynthia roretzi and Ciona intestinalis. *Dev. Gene Evol.* 210: 162 – 5.

[76] Good P, Yoda A, Sakakibara S, Yamamoto A, Imai T, Sawa H, Ikeuchi T, Tsuji S, Satoh H, Okano H 1998 The Human Musashi homolog1 (MSI1) gene encoding the homologue of Musashi/Nrp-1, a neural RNA-binding protein putatively expressed in CNS stem cells and neural progenitor cells. *Genomics.* 52: 382 – 384.

[77] Okabe M, Imai T, Kurusu M, Hiromi Y, Okano H 2001 Translational repression determines a neuronal potential in Drosophila asymmetric cell division. *Nature.* 411: 94 – 98.

[78] Ito K, Hotta, Y 1992 Proliferation pattern of postembryonic neuroblasts in the brain of Drosophila melanogaster. *Dev. Biol.* 149: 134 – 48.

[79] Kaneko Y, Sakakibara S, Imai T, Suzuki A, Nakamura Y, Sawamoto K, Ogawa Y, Toyama Y, Miyata T, Okano H 2000 Musashi1: an evolutionally conserved marker for CNS progenitor cells including neural stem cells. *Dev. Neurosci.* 22: 139 –53.

[80] Johansson CB, Momma S, Clarke DL, Risling M, Lendahl U, Frisen J 1999 Identification of a neural stem cell in the adult mammalian central nervous system. *Cell.* 96: 25 – 34.

[81] Doetsch F, Caille I, Lim DA, Garcia-Verdugo JM, Alvarez- Buylla A 1999 Subventricular zone astrocytes are neural stem cells in the adult mammalian brain. *Cell.* 97: 703 – 16.

[82] Pincus DW, Keyoung H, Restelli C, Goodman RR, Fraser RAR, Edgar M, Sakakibara S, Okano H, Nedergaard M, Goldman SA 1998 FGF2/BDNF-responsive neuronal progenitor cells in the adult human subependyma. *Ann. Neurol.* 43: 576 – 85.

[83] Okano H, Kawahara H, Toriya M, Nakao K, Shibata S, Imai T 2005 Function of RNA-binding protein Musashi-1 in stem cells. *Exp. Cell Res.* 306:349-56.

[84] Zhong W, Feder JN, Jiang MM, Jan LY, Jan YN 1996 Asymmetric localization of a mammalian numb homolog during mouse cortical neurogenesis. *Neuron.* 17: 43 – 53.

[85] Berdnik D, Torok T, Gonzalez-Gaitan M, Knoblich JA 2002 The endocytic protein alpha-Adaptin is required for numb-mediated asymmetric cell division in Drosophila. *Dev. Cell.* 3: 221 – 231.

[86] Imai T, Tokunaga A, Yoshida T, Hashimoto M, Weinmaster G, Mikoshiba K, Nakafuku M, Okano H 2001 The neural RNA-binding protein Musashi1 translationally regulates the m-numb gene expression by interacting with its mRNA. *Mol. Cell Biol.* 21: 3888 – 39000.

[87] Nakamura Y, Sakakibara S, Miyata T, Ogawa M, Shimazaki T, Weiss S, Kageyama R, Okano H 2000 The bHLH gene Hes1 as a repressor of neuronal commitment of the CNS stem cells. *J. Neurosci.* 20: 283 – 93.

[88] Hitoshi S, Alexson T, Tropepe V, Donoviel D, Elia AJ, Nye JS, Conlon RA, Mak TW, Bernstein A, van der Kooy D 2002 Notch pathway molecules are essential for the

maintenance, but not the generation, of mammalian neural stem cells. *Genes Dev.* 16: 846 – 58.

[89] Tokunaga A, Kohyama J, Yoshida T, Nakao K, Sawamoto K, Okano H 2004 Mapping spatio-temporal activation of Notch signaling during neurogenesis and gliogenesis in the developing mouse brain. *J. Neurochem.* 90: 142 – 154.

[90] Reya T, Duncan AW, Ailles L, Domen J, Scherer DC, Willert K, Hintz L, Nusse R, Weissman IL 2003 A role for Wnt signalling in self-renewal of haematopoietic stem cells. *Nature.* 423: 409 – 14.

[91] Lee SM, Tole S, Grove E, McMahon AP 2000 A local Wnt-3a signal is required for development of the mammalian hippocampus. *Development.* 127: 457 – 67.

[92] Marshman E, Booth C, Potten CS 2002 The intestinal epithelial stem cell. *BioEssays.* 24: 91 – 98.

[93] Barker N, Huls G, Korinek V, Clevers H 1999 Restricted high level expression of Tcf-4 protein in intestinal and mammary gland epithelium. *Am. J. Pathol.* 154: 29 – 35.

[94] Ishizuya-Oka A, Shimizu K, Sakakibara S, Okano H, Ueda S 2003 Thyroid hormone-upregulated expression of Musashi-1 is specific for progenitor cells of the adult epithelium during amphibian gastrointestinal remodeling. *J. Cell Sci.* 116: 3157–64.

[95] Asai R, Okano H, Yasugi S 2005 Correlation between Musashi-1 and c-hairy-1 expression and cell proliferation activity in the developing intestine and stomach of both chicken and mouse. *Develop. Growth Differ.* 47: 501–10.

[96] Nagata H, Akiba Y, Suzuki H, Okano H, Hibi T 2006 Expression of Musashi-1 in the rat stomach and changes during mucosal injury and restitution. *FEBS Letters.* 580: 27–33.

[97] Ohtsuka T, Ishibashi M, Gradwohl G, Nakanishi S, Guillemot F, Kageyama, R 1999 Hes1 and Hes5 as notch effectors in mammalian neuronal differentiation. *EMBO J.* 18: 2196–207.

[98] Stemmermann GN, Hayashi T 1968 Intestinal metaplasia of the gastric mucosa:a gross and microscopic study of its distribution in various disease states. *J. Natl. Cancer Inst.* 41: 627–34.

[99] Morson BC 1955 Carcinoma arising from areas of intestinal metaplasia in the gastric mucosa. *Br. J. Cancer.* 9: 377–85.

[100] Correa P 1992 Human gastric carcinogenesis: a multistep and multifactorial process—First American Cancer Society Award Lecture on Cancer Epidemiology and Prevention. *Cancer Res.* 52: 6735–40.

[101] You WC, Blot WJ, Li JY, Chang YS, Jin ML, Kneller R, Zhang L, Han ZX, Zeng XR, Liu WD 1993 Precancerous gastric lesions in a population at high risk of stomach cancer. *Cancer Res.* 53: 1317–21.

[102] Kawachi T, Kogure K, Tanaka N, Tokunaga A, Sugimura T 1974 Studies of intestinal metaplasia in the gastric mucosa by detection of disaccharidases with "Tes-Tape." *J. Natl. Cancer Inst.* 53: 19–30.

[103] Matsukura N, Suzuki K, Kawachi T, Aoyagi M, Sugimura T, Kitaoka H, Numajiri H, Shirota A, Itabashi M, Hirota T 1980 Distribution of marker enzymes and mucin in intestinal metaplasia in human stomach and relation to complete and incomplete types of intestinal metaplasia to minute gastric carcinomas. *J. Natl. Cancer Inst.* 65: 231–40.

[104] Inada K, Nakanishi H, Fujimitsu Y, Shimizu N, Ichinose M, Miki K, Nakamura S, Tatematsu M 1997 Gastric and intestinal mixed and solely intestinal types of intestinal metaplasia in the human stomach. *Pathol. Int.* 47: 831–41.

[105] Inada K, Tanaka H, Nakanishi H, Tsukamoto T, Ikehara Y, Tatematsu K, Nakamura S, Porter EM, Tatematsu M 2001 Identification of Paneth cells in pyloric glands associated with gastric and intestinal mixed-type intestinal metaplasia of the human stomach. *Virchows Arch.* 439: 14–20.

[106] Yuasa H, Inada K, Watanabe H, Tatematsu M 2002 A phenotypic shift from gastric-intestinal to solely intestinal cell types in intestinal metaplasia in rat stomach following treatment with X-rays. *J. Toxicol. Pathol.* 15: 85–93.

APPENDIX - FIGURES

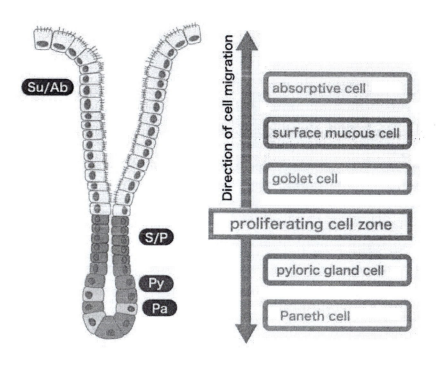

Figure 1. Schematic view of the cell differentiation (left panel) and direction of cell migration (right panel) in gastric glands. Su, surface mucous cells; Ab, absorptive cells; Su/Ab, absorptive cells retaining mucin of surface mucous cells; S/P, stem cells and proliferating cells; Py, pyloric gland cells; Pa, Paneth cells.

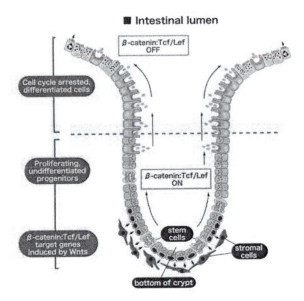

Figure 2. β-catenin and the biology of colonic crypts. The colonic crypt contains replicating stem cells near the bottom, which contain high levels of β-catenin (small red arrows). In the cells located near the bottom of the crypts, intracellular β-catenin levels are high because these cells are receiving Wnt signals from the stroma. These β-catenin molecules migrate to the nucleus and associate with Tcf/Lef transcription factors; this derives increased proliferation of these cells and prevents their differentiation. In the normal intestine, many of the progeny of these stem cells migrate upward toward the lumen. As they do so, stimulation by Wnts decreases; this leads to increased degradation of β-catenin, which results, in turn, in cessation of proliferation and increased differentiation as these cells approach the lumen.

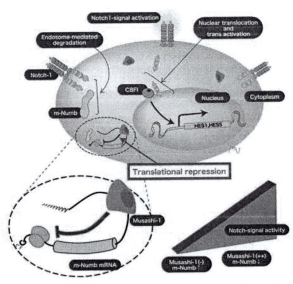

Figure 3. Mechanism of Notch-1-signal activation by Musashi-1 protein. Musashi-1 protein binds to the 3'-UTR of m-Numb mRNA and inhibits its translation [86]. On the other hand, m-Numb protein binds to the intracellular domain of Notch-1 protein and inhibits the activation of the Notch-1 pathway, putatively by guiding Notch-1 protein from the cell surface to the endosome-mediated degradation pathway [85]. Consequently, Musashi-1 protein augments the Notch-1 signaling pathway.

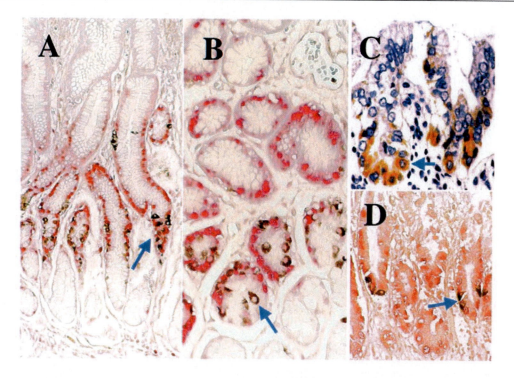

Figure 4. A, Double-staining for PCNA and Msi-1 in the gastric glands of the antral mucosa. In the antral mucosa, PCNA-positive nuclei (red labeling) are distributed throughout the epithelial cells in the isthmus/neck region. Msi-1-positive cells (brown labeling; arrow) are intermingled with the PCNA-positive cells and are present in the lower part of the isthmus/neck region. B, Higher magnification of Msi-1-positive cells within the proliferative region. Msi-1 reactivity (brown labeling) is present in the cytoplasm, while PCNA reactivity (red labeling) is restricted to the nucleus. The arrow indicates cells with an Msi-1-positive cytoplasm but devoid of nuclear PCNA staining. C, Msi-1 expression in the fetal human antrum. By the 14th week of gestation, the pit/gland structure has elongated, while the surface columnar epithelial cells have differentiated and exhibit cytoplasm with basal nuclei. Msi-1 expression (brown labeling; arrow) is concentrated in the basal regions of the pyloric glands. D, Double-staining for PCNA and Msi-1 in the gastric glands of the antrum at the 22nd week of gestation. Along with a concomitant increase in the heights of the pits and glands, the PCNA-positive cells (red labeling) are concentrated in the epithelial cells in the pit regions of the glands. By the 22nd week of gestation, most cells with PCNA-positive nuclei have moved to a higher position than cells with Msi-1-positive cytoplasm (brown labeling). The arrow indicates cells with an Msi-1-positive cytoplasm but devoid of nuclear PCNA staining.

Index

B

C

D

H

I

M

N

O

Q

R

S

U

V

W

X

Y

Z

β